VETERINARY ASPECTS
OF
CAPTIVE BIRDS OF PREY

1985 Supplement as tinted section
at the rear of this book

Preface to the 1985 Edition

The binding of the last thousand copies of the 1978 edition of "Veterinary Aspects of Captive Birds of Prey" has permitted the inclusion of an Addendum. This 1985 edition will, therefore, provide the reader with the original text together with additional and more up-to-date information on a chapter to chapter basis. I cannot claim that the latter is comprehensive. Nevertheless, it should help to alert the reader to the many new, and often exciting, advances that have been made since this book first appeared.

Raptor diseases have now become a respectable and *bona fide* field of study and many disciplines, in addition to the veterinary profession, can and do have an important part to play. Indeed, it might be argued that no longer is it realistic for one person to write a volume on the subject singlehanded. Certainly, as chapters on raptor medicine and pathology in other books have illustrated, there is merit in inviting specialists to contribute sections on their own subject and this approach may well be emulated when a further edition of "Veterinary Aspects of Captive Birds of Prey" appears sometime in the future.

I must express my thanks to those people, many of them referred to personally in the 1978 edition, who have continued to collaborate with me in my studies on birds of prey and their diseases. I owe a particular debt of gratitude to friends and colleagues who have referred cases, submitted pathological material or permitted me to have samples for research. Many other people supported and helped me, especially by providing second opinions on cases or specimens, identifying parasites or analysing carcases. My special thanks in this respect are due to Malcolm Brearley, John Eley, Dermod Malley, Martin Lawton, Eileen Harris and Michael French. Simon Rolfe has assisted me on many occasions with clinical procedures and other tasks and Sally Dowsett has dealt cheerfully with the typing of manuscripts and reports. Colleagues and staff at the Royal College of Surgeons have given me support and encouragement in my studies.

Finally, as before, I must thank my family for their long-suffering support and forbearance and, in particular, my wife who, in addition to assisting with the care of birds and protecting me from the telephone, has enthusiastically developed her own interest and expertise in the law so that we are able to work as a team – with a remarkable degree of synergism – on both a professional and domestic level.

London   *J. E. Cooper*
    October 1985

VETERINARY ASPECTS
OF
CAPTIVE BIRDS OF PREY
WITH 1985 SUPPLEMENT

by

J. E. COOPER,
BVSc DTVM MRCVS FIBiol

Line drawings by
THEA LLOYD

With a Foreword by the late
LESLIE BROWN

THE STANDFAST PRESS

First published by The Standfast Press, 1978
2nd edition with revisions 1985
Reprinted 1987

Published by The Standfast Press, The Old Rectory,
Cherington, Tetbury, Gloucestershire

ISBN 0 904602 04 4

Text set in 11/12 pt Photon Times, Printed by photolithography
and bound in Great Britain at The Bath Press, Avon

TO

Margaret, Vanessa and Maxwell

"Call down the hawk from
the air;
Let him be hooded or caged."

W. B. Yeats

Preface

This book first appeared, as a limited edition, in 1973 and was published by the Hawk Trust. The second edition differs in many ways from its predecessor and I discuss this in more detail at the end of Chapter 1. Basically the aim of the book is to bring together in one volume much of the information available on the veterinary care of birds of prey which are maintained in captivity. After considerable thought I decided to write in the first person throughout in preference to the rather cumbersome third person which is prevalent in scientific publications. In so doing I hope I have made the book more readable and less impersonal. For the same reason the References are listed at the end and only referred to by number in the text.

I should like to acknowledge the many colleagues and friends who have assisted over the years in my investigations into the diseases of birds of prey, especially by submitting sick or dead birds to me for examination.

Many veterinary surgeons, both in Britain and overseas, have been most helpful in referring birds to me, by providing access to their records or correspondence and by commenting on my own cases. Having expressed my thanks to many of them in the first edition I trust they will understand if I do not list them again here. Michael Williams, who wrote a kind and complimentary Foreword to the first edition, has continued to collaborate closely and I must repeat my gratitude to him.

I am indebted to North American colleagues on the Pathology Committee of the Raptor Research Association for advice and opinions provided by them on many occasions; and likewise to the Hawk Trust and British Falconers' Club for their encouragement with my work. Both the latter two organisations permitted me to include in this book parts of articles which previously appeared in their publications. The Hamlyn Group granted me permission to use material in Chapter 9 from "Eagles, Hawks and Falcons of the World" by L. H. Brown and D. Amadon while the Post Office allowed me to reproduce the part of their Regulations relating to the submission of material for laboratory examination.

I have been fortunate in having the assistance of many competent and enthusiastic people with my surgical and *post-mortem* work and I must mention in particular Keith Bolton, David Evans and, while I was in Kenya, Alfred Odingo and Sammy Njengi. I owe particular thanks to Jeffrey Needham for his support in my work and his co-operation with bacteriological examinations on many occasions.

I am especially grateful to Dr W. M. (now Sir William) Henderson, Mr John Tremlett and Dr Charles Coid for their encouragement and tolerance of my extra-mural studies while I was a member of their staff. Dr Ariela Pomerance has been most generous with her time and contributions to our joint study of cardiovascular lesions in non-domesticated species. Much of the radiology reported in this book and in papers elsewhere would have been impossible without the enthusiasm of Dr. Louis Kreel and his staff at the Clinical Research Centre and, more recently, the co-operation of Mr David Soldan and his colleagues in Huntingdon. Ian Jebbett, Graeme Backhurst and the staff of the Medical Illustration Department at the Clinical Research Centre assisted with the photography of specimens. While I was in Kenya, Dr Leslie Brown gave me great encouragement and invaluable advice on the biology and management of my captive birds.

The following very kindly read and criticised parts of this book prior to publication: M. Allen, D. M. Bird, M. Böttcher, G. Clayton-Jones, M. E. Cooper, A. G. Greenwood, P. E. Holt, P. N. Humphreys, L. H. Hurrell, C. Jones, R. E. Kenward, J. Kirkwood, D. J. Lewis, J. W. Macdonald, J. R. Needham, M. A. Peirce, A. Pomerance, P. T. Redig and R. Scammell.

A number of people assisted with typing but Anita Whittaker and Mrs. D. Suttie bore the brunt of this in the later stages. I must thank Murielle John for her help in this respect as well as for technical support with clinical and *post-mortem* cases. I am greatly indebted to the library staff at the Clinical Research Centre, Huntingdon Research Centre, Houghton Poultry Research Station and the Royal College of Veterinary Surgeons for their research on many occasions.

Parasites were very kindly examined and identified by members of staff at the British Museum (Natural History) to whom I am most grateful. Blood smears were examined (or, in some cases, re-examined) by Michael Peirce with whom I have been fortunate enough to collaborate for some years. Mr. Ian Prestt, formerly of the Nature Conservancy (Monks Wood) and now Director of the Royal Society for the Protection of Birds, very kindly analysed tissues from a number of cases where pesticides were suspected. Staff of many other establishments have advised me on numerous occasions and continue to do so; their advice and support are greatly appreciated.

I am particularly indebted to Leslie Brown for his Foreword, Thea Lloyd for her drawings, to my wife for the Appendix on the relevant law and to them and Captain Richard Grant-Rennick for their help with the production of this edition.

I should like to take this opportunity of expressing my debt of gratitude to the late Major Maxwell Knight, the naturalist and broadcaster, my friend and mentor for many years. Were it not for his interest in my first injured kestrel, I should not have had a glimpse of the world of hawks and falconry and this book might never have been written. In the same context it gives me great pleasure to thank Mr. Paul Jacklin for his tuition and encouragement and for entrusting me with his hawks on so many occasions.

Finally, I must thank my parents for their constant encouragement and my wife for her invaluable assistance and advice, in particular in checking manuscripts and in the post-operative care of patients. Sick and injured birds of prey have shared our home for nine years and will undoubtedly continue to do so!

Huntingdon   *J. E. Cooper*

January 1978

Contents

Foreword

Mystery enshrouds the causes of death in most wild birds—including birds of prey—unless they are shot or electrocuted or run down by cars. In a few cases we know that they die of disease, and often, we assume, of starvation. However, the really well-documented causes of death or illness, other than by unnatural means such as shooting, are few; and will probably remain so.

We may assume, however, that some of the ailments that affect wild birds of prey also affect captives. Here we have a solid, thoroughly researched and abundantly documented treatise on the diseases and accidents that may affect captive birds of prey, both diurnal species and owls, by an expert veterinarian with deep and long practical experience of such matters. I knew John Cooper when he was in East Africa and his house was then full of sick or damaged raptors, apparently is so still, and is, according to him, likely to remain so. It is very doubtful if they could have the fortune to fall into better hands.

Mr. Cooper firmly removes the treatment of sick or injured birds of prey from the hocus-pocus and abracadabra of old wives' tales and obscure remedies, right into the twentieth century. But he does not neglect to pay tribute to an older generation of falconers, who from practical necessity found ways to cure or ease some of the ills from which their prized birds suffered. Falconers, apparently, used to be reluctant to consult veterinarians who perhaps knew less about it than they did. Here is a book that shows conclusively that any such attitude is out of date: the treatment of birds of prey, sick or injured, has been modernised, and is thoroughly described herein, with details of how to do it, using many of the modern techniques applied in human medicine.

Arabs used to equate the value of a fine falcon with that of a good horse. A good falcon might now be the more valuable of the two, and is certainly a very valuable bird. Some rare specimens in zoos may be priceless, for restrictions on the capture of threatened species such as the Philippine monkey-eating eagle will ensure that no more can be obtained. For such birds it is necessary to have the service of a skilled veterinarian, who knows what he is talking about: and in this book you can find how to look after an injured or sick bird until such a skilled veterinarian can be found, so that he has a better chance of saving its life.

Falconers use many queer but ancient terms for the condition and ailments of birds of prey. Mr. Cooper makes simple sense out of all that. "Snurt" seems to me an entirely appropriate name for a runny nose, or rhinitis, an affliction I often suffer from myself. When next I am constipated I shall complain that I have something wrong with my tewel. We move here straight from the middle ages, and earlier, to the twentieth century.

The twelve chapters explain everything from nomenclature, investigation and treatment to nervous disorders, anaesthesia, and surgery. You need not give up hope if your bird has a simple fracture: there is quite a chance that it may fly again. Mr. Cooper sums it all up in a valuable chapter on discussion and conclusions and provides many appendices, line drawings by Thea Lloyd and photographs.

He has gathered his information from several hundred references, old and modern. This is a very thoroughly researched book indeed. It will be indispensable not only to those who keep falcons or birds of prey in zoos, but to students of the wild species in the field.

JUNE   LESLIE BROWN
1978

CHAPTER 1

Introduction

In the first edition of this book I expressed surprise at the paucity of scientific information on the diseases of birds of prey in view of the fact that the sport of falconry has been practised for over 2,000 years. This was not to suggest, however, that nothing was known of the subject. Early writings show that many diseases of trained falcons were recognised by the Arabs 1,000 or more years ago and there is a wealth of information in such literature. In a lecture at the International Conference on Falconry in Abu Dhabi in 1976 Möller (300) discussed Arabic treatises on falconry and drew attention to the many references to diseases of the birds and their treatment; amongst works he reviewed were some dating from the 9th century AD. In a paper on "Diseases of the falcon and their treatment" (425) Shaikh Zaid Bin Sultan Al Nahayan, President of the United Arab Emirates, emphasised the number of traditional cures known to the Bedouin. A detailed modern work on Arab falconry is urgently needed and it is hoped that this will bring together some of the scattered information on disease.

One of the first printed books in English on falconry, "The Boke of Saint Albans" (30), appeared in 1486 and this contained a considerable amount of data on the then known diseases of hawks. An earlier work on hunting, by William Twiti, has recently been edited by Daniellson (124) and later volumes, not yet published, include sections on diseases of birds used in falconry. It will be of great interest to compare these with other works.

A large number of other books on falconry appeared between the fourteenth and sixteenth centuries and in the majority of these information was given on the diseases of hawks, their prevention and cure. There is a need for a full account of the history of hawk medicine since, as Comben (78) pointed out in a review of early literature on bird diseases, several of the conditions of trained hawks diagnosed centuries ago, such as "frounce" and "cramp", are still recognisable today.

The important names in hawk medicine in the 16th and 17th centuries were probably Turbervile (395), Latham (269) and Bert (32), all of whom published books on falconry. Bert appears to have been something of a veterinary consultant for in his book "An Approved Treatise of Hawkes and Hawking" he introduced the section on disease as follows:—

> "Wherein is contained cures for all known diseases, all of which have been practised by my selfe more upon worthy mens Hawkes that have be sent unto me . . .".

Although much of the information in these books is anecdotal, some techniques are worthy of note. Attention will be drawn later to Latham's recommended treatment for bumblefoot; his description differs very little from modern surgical techniques and I think we can assume that Latham and his contemporaries achieved some success with the method.

Richard Blome is worthy of mention even though he openly published other men's work under his own name. From the veterinary point of view, his publications are of interest. He depicted surgical (cauterising) instruments in his book "The Gentleman's Recreation" (46) and in the same volume included the following very important maxim:

> "Diseases are easier prevented than cured; everyone therefore that intends to keep Hawks should be well advised in the first place how to preserve them from Sickness and Maladies, which is of greater concern than to cure them when distempered".

For all his shortcomings, Blome can be considered one of the earliest proponents of preventive medicine!

Little was then published of an original nature for over 150 years. Harting's "Hints on the Management of Hawks and Practical Falconry" (200) appeared in 1898 and it is of interest to note that he had little time for the ancient remedies for treating hawks: he stated that "No English falconers of the present day believe in them, and there can be no doubt that the less medicine given the better". In 1891 Harting produced his "Bibliotheca Accipitraria" (199) which reviewed the literature on hawks and falconry and it is of interest to note that, by that date, 82 such works had appeared in English and many of these dealt in whole or in part with disease. Nevertheless, with the advent of the gun and the enclosure of land, interest in falconry had waned in Britain and the status of the bird of prey had declined from that of a strictly protected bird (with severe penalties for those who killed or took one) to the stage where every bird with a hooked beak was shot mercilessly by landowners and gamekeepers.

Falconry, however, never completely died out and a small band of enthusiasts, first named The Old Hawking Club and later the British Falconers' Club, sustained the sport during the difficult period of the late 19th and 20th centuries. Books continued to appear in small numbers but these mainly repeated many of the age-old remedies and it is obvious that knowledge of hawk pathology did not advance at the same rate as other spheres of veterinary medicine. For example, in his book "The Art and Practice of Hawking" (299) in 1900 Michell described a number of diseases but his suggested remedies were almost entirely taken from the older texts. For "snurt" (cold in the head), for instance, he referred his readers to Bert's recipe of "root of wild primrose dried in an oven and powdered". Blaine (44), in his book "Falconry" (1936), showed a rather more enlightened approach, in that he described some of the ailments of hawks in twentieth century English. He retained faith in many of the old falconers' medicines, however, and stated "For my own part, I feel that great benefit might accrue from the use of many of their quaint remedies, if we only knew how to concoct and apply them".

The first real scientific advance in raptor medicine was probably in the 1930's when Dr Tom Hare, a veterinary surgeon who was also medically qualified, began to examine birds for the British Falconers' Club. I have been fortunate enough to be given, by Mr J. G. Mavrogordato, some letters which he received from Dr Hare and the latter's enthusiasm for the subject ("Many thanks for the specimens – send lots more") is very apparent. Hare was preoccupied with certain conditions, for example capillariasis and coccidiosis (198), but this in no way detracts from his reputation as the first to utilise modern laboratory techniques, such as parasitology, for the diagnosis of hawk diseases.

The 2nd World War delayed further progress but advances were made in the succeeding years. Falconers in particular began to realise that veterinary attention for hawks might prove profitable and there was renewed interest in having *post-mortem* examinations carried out – ". . . we might even get to the point of curing some at least of these sick hawks" stated one contributor to "The Falconer" (3). In 1954 Stabler (382) elucidated the cause of "frounce" and was able to recommend a modern antiprotozoal drug for its treatment; this and other scientific contributions were quoted in Woodford's "A Manual of Falconry" (422) in 1960. Woodford's book was one of a number to appear in the 1960's but its approach to disease was a scientific one and, while some caution was urged, the use of modern drugs and techniques was unequivocally recommended. Other authors were less than enthusiastic, however, and ap Evans (138), also writing in 1960, went so far as to state that:

". . . there is no doubt it is far better (except in cases of Frounce) to stick to the natural physics which are the basis of these old recipes. Only if they fail should the falconer subject his hawk to the mercy of laboratory remedies".

With the passing of The Protection of Birds Act, 1954, and subsequent legislation the survival of falconry in Britain was assured and its popularity began to increase. Soon after this time a drastic decline in numbers of certain birds of prey in Europe and America was noted (205, 347, 348) and investigations at that time, and subsequently, indicated that pesticides, particularly the chlorinated hydrocarbons, might be responsible (230, 350). Further work suggested that one effect of such chemicals was a decrease in eggshell weight and hence reduced hatching success (349, 350) although other factors involved probably included failure to lay, desertions and embryonic deaths (319). Later investigations suggested that the polychlorinated biphenyls (PCB's) might also be contributing to the decline of some species (275). A useful review of the role of pesticides was the article in the "Canadian Field-Naturalist" in 1976, by Peakall (330) and the reader is referred to that and other papers in the same edition. It is important to remember that certain species have also become threatened due to destruction of habitat and persecution by man; an indication of the status of some is given in the IUCN "Red Data Book" (401).

In the 1960's and 1970's progressive restrictions were imposed on the use of DDT and certain other pesticides in European countries, the United States and Canada and these appeared to reverse the trend. However, the status of some species is still precarious and has not been helped in recent years by an increase in thefts of eggs and young. As a result the future of falconry at present is in doubt, there being many enthusiasts but few suitable birds available, and a number of falconers have turned their interest towards conservation and the breeding of hawks in captivity, fields in which they have made great advances.

The risk of extinction which threatens many free-living predatory species has resulted in considerable interest amongst biologists in the behaviour, physiology and ecology of birds of prey and increasingly large numbers are now being maintained and, in some cases, bred in captivity for study purposes. In the United States of America, for example, a colony of American kestrels was established some years ago to study the effects of various pesticides (341). Serious attempts to breed the peregrine commenced in North America in 1970 and met with great success (64) permitting birds to be used for a variety of purposes. Such work could conceivably have far-reaching implications for man since considerable concern has been expressed over the build-up of insecticide residues in the environment, and the role of these and other pollutants in man himself (9, 222, 285).

There are also possible conservation reasons for breeding predators in captivity. The most acceptable of these is that, by breeding birds in captivity and making them available to falconers and zoological collections, one is able to reduce pressures on those in the wild. This was the point made in the following Recommendation of the European Section of the International Council for Bird Preservation in 1976:

> "That the avicultural societies of Europe promote and encourage breeding programmes in order to lessen the drain of taking birds from wild populations".

The second reason is the possibility of releasing captive bred birds to the wild, but this is more controversial. The mortality rate of most first-year birds in the wild is very high (59, 381) and many people have suggested that the wild populations could be augmented by breeding, or rearing, young hawks in captivity for their first year and subsequently releasing them. In Britain this proposition has encountered considerable opposition from many conservation bodies but elsewhere, particularly where free-living populations are at risk, the reception has been generally favourable. For example, in an editorial on raptor research and conservation in the "Canadian Field-Naturalist" mentioned earlier, Dr Ian Newton (318) (himself British) said:

> "Another welcome development of the last five years has been the successful breeding of peregrines in captivity, not just a few birds, but on a scale sufficient for release projects".

Newton went on to argue that such work had at least ensured the survival of endangered genotypes, albeit in captive populations, and this alone could be an important argument for captive breeding. However, in North America reintroduction of such birds to the wild has already commenced and encouraging results have been obtained (267). Work on captive breeding has been extended to other species, amongst them the endangered Mauritius kestrel, and at the time of writing a pair of this species is being maintained in the hope of breeding them for ultimate release.

It will be apparent from the foregoing that, since the first edition of this book appeared, there have been dramatic advances in captive breeding. The significance of such work is enormous, not only to falconry but also to all aspects of raptor biology; the emphasis, therefore, in many sections of this edition is on the health problems of captive bred birds.

The relevance of birds of prey to the veterinary profession was at one time only minimal but has increased greatly in recent years. The veterinary surgeon may be involved in four main fields, these being falconry, aviculture, wild bird casualties and research.

With the upsurge of interest in falconry, many practising veterinary surgeons find they are consulted on sick or injured hawks. A well-trained bird is valuable and the genuine falconer will go to much trouble and expense to obtain help or advice; less experienced falconers may need guidance on management from the point of view of health and preventive medicine.

Large numbers of birds are maintained in captivity in zoos, safari parks and private collections and these often include birds of prey. Veterinary advice on such collections is increasingly being sought. Captive breeding in particular is very much in vogue and birds of prey that are "close-ringed and bred in captivity" are now a recognised part of the avicultural scene. Captive breeding does, however, bring with it many problems related to health. Recent legislation in Britain has helped increase the participation of the veterinary profession in work with birds kept for exhibition, aviculture or pets. The Importation of Captive Birds Order 1976 requires all incoming birds, including raptors, to be quarantined and the veterinary surgeon who is a Local Veterinary Inspector may find himself involved in the regular inspection of birds in quarantine. Such duties are greatly facilitated by an interest in, and understanding of, avian diseases.

There has always been great concern amongst the public in Britain and elsewhere over the plight of wild bird "casualties" and many species, including raptors, may be presented for veterinary attention (101). Such care can certainly be justified on humanitarian grounds and, in some cases, may be significant in terms of conservation. From the scientific point of view work with casualties can yield useful information on causes of disease and death in wild populations. Involvement in the care of such birds will certainly offer the veterinary surgeon a unique opportunity to deal with unusual species and to gain expertise in surgical and medical techniques.

As a result of increased interest in the biology of predatory birds veterinary advice on such subjects as immobilisation, surgery and pathology is proving of increasing value to the scientists engaged in such studies. For example, while in Africa I was frequently asked to assist zoological colleagues at a number of institutions in their work with free-living and captive birds. Similar liaison occurs elsewhere including Europe and North America; for example Ratcliffe (350) consulted avian pathologists on possible differential diagnoses for eggshell thinning in British raptors when carrying out his famous work on pesticide residues. Under this same heading one can include birds of prey maintained for experimental purposes; they have been used for bacteriological (45) and toxicological studies (146, 342), and for more basic research, such as work on metabolism (167), pellet formation (182) and vision (291, 292).

When the first edition of this book appeared, I pointed out how little scientifically based literature on raptor disease was available to the veterinary surgeon with the exception of scattered papers, data in the 1955 bibliography by Halloran (190) and certain articles in falconry books and journals. Indeed, it was largely on account of this dearth of information that the book was originally launched.

In the last five years however, the situation has improved enormously. In particular it has been encouraging to note the inclusion of raptors in books on avian, and even poultry, health. The book "Bird Diseases" by Arnall and Keymer (15) includes data on birds of prey as does "Poultry Diseases" edited by Gordon (170). In addition, there has been a great increase in relevant papers in veterinary, ornithological and falconry journals. The majority of these have dealt with specific diseases or case histories but there have also been useful reviews and surveys. For example, Keymer (249) examined 125 captive birds of prey *post mortem* and compared his results with those of other workers. Some indication of fatalities in captive birds was given by Kenward (245) who estimated the first year mortality using a questionnaire distributed to falconers. Papers have also continued to appear on causes of death in free-living birds, amongst them raptors.

Certain zoological publications, for example, the "International Zoo Yearbook", regularly include contributions that are relevant to birds of prey. Pathological reports from veterinary laboratories and zoological collections, in particular the Zoological Society of London, are useful sources of information on causes of death of captive species. "Index Veterinarius", which lists publications on various veterinary topics each year, is of particular value. Birds of prey are now allotted their own heading in the Index and between 1972 and 1975 there were 94 papers dealing specifically with them, and a number of others which had some relevance to their biology or diseases.

In languages other than English, progress has also been made; some early useful additions to the literature included theses in German by Gerdessen (168) and Stehle (385), and in French by Bougerol (51), all of which discussed diseases of birds of prey and supplied a number of references. These works were valuable contributions but Bougerol did not, on his own admission, give detailed clinical or pathological data on the conditions discussed. There have also been scientific papers on raptor disease in German in recent years, for example by Kaleta and Drüner (241) and Kösters (265).

An important factor in the accumulation of data on diseases of birds of prey has been the co-operation of falconers and aviculturists who have increasingly sought professional advice over sick and dead birds. There has been a refreshingly new approach to disease and the majority of falconers, in particular, no longer seek to withold information on their birds and are generally willing to permit modern medical and surgical techniques to be used on them. In this context one should note the comments made by the ornithologist Dr Leslie Brown in his book "British Birds of Prey" (57). While complimentary about falconry and the past and present role of falconers as champions of birds of prey, Brown says

"I could wish that falconers kept better records of such details as moult to adult plumage, the age to which their hawks survive, disease problems, amount of food consumed, and survival rates of captive as opposed to wild hawks, for in these ways they could add considerably to our knowledge of birds of prey . . ."

Although undoubtedly true some years ago, this statement does not take into consideration the great advance made in bird of prey pathology in the past ten years through the efforts of European and North American falconers, many of them professionally involved in veterinary medicine or avian biology. Such work is exemplified by the papers of high quality presented in recent years at the meetings of the Raptor Research Foundation in the United States, many of which are published in the journal "Raptor Research" and the interest shown in Britain in British Falconers' Club Conference sessions on diseases of birds of prey (177, 107).

The second edition of this book has a rather different approach from the first. I hope that it will prove to be a useful, and practical, handbook for veterinary surgeons and others who deal with the health and welfare of birds of prey. It should particularly be noted that no attempt has been made to mention all recorded diseases of raptors and there are some omissions, especially amongst those conditions reported only from free-living birds. A number of other books on avian diseases, while providing ample text, have tended to give few supporting references. In this book, therefore, I have referred to a wide variety of published works and it is hoped that the journals and books listed at the back will prove a useful guide to the scientific and lay literature. Every effort has been made to provide a reference when an unusual or poorly documented subject is under discussion or when it is probable that the reader will need further information.

Another important point concerns the subject matter and the arrangement of chapters. The layout of the book does not always correspond closely to that in more conventional books on veterinary medicine. Instead prominence has been given to topics of practical or potential importance, and, where appropriate, a chapter or section has been devoted to these in preference to subjects of more academic interest only. Other conditions may be mentioned only briefly or, perhaps, discussed under a less familar heading. For example, stomatitis is covered in the chapter on parasitic diseases since the most common (or most widely recognised) form of stomatitis is that due to a protozoan parasite; the causes of regurgitation are discussed under infectious diseases for similar reasons. The reader is advised, therefore, to refer to the index at the back of the book since a particular topic may be covered under a number of different subjects.

In the first edition I included clinical and pathological data on all the cases that I had personally treated or examined. These are omitted from this edition and, instead, the accumulated data have been used to compile a general guide. Those readers who require such detailed information can best be advised with the words of Markham (287) in 1631:

> "All which forasmuch as I have shewed the Medicines and cures thereof in the former treatise . . . I will refer you unto the same, and not doubt but it will give you satisfaction".

CHAPTER 2

Nomenclature

Falconry abounds in unusual terminology, much of which has been in use for centuries and some of which has crept into work with raptors kept for exhibition and breeding. A summary of the more relevant terms was given in an article I wrote in the "Journal of Small Animal Practice" in 1968 (82) while comprehensive lists are to be found in most falconry books. "A Manual of Falconry" by Woodford (422) is particularly recommended since it reprinted Harting's glossary and vocabulary (199) and gave the origins of such words. It also provided a list of falconry terms in other languages.

In this book I have avoided such words except where they are either commonly used or are pertinent to veterinary work and in such cases an explanation will be given. As was pointed out in the first chapter, very many diseases of hawks were known centuries ago and the terminology was often fascinating – for example, Markham (287) wrote in 1631:

> "Hawkes have divers infirmities and diseases, as Feavers, Palsey, Imposthumes, Sore eyes, and Nares, Megums, Pantas, casting her Gorge, fouleness of Gorge, Wormes, Fillanders, ill liver, or Goute, Pinne in the foot, breaking the pounce, Bones out of ioynt, Bones broken, Bruises, Lice, Colds, Frounce, Fistulaes, Stone, much gaping, more foundring, privy evill, taint in the feathers, loste of appetite, broken wind, blow on wing, wounds, swellings, eating their owne feet, taking up of veines in Hawkes, Crampe, and a world of others".

Examples of ancient and modern terms for some hawk diseases are given in Table I. Falconers will still use words such as "croaks", "cramp" and "frounce" and it is important that the veterinary surgeon is aware of them and their probable meaning.

A knowledge of falconry terms for parts of the hawk's body can also prove useful; reference should be made to Figure 1 which depicts both falconers' and "scientific" terms for various structures. Internal anatomy cannot be considered in detail in this book but it is important that anyone dealing with birds of prey has an understanding of it. Of particular importance in surgery is the skeletal structure of the limbs and the relative positions of visceral organs. Much useful information on this can be obtained from poultry textbooks and from the chapter on anatomy by Evans in "Diseases of Cage and Aviary Birds" (139). The physiology of birds is also important and reference will be made to various aspects of this later in the book. Again there is specialised and technical language and the reader is advised to consult relevant books and papers; a useful review of raptor energetics is that by Mosher (304), while the volumes on "Avian Biology" edited by Farner and King (142) cover a wide range of subjects.

Table 1

SOME ANCIENT CONDITIONS OF HAWKS AND THEIR POSSIBLE MODERN EQUIVALENTS

Old name	Usual description	Possible modern equivalent	Comments
"Blain"	Watery blister on second joint of wing. Later the joint may stiffen.	Bursitis of carpus followed by arthritis and ankylosis.	A word still used by falconers. Sporadic cases are still seen. See Chapter 5.
"Craye" or "Cray"	Stoppage of the "tewel" (lower bowel).	Constipation or impaction of intestine.	Regularly seen. Some old fashioned remedies are still in use.
"Crampe" or "Cramp"	Stiffness, especially of legs; spontaneous fractures may occur.	Osteodystrophy (and possibly other causes).	A word still used by falconers. Osteodystrophy is very important in young birds. See Chapters 9 and 11.
"Croaks", "Kecks" or "Pantas"	Difficult and noisy respiration.	Various respiratory infections.	The word "croaks" is still used by falconers. Respiratory diseases are very important. See Chapter 5.
"Fellanders" or "Fillanders"	Intestinal worms.	Capillariasis.	A term now rarely used by falconers. See Chapter 6.
"Frounce" or "Frownce"	Debris in mouth, especially palate and tongue.	a) Trichomoniasis b) Stomatitis (various aetiologies).	A word still used by falconers. Very important. See Chapter 6.
"Pinne in the foot"	Swelling of the foot.	Bumblefoot.	Very commonly seen. See Chapter 7.
"Rye"	A swelling in the head.	Sinusitis.	Regularly seen. See Chapter 5.
"Snurt" or "Cold"	Nasal discharge and sneezing.	Rhinitis.	Regularly seen. Still sometimes treated by falconers with intra-nasal oil of eucalyptus. See Chapter 5.
"Vertego"	A swimming of the brain.	Nervous disease.	Many nervous diseases are now recognised. See Chapter 8.

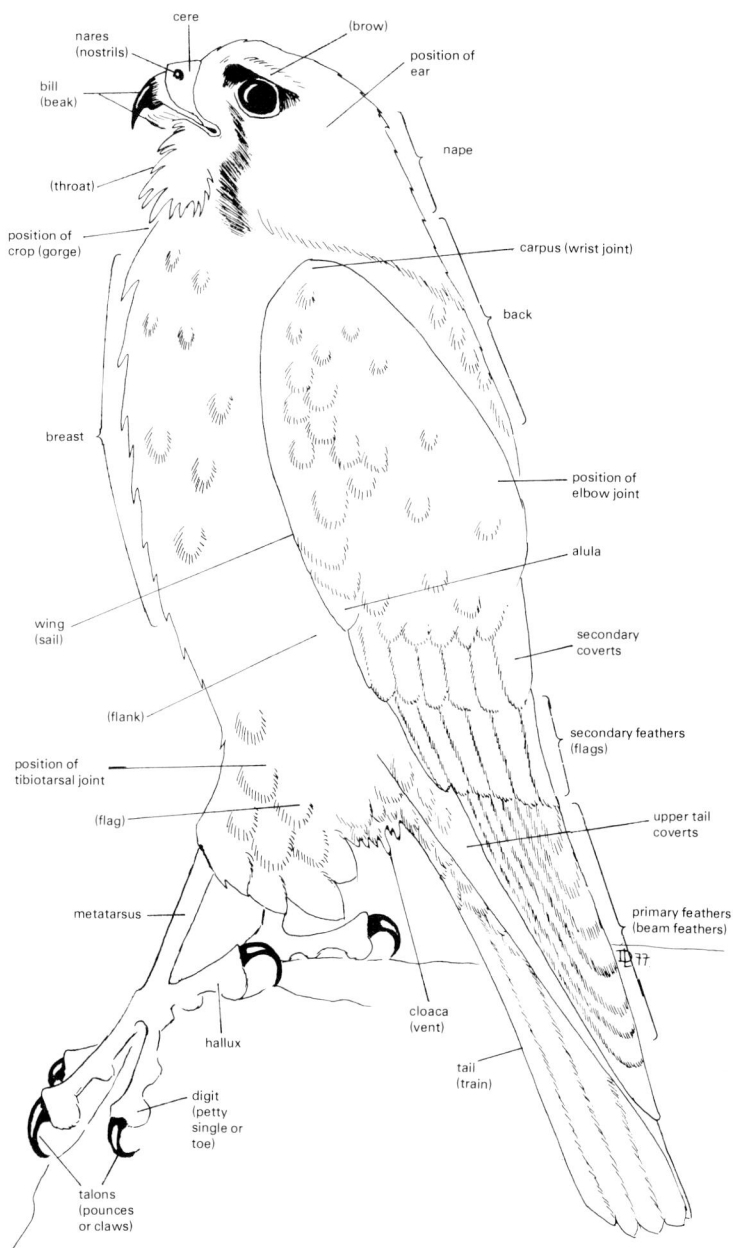

Fig. 1   External features of a falconiform bird of prey. Falconers' or laymen's terms are given in brackets

The birds covered in this book are those in the Order Strigiformes, the owls, (Families Strigidae and Tytonidae), and the Order Falconiformes which includes the Families Cathartidae (New World vultures), Accipitridae (kites, hawks, eagles and Old World vultures), Falconidae (falcons), Pandionidae (ospreys) and Sagittariidae (secretary birds). For more detailed information on taxonomy the reader is referred to the standard volumes by Brown and Amadon (59) for the Falconiformes and Peters (338) for the Strigiformes. Other terminology relating to birds of prey may also be found in ornithological texts, including "Birds of Prey of the World" (183) which includes an interesting chapter on birds of prey and man, and the recent book by Brown (58). The word "free-living" is used to distinguish those raptors in the wild from their captive counterparts: all birds of prey are, strictly, "wild" birds although after several generations in captivity they will probably be justifiably termed "domesticated".

Various falconry words refer to the different species and sexes of birds of prey and these can be confusing to the uninitiated. For all falconiform birds of prey, of either sex, therefore, the comprehensive word "hawk" will generally be used in this book and for all strigiform species, "owl". "Raptor" is more often heard in North America than Britain, but will be used here for any type of bird of prey. The word "falcon" will be used in the ornithological sense (i.e. a member of the Family Falconidae) and not, as in falconry parlance, for the female bird alone. The term "tiercel" (a male bird) will not be mentioned. When a specific bird is discussed the English name will be employed and a list of English and scientific names of all birds of prey mentioned in the text is given in Appendix I.

Other problems of falconry nomenclature concern management since trained hawks are kept rather differently from those in a collection. Many such terms have also crept into captive breeding. The management of trained hawks was outlined for the veterinary surgeon in the paper mentioned earlier (82) and will not be repeated in detail. Useful notes were also given by Greenwood (177) in his report of a British Falconers' Club Conference; he dealt with raptors in aviaries and breeding lofts as well as those kept for falconry. Suffice it to say that a trained hawk is kept tethered other than when it is being flown. It has a pair of leather jesses tied to its legs and except when flying these are attached by a swivel to a leash. The hawk is carried on a leather glove on the falconer's left hand.

It may or may not be "hooded" in order to quieten it. It is flown by reducing its food intake so that it is "keen" but not starved. During the day it is perched on a "block", a "ring perch" or a "bow perch" (depending on species and size) and, at night, indoors on a "screen perch". It may be carried – for example, to a veterinary surgery – on a portable perch called a "cadge". The building in which the bird is housed is called a "mews" and the droppings of a hawk (which contain both faecal and urate portions) are commonly called "mutes". The latter term will be used from time to time in this book. The droppings of short-winged hawks, such as goshawks, are called "slices" since they are shot with considerable force away from the bird's perch. A hawk "bates" when it tries to fly off the fist or perch, but remains held by its jesses. Other terms are explained elsewhere in the book.

A brief explanation of some scientific terms may also prove useful to those readers who are not veterinary surgeons or otherwise familiar with medical language. Anatomical terminology will not be covered; for this I would refer the reader to standard texts such as "Outlines of Avian Anatomy" by King and McLelland (256). Information on medical words not explained in this Chapter can be obtained from standard medical or veterinary dictionaries.

Insofar as clinical descriptions are concerned, "clinical signs" can be equated with "symptoms"; the latter word is now rarely used in veterinary medicine. Some important clinical signs described in the book include "anorexia" (absence of appetite), "dyspnoea" (difficult breathing), "tachypnoea" (rapid breathing), "dysphagia" (difficulty in swallowing), "diarrhoea" (loose faeces), "dysentery" (blood in faeces), "oedema" (abnormal accumulation of fluid), "hyperaemia" (increase in blood supply), "atrophy" (decrease in size of a tissue or organ) and "hypertrophy" (increase in size of a tissue or organ). Clinical diseases may be described as "peracute", "acute", "subacute" and "chronic" depending upon their duration while the forecast of the probable course of a disease, regardless of its cause, is the "prognosis".

Pathology is "the study of disease" but usually implies the examination of dead tissues, or samples taken from clinical cases. Some of the terms used in pathology are worthy of mention although many of the words mentioned earlier are also used in a pathological context. The "aetiology" of a disease is "the study of the cause" of that disease. There are many definitions of "disease" but the one I favour is that in the Oxford Dictionary – "disordered state of an organism or organ". Insofar as "infection" is concerned, this is different from disease since an infection implies the entry of an organism into a susceptible host, in which it may persist, but detectable clinical or pathological effects may or may not be apparent. Thus, for example, a bird of prey can be *infected* with coccidia but not necessarily suffering from coccidiosis. An "infectious disease", on the other hand, implies a disease caused by the actions of a living organism as opposed to physical injuries or endocrinological disorders or genetic abnormalities. In a "latent infection" there is an inapparent infection in which the pathogen persists within a host, but may be activated to produce clinical disease by such factors as stress or impaired host resistance. A "pathogen" is an organism capable of producing disease; the term can be used for organisms as diverse as viruses, bacteria and parasites and the adjective describing such agents is "pathogenic". A "lesion" is an abnormality caused by disease of a tissue; usually it is characterised by changes in appearance of that tissue. A "focus" (plural "foci") is a small, usually distinct, lesion, such as a micro-abscess in the liver. The word is also used clinically to imply the principal seat of a disease – for example, "a focus of tuberculosis in the thorax".

Words with the suffix "-aemia" imply an abnormality, or presence of an obnoxious agent, in the blood. Thus "toxaemia" is a condition in which a toxin (poison) is present in the blood and the terms "bacteraemia" "viraemia" and "parasitaemia" are self explanatory. The multiplication of organisms in the blood, usually with pathological effects on organs, is called a "septicaemia".

In epidemiological parlance the "incubation period" is the time between infection and clinical signs. "Mortality rate" refers to the proportion of deaths during a given time and "morbidity rate" to the proportion of cases of a particular disease during a given time.

Two terms which are often misused – and here I make no apology to veterinary colleagues for referring to them – are "incidence" and "prevalence". The former is "the number of new cases of a particular disease during a stated period of time, in a population under study" whereas "prevalence" means "the total number of cases of a particular disease at a given moment of time, in a population under study".

In publishing these definitions I realise that I lay myself open to accusations of being too brief and inaccurate and of attempting to make the book readable to the layman at the expense of the reader with a veterinary or medical background. Likewise my falconer friends will insist that my description of falconry terms is far from adequate and, in places, open to wider interpretation. Nevertheless, in a book such as this, which is likely to be used by people from a wide range of disciplines, it seems important to include some mention and interpretation of technical terms, whether relating to the birds or their diseases.

CHAPTER 3

Methods of investigation and treatment

The species covered in this book are the "diurnal" birds of prey (Falconiformes) and "nocturnal" ones (Strigiformes) and the classification of these was discussed briefly in the previous chapter.

There are two main aspects to veterinary work with birds of prey:

(1) Clinical – clinical examination, clinical aids and laboratory tests,
(2) *Post mortem* – macroscopical examination and laboratory tests.

In addition to my own work I shall be referring to correspondence and discussion with other veterinary surgeons, zoologists, falconers and aviculturists and, in some cases, quoting their records. Much of the original work on which this book was primarily based was carried out in conjunction with the British Falconers' Club and Hawk Trust.

Members of these organisations (and others) submit live birds for treatment, specimens for laboratory investigation and carcasses for *post-mortem* examination. In addition, many patients owned by private individuals, zoos and scientific establishments are referred to me by veterinary colleagues.

Although free-living birds of prey are excluded from the general terms of reference of this book some mention is made of their treatment since, at a certain stage, wild raptor casualties can be assumed to have become "captive". If treatment of such birds is successful they will usually be returned to the wild. The assessment of the health of these and other captive birds intended for release is likely to become increasingly important and it is therefore wise not to divorce too drastically care of captive birds from that of their wild counterparts. There is also the important point that a falconer's hawk which is being flown is exposed to many of the same potential hazards as a free-living bird.

Since most of my study has been performed in Britain the main emphasis in the book will be on work in this country. Nevertheless, reference will also be made to cases examined in East Africa (Tanzania and Kenya) in 1966–67 and 1969–73 and in the United States and United Arab Emirates during short visits in 1974, 75 and 76. However, there is no reason to suppose that the value of the book will be restricted to these countries since many of the species examined came from other parts of the world and I have referred to other people's publications from a number of areas overseas.

Source of material

The main potential sources of clinical and pathological material were outlined in Chapter 1. Birds of prey are primarily kept in captivity for the following purposes:

(1) falconry
(2) aviculture
(3) captive breeding
(4) zoological display
(5) scientific research

There is, of course, considerable overlap between these groups, especially since captive breeding has now become a feature of other disciplines as well as being a subject in its own right. I do not intend to discuss these methods of management in any detail not to justify them, other than to emphasise that in each discipline there are persons of tremendous experience and integrity and to urge closer cooperation between them. An important point to remember, however, is that birds used for falconry are almost exclusively diurnal (falconiform) species and not owls. I should also mention that falconry is essentially a sport; the breeding of hawks in captivity and their maintenance in aviaries is a new (and not universally welcomed) development.

It is difficult to be certain how many birds of prey are maintained in captivity since, in addition to those taken or imported legally, there are others bred in captivity or being tended on account of injuries. In a paper presented at a Hawk Trust Conference in 1976 Kenward (246) gave a figure of 621 birds possessed by falconers in Britain on 31st December 1975. Data on birds of prey kept for purposes other than falconry appear not to be available but some indication of breeding success can be obtained from aviculture journals and reports; for example, in a recent Avicultural Society Register (17) it was reported that ten falconiform and 18 strigiform species or subspecies were bred in captivity in 1976. Thacker (391), in 1971, estimated that a total of between 4,600–5,800 birds of prey (strigiforms and falconiforms) were in captivity in the United States.

Insofar as mortality rates in captive birds of prey are concerned, Kenward (245) presented figures for first year birds kept by falconers and these ranged from 11% for 89 kestrels to 53% for 36 sparrowhawks. It is of interest to note that the first year mortalities in captivity of peregrines, kestrels and goshawks were considered to be substantially lower than those of wild birds ringed in the nest. Morbidity rates are more difficult to obtain although a number of the publications cited in this book give some indication of the prevalence of certain diseases in different species.

Space does not permit detailed discussion of the different types of management used for captive birds of prey, and the reader is advised to consult appropriate publications, some of which are listed at the end. The veterinary surgeon who hospitalises birds of prey for treatment may have to modify his premises to suit these patients, especially if they are falconers' birds. Kennels can be adapted fairly well to accommodate raptors. Alternatively, a wooden "hospital cage" can be constructed so that the bird is kept warm, in subdued light if necessary, and yet under regular observation. For short-term accommodation cardboard boxes are ideal. They enable the bird to be kept in the dark–which will reduce its activity– and the box can be burned after use. However, the person who is regularly treating raptors is advised to use purpose-built accommodation and advice on its design can usually be obtained from a falconer or aviculturist experienced in birds of prey.

There are, as yet, no guidelines as to size or construction of accommodation for captive birds of prey. However, it should be noted that recent legislation in the United States requires falconers to pass a "qualifying examination" for a falconry permit and part of this involves inspection of their facilities. There are certain minimum rules relating to the mews, weathering area, environmental protection and equipment. In Britain no such legal control over falconry yet exists but, as was mentioned earlier, under the Importation of Captive Birds Order 1976, incoming birds, including raptors, have to be quarantined and strict regulations govern the quarantine premises. Veterinary staff involved in inspections should have some knowledge of the management of birds of prey, particularly if falconers' birds are kept. Increases in legislation are likely to lead to tighter control over captive birds of prey and it has even been suggested that in Britain licences to "possess" a raptor may, in due course, be necessary (228, 302). Should this become the case, it is probable that a future edition of this book will include data on size and construction of facilities and will offer guidance to those involved in inspections.

The legal situation is also important. In Britain it is a contravention of the Veterinary Surgeons Act for an unqualified person to diagnose or treat disease. For this reason all problems relating to a captive bird must be referred to a veterinary surgeon. There is, however, no objection to emergency or first aid treatment being offered by an unqualified person so long as no charge is made for the advice. Treatment of a bird by the owner is also permitted but may lay the person open to prosecution under the Protection of Animals Act, 1911 if unnecessary suffering is thereby caused. My own approach in recent years has been to encourage falconers and others who keep birds of prey to consult and use a local veterinary surgeon. He or she may have little experience of birds but has the medicines, equipment and expertise that are so often needed to make an accurate diagnosis and initiate treatment. If encouraged the veterinary surgeon will usually develop an interest in the subject and a valuable relationship can result. Particular problems can always be referred to those colleagues who are active in raptor medicine and it is desirable that the veterinary surgeon, rather than the owner, should consult them. I should mention here that, in Britain at least, the veterinary profession is bound by ethics which should be respected. For example, if one veterinary surgeon is already dealing with a case, it must not be referred to another without his (the first veterinary surgeon's) knowledge. Such rules may appear tiresome but in the long run they benefit both animal and client.

Nowadays it is usual for a client to be asked to sign an anaesthetic and surgery consent form before hospitalisation and treatment of his animal; an example of a suitable form for birds of prey is given in Appendix XII. This authorises the giving of an anaesthetic and surgical procedures but in no way reduces the professional responsibilities of the veterinary surgeon.

A list of British laws and regulations which may be relevant to veterinary work with birds of prey is given in Appendix XI.

Clinical investigation

The first step in the clinical examination of a bird is to obtain as much history as possible. In some cases this will pose no problems but in others there may be little information available. An example of a clinical examination form is given in Appendix III; many people prefer to have a "check-list" of background data (for example, length of time in captivity, previous diseases etc.) and to work through

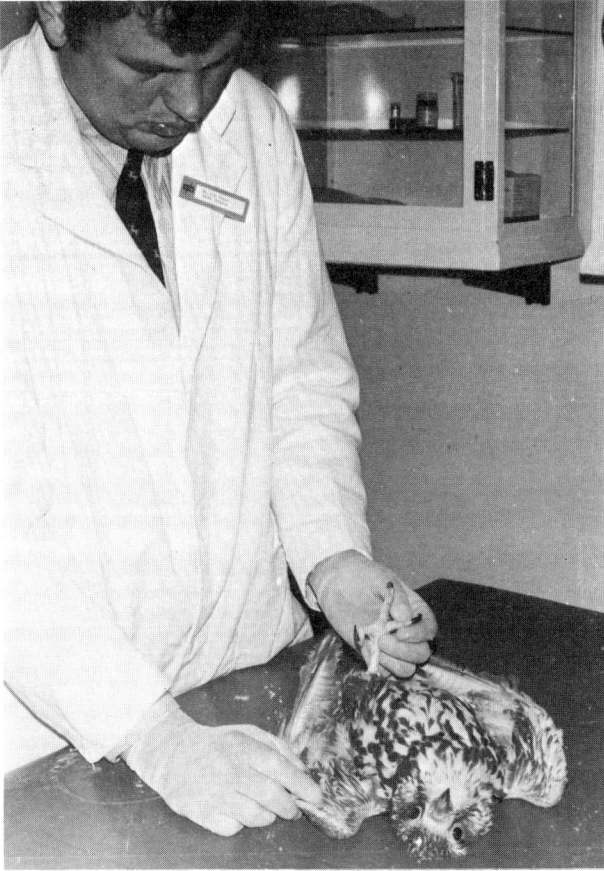

Photo 1.   A lightly anaesthetised saker is examined clinically

this rather than compile their own history. It is useful to ask the owner of the bird to bring with him notes of its previous history or, in the case of zoological specimens, to supply a copy of the bird's records. These can be appended to the clinical examination sheet.

Although it is generally true that all raptor patients should receive a full clinical examination, special techniques are needed when a neurological disorder is suspected. The examination of such a patient is described in Chapter 8. The description that follows refers to general examinations.

In the first instance a bird should be observed from a distance. This enables an assessment to be made of its general condition, respiration rate and obvious clinical signs of disease before it is unduly perturbed. In the case of birds in breeding condition, especially in "skylight and seclusion aviaries" (224), further disturbance is often not possible and a provisional diagnosis may have to be made on such an examination alone, coupled with whatever information may be available on food consumption and other activity. It must be stressed that, as in other branches of veterinary work, regular inspection of a bird by the owner is very important; some conditions, for example foot lesions, may be diagnosed early if the bird is subjected to careful daily observation.

Some useful indicators of health (or lack of it) were given in the chapter on disease that I revised for my friend Jack Mavrogordato's book "A Hawk for the Bush" (94). A full round eye is an important sign; in a hawk that is unwell, or perhaps excessively low in condition, it tends to be slightly oval. The colour of the feet and nares is not particularly significant – a yellowish orange colour usually indicates that day-old chicks have been fed – but *pale* colouration on such a diet may be indicative of some metabolic disturbance. Other examples of health include the use of only one leg when at rest and well formed mutes and castings (pellets). One must not be misled, however, into assuming that a hawk showing these and other "healthy" signs is necessarily clinically well, since some conditions manifest themselves very subtly. Owners, particularly falconers, will often spot early signs of disease; it is then up to the veterinary surgeon to perform a thorough examination. Some of the more important clinical signs are listed in Appendix VI and this may prove a useful guide. It is not intended to be comprehensive and usually a definitive diagnosis needs detailed examination and laboratory tests.

For a full clinical examination it is necessary for a bird to be handled. In the case of a falconer's bird this poses few problems since the hawk will usually be presented on the fist and is likely to be relatively amenable to contact, especially if hooded. A hood prevents the bird from seeing and can also be used on birds which are not trained for falconry. The effect is often spectacular, even on a wild casualty; as a result of being hooded the bird lies still and may permit minor procedures to be carried out. A similar, though less marked, effect can be obtained by covering the bird's head with a piece of cloth or canvas. It is also useful to carry out handling in a darkened room, using a lamp for subsequent examination. The veterinary surgeon who is examining raptors regularly will find it useful to have a "dimmer" switch on his light so that he can vary the intensity.

Handling a raptor in an aviary presents a bigger challenge since the first problem is how to capture it. If circumstances permit it is often best to catch diurnal birds at night, with the aid of a small torch, and nocturnal species by day. If a raptor cannot be easily grasped and held it may be necessary to resort to a net or piece of cloth which can be thrown over it. Gloves do not need to be worn for handling birds of prey but may reassure the handler and are often helpful during the act of capturing the bird, even if subsequently discarded. I have a pair of thin, but strong, industrial gloves which also cover the elbows and these are ideal for handling a variety of species.

Whether gloves are worn or not, it is vital to ensure that the bird's wings are held close to the body and not allowed to flap; uncontrolled wing movements can damage the plumage and are distressing to both bird and owner. Handling techniques are shown in Figures 2a, b and c and it should be noted that it is possible to hold a bird firmly (yet gently) in such a position that one cannot be reached by either feet or beak.

Once the bird has been grasped it should be cast, on its breast, on to a soft towel or blanket. If a hawk is wearing jesses these should be pulled backwards so that the feet are visible on either side of the tail. The provision of a soft cloth for the bird to grasp with its talons is often a worthwhile precaution; it helps calm the bird and reduces the possibility of self-inflicted foot damage. Laymen tend to be wary of the beaks of raptors but it is often the feet which cause the greater damage; in small birds in particular they can be extended at great speed enabling the talons to embed in the hands. Clipping the talons of birds received for treatment is, with the possible exception of wild casualties destined for early release, a wise precaution; it serves to protect the handler as well as the bird!

Examination of a bird of prey that has been cast usually requires two people since one must restrain the patient. In some cases it may be desirable to anaesthetise the bird lightly and this certainly facilitates examination (Photo 1). Alternatively, a self-adhesive wrap can be tried as described by Fuller (163). This enables

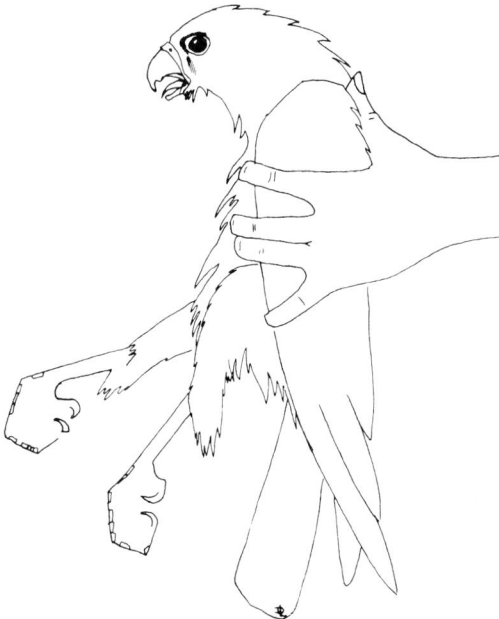

Fig. 2a   Handling a bird of prey. Note how the wings are restrained

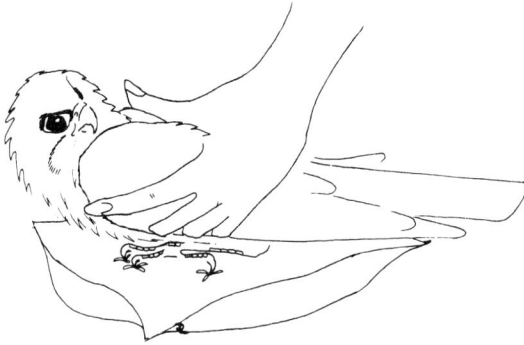

Fig. 2b   A bird of prey is cast on to a cushion for examination

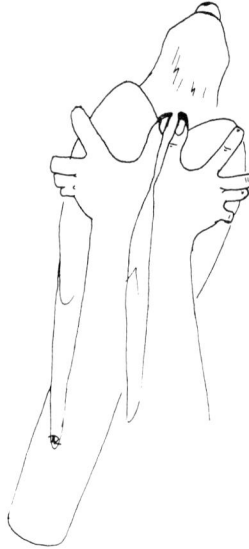

Fig. 2c   Position of the hands when casting a bird

one person to secure the bird and then have both hands free. Fuller used a proprietary bandaging tape which can be cut to different sizes and which will adhere to itself but not to feathers, skin or vegetation.

Each veterinary surgeon has his own method of investigation and it is advisable that he adheres to it. For my own part, I start at the head and work down the body; some important features are as follows:

Eyes – examine grossly and with ophthalmoscope.

Head – palpate and assess calcification by slight digital pressure on the cranium.

Cere and nostrils – observe for injury, asymmetry or blockage of nares.

Beak – examine externally and then open (artery forceps can be used) in order to inspect mucous membranes for colour, lesions, presence of parasites, etc. Observe glottis for respiration rate or lesions and trachea for presence of parasites. A finger can be inserted down the oesophagus to search for foreign bodies or lesions while the use of a small torch will facilitate examination of the trachea.

Neck – palpate externally and auscultate trachea and interclavicular air sac with stethoscope. Particularly check crop for evidence of food or air.

Body – palpate. The sharpness of the "keel" (sternum) is an aid to assessment of condition. Disparity in the size of the pectoral muscles can be indicative of muscle atrophy of one side (for example, wing injury) or inflammation (for example, irritant injection) of the area. The keel and overlying skin may have been damaged in recently imported birds. Auscultate heart in interclavicular space and lungs and air sacs along lateral aspects of body. Gently palpate abdomen for evidence of body fat, food in stomach or space-occupying lesion. Examine uropygial (preen) gland at base of tail; ensure it is normal in appearance and that the feathers around the external orifice are slightly oily. Palpate cloaca externally but also use lubricated gloved finger to examine interior for calculi, blood or other pathological signs. In addition the cloaca may be examined with a speculum or auroscope.

Wings and legs – palpate all bones and all joints; where possible compare with corresponding member on other side. Assess muscle tone and relative size of muscle masses. Flex and extend joints – feel and listen. Check for areas of feather loss, swelling or deformity. Examine legs and feet carefully for lesions; pay particular attention to the plantar surfaces of the feet. Check how sharp are the talons.

Tail – examine and count feathers, note presence of "hunger traces" or other feather lesions.

At some stage of the clinical examination the bird should be weighed. Falconers usually know the weight of their hawk but it is wise to check it; the bird can be made to step on to suitably padded scales and allowance must be made for the weight of jesses, bells and other equipment. Birds which will not stand on the scales, even if hooded or in subdued light, must be weighed following casting. It may be possible to lay them on the scales for a few seconds, failing which they should be weighed in a cloth bag.

When searching for *minor* wing injuries, my friend Dr Leonard Hurrell recommends holding the bird up for a few seconds by its feet; comparison of the positions of the wings will help reveal any weakness or abnormality. Such a technique should only be used after the legs have been checked and if the bird is not shocked or in low condition.

The stethoscope can play an important part in clinical examination but some experience is needed of its use with avian patients.

In the case of a falconer's bird with clinical signs suggestive of respiratory disease, examination can resemble that for soundness in a horse in that it is advisable to examine the bird at rest and then following a short flight of about 10–15 yards to the fist or lure.

The respiration rate of raptors below 2000 grammes in weight is usually between 15 and 30 per minute although in very small species, such as merlins, it may reach 50. Larger birds, such as vultures, usually respire 10–15 times per minute. There is, however, often much variation.

Although the stethoscope can be used to monitor heart rate, the latter is likely to increase as a result of examination. In my experience it is almost impossible to count the beats accurately but approximate figures for falcons are 200–350 beats per minute.

Aids to clinical investigation

In addition to the above examination a number of aids to clinical investigation are available. The use of the stethoscope has been mentioned. Other techniques range from the passing of a piece of tubing down the oesophagus or the oral administration of carmine powder (to assess patency of the gut) to the use of a clinical thermometer, electrocardiography, ophthalmoscopy and radiography. Investigation of nervous diseases will involve the use of a needle to assess pain and a pinpoint source of light to check the pupillar reflex. Most of these examples are discussed elsewhere in the book and attention will be drawn to the need for more investigation of modern techniques.

I do not regularly use a thermometer myself but it is advocated by some colleagues as a routine part of examination. The metabolic rate (and hence body temperature) of raptors is inversely proportional to size and figures for cloacal temperature range from 39·5°C for many of the larger vultures to 41°C for the kestrel. However, in my experience, there are variations within a species and even individual birds may give different figures on different occasions. A drop in body temperature at night is a recognised physiological feature of certain owls (226). There is need for more work on the body temperature of birds of prey and its response to disease, physical injury and restraint, as well as the development of thermoregulation on the young bird.

Radiography

Radiography cannot be discussed in detail. However, it is increasingly realised that it has a valuable role to play in raptor work (108). Whilst it should be used primarily to confirm or elucidate a diagnosis it frequently has to be employed as a diagnostic tool *per se*. Radiographic examination will help diagnose fractures, dislocations, foreign bodies and respiratory conditions; it will also reveal lead shot and non-palpable soft tissue lesions and give valuable information on the severity of tissue damage in bumblefoot or joint infections. Examples will be given later in the book. I have not personally used barium sulphate in birds of prey but it has been used experimentally, for example in studies on pellet formation in owls (182).

If a raptor is hooded it may be possible to perform limited radiography without further restraint. I personally prefer to anaesthetise my birds, however, and suitable anaesthetics are CT 1341 by injection or halothane or methoxyflurane by inhalation. It is advisable to take both lateral and ventro-dorsal views, and the bird must be carefully positioned using sandbags and sticky tape.

Examples of exposures used for birds of prey would serve little purpose since each X-ray machine has its own characteristics and output dependent upon age, model and design.

Much of my own early work was carried out at the Clinical Research Centre employing a sophisticated Siemens Triplex Optimatic 723 machine, fine focussing and a Kodak film. This equipment gives a high mA enabling a very short exposure time to be used. Smaller equipment usually needs a longer exposure.

All types of X-ray machine can be used for avian work although those with a fine focus will give the best results. However, there are many variables and the veterinary surgeon who anticipates dealing with birds of prey is advised to try a few test exposures, using a dead bird (a pigeon, *Columba livia*, if a raptor is not available) before his first case arrives on the doorstep.

Radiography of dead birds is also often advisable, particularly when traumatic injuries or lead shot (which is notoriously difficult to find on dissection) is suspected. At the Clinical Research Centre, Dr Louis Kreel and I radiographed a number of dead birds using a Chirana Dental Unit. This small, relatively inexpensive, piece of equipment was found to give good results, with excellent contrast. A fixed KV of 55 KV and fixed FFD of 75 cm were used and a variable exposure time, depending upon the size of the bird, from 5–10 seconds. This long period of exposure would preclude its use with live birds but for *post-mortem* investigation the method was ideal.

Good detail is essential for avian radiopathology and this can be achieved by the use of non-screen film or cassettes that are fitted with detail intensifying screens. For very small areas and for use in the investigation of *post-mortem* material industrial X-ray film is of value.

Certain features of normal anatomy must be borne in mind when interpreting radiographs of birds, whether alive or dead. In raptors bones are frequently seen in the crop and gizzard, in contrast to poultry and many other non-carnivorous species whose gizzards contain stones. Such bones should not be confused with foreign bodies.

For the investigation of respiratory lesions the lungs are best visualised by a lateral view, with the wings folded back above the bird's body (Photo 2). However, for examination of the air sacs a ventro-dorsal view should be obtained so that comparisons of the two sides of the patient can be made. Careful positioning is particularly important in this case.

For casualties a routine whole body radiograph is a valuable diagnostic aid. Not only will this demonstrate major skeletal injuries but it will also help elucidate some soft tissue lesions.

Clinical samples

The taking of specimens for laboratory investigation is an important part of clinical examination. In view of the difficulties inherent in handling a raptor it is important to ensure that collecting equipment is available before the bird is cast.

Feathers can be plucked; if primaries or secondaries are to be taken the bird should be lightly anaesthetised. Removal of feathers may be necessary in order to investigate plumage abnormalities, to search for parasites or in analysis for mercury. The last named technique has been used extensively in Sweden (28).

Skin scrapings can be removed easily although it should be noted that a bird's skin is thin and easily damaged. Swabs of external lesions should be moistened beforehand in sterile saline. Swabs of pharynx, trachea and cloaca can be taken relatively simply; it is wise to use narrow (human nasopharyngeal) swabs and again they should be moistened.

Air sac aspiration through the last intercostal space can be used to aid the diagnosis of air sac infections; Redig (351) recommended lavage, using saline.

Biopsies can play an important part in diagnosis and are discussed later in Chapters 7 and 10; Redig (351) recommended biopsy of the lung in respiratory cases, using a 25 gauge needle and 10 ml glass syringe. The needle is thrust

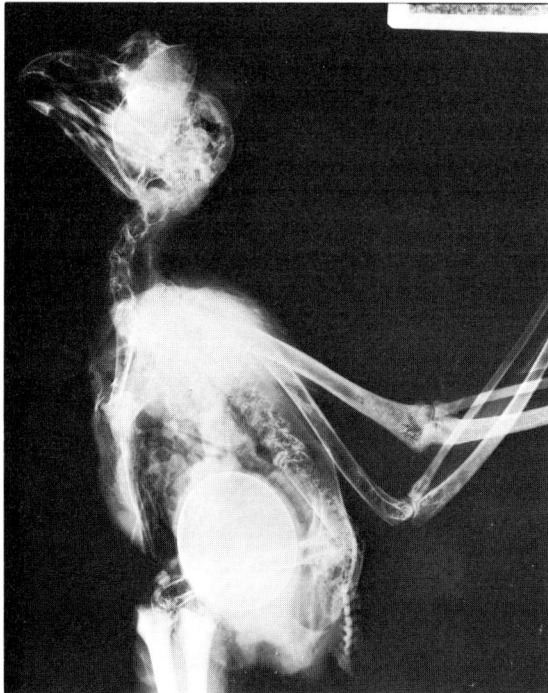

Photo 2.   Lateral radiograph of a spectacled owl. In this case there is a fully formed egg in the oviduct

through the penultimate intercostal space to a depth of up to 2/3 of the distance to the midline. The material thus obtained is sprayed on to a slide, stained and examined microscopically.

Although a mute sample can sometimes be removed from the cloaca it is usually more satisfactory to collect a freshly voided specimen from the bird. A bird of prey defaecates regularly and will often do so when first handled: owls in particular tend to produce large quantities when cast. It is, of course, the dark (faecal) portion that is required for parasitological examination. Ideally two days' pooled samples should be taken and examination for parasites repeated after 7–10 days. When submitting faecal samples for sexing (see Chapter 11) the material should be deep frozen. Castings (pellets) will not usually be produced in the surgery; the owner should be asked to bring a specimen with him. "Normal" droppings and a pellet are shown in Figures 3a and b. Blaine (44) provided a useful description of the former:

> "Perfect mutes should be pure white of the consistency of thin cream, with a few small lumps of black in the centre".

Blood samples for haematology and clinical chemistry should be taken from the brachial vein, with the bird cast on its back. The vein lies just distal to the elbow joint (Figure 4) and is easily exposed if a few feathers are plucked and the area dampened with alcohol. The vein is best raised by applying pressure on the lateral aspect of the humerus. For small birds (500 grammes in weight or less) a 25 gauge needle and 1·0 ml (tuberculin) syringe should be used, though the use of a "butterfly" attachment will lessen the chance of the needle coming out of the vein when the bird moves. Alternatively the jugular vein can be used or, if the bird is to be killed, the heart – using the same technique as for chickens. Cutting one or more talons short may also yield enough blood for tests but this method should be avoided if possible since not only is it probably painful but it may permit infection to enter the foot.

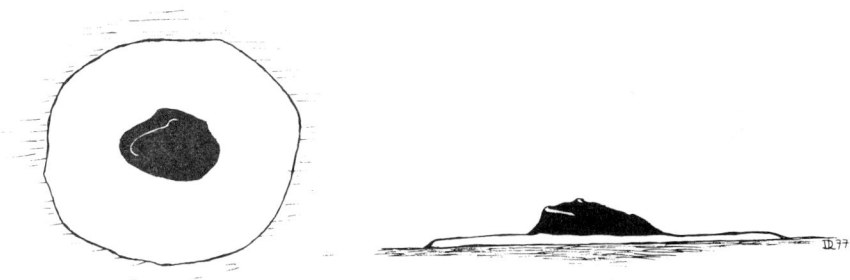

Fig. 3a   A normal dropping ("mute") sample. The central portion consists of faecal material.

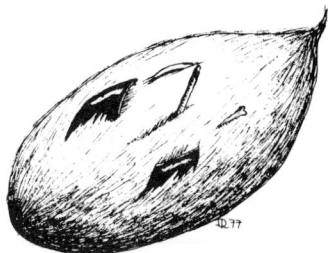

Fig. 3b   A normal casting (pellet) containing rodent hair, bones and portions of chitin from beetles

For blood smears, only small samples are required; the brachial vein can be pricked or one talon cut slightly short.

Aspiration of fluid or pus should be preceded by thorough cleansing of the area. Surgical spirit or a proprietary disinfectant can be used but the latter may persist and destroy organisms on the swab. For foot lesions I usually scrub the area with soap and water, rinse with warm water and dry before inserting a 23 or 25 gauge needle and attempting to aspirate material. Swabs for bacteriology should either be cultured within 6 hours or stored in Stuart's Transport Medium while those for mycoplasmology should be placed immediately in liquid medium.

Screening

The value of screening captive raptors at intervals will be emphasised later in the book. It should be a regular procedure in all establishments where birds of prey are maintained in relatively large numbers, particularly if several birds share an

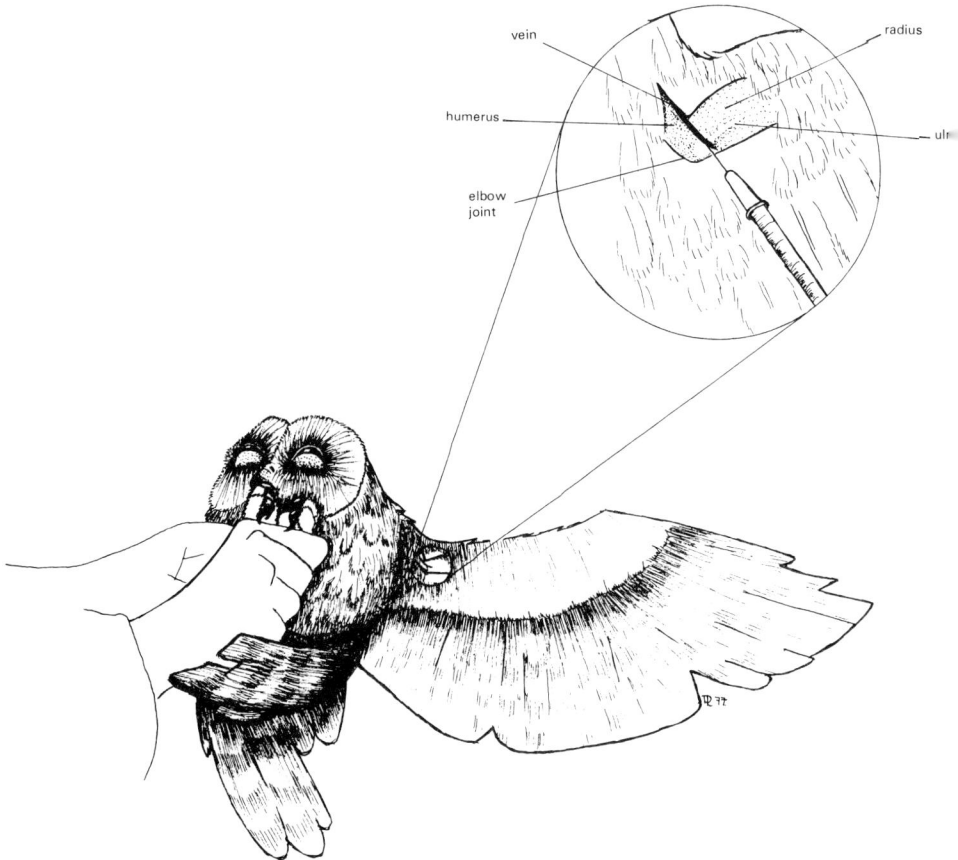

Fig. 4　Taking a blood sample from the brachial vein of an owl

aviary or enclosure. At the Hawk Trust aviaries in Hungerford, England, for example, regular screening of faeces for parasites and bacteria has been practised for over two years. In addition, once a year (after the breeding season) all birds are caught, examined clinically and bled. Haematology is performed on the blood samples and smears are examined for parasites. The protocol followed at Hunger-

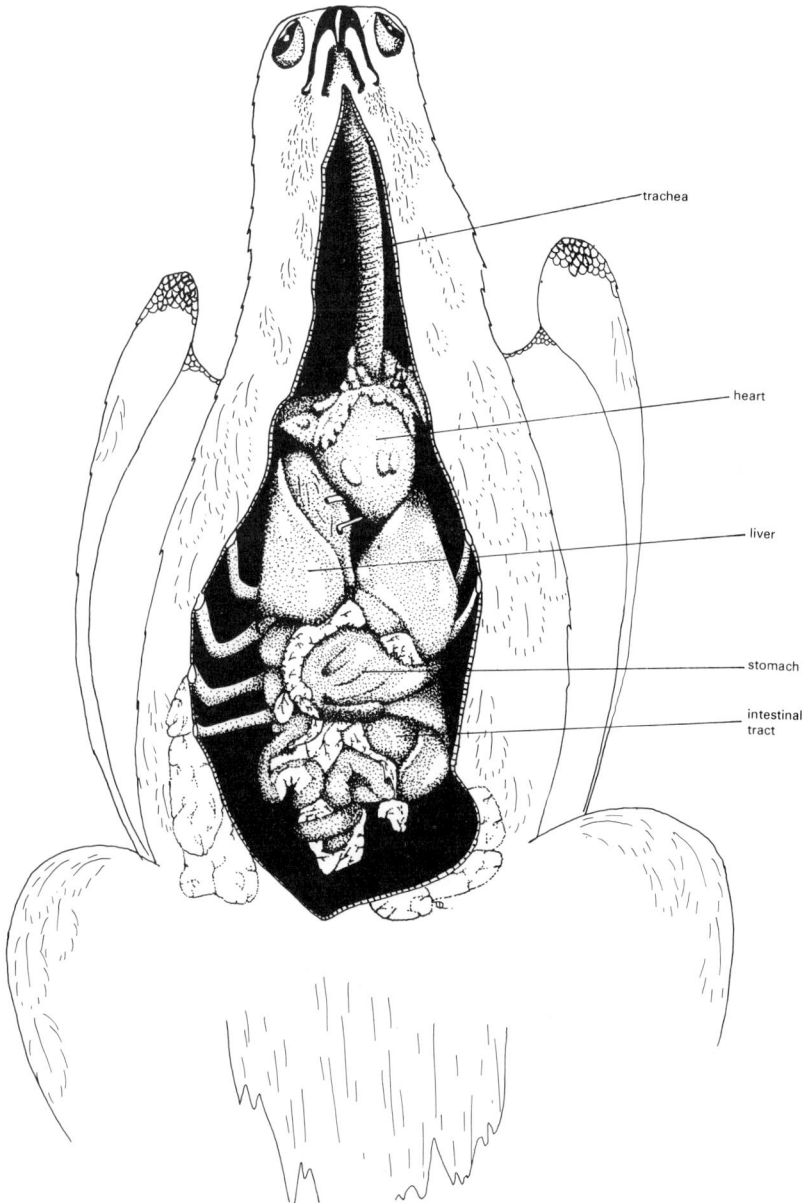

Fig. 5a   Internal organs of a buzzard as seen when first opened for *post-mortem* examination

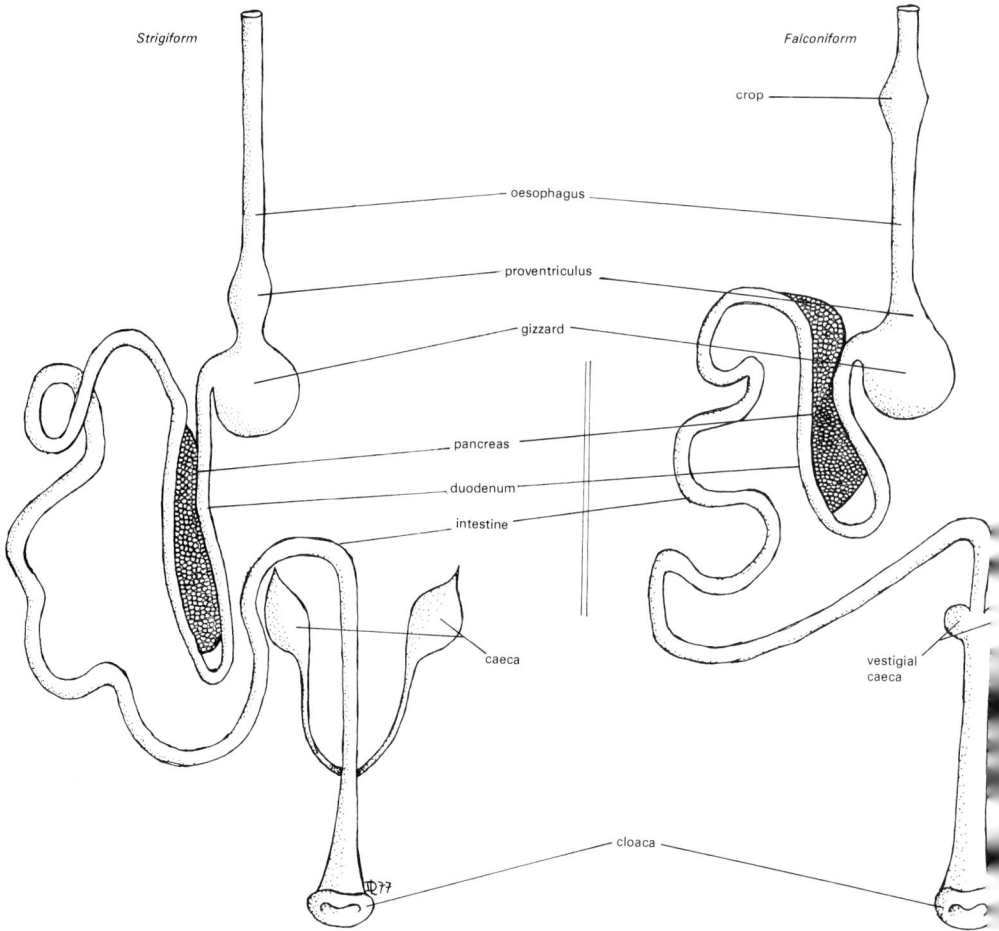

Fig. 5b   Structure of the intestinal tracts of strigiform and falconiform birds of prey

ford was discussed in an article in the Trust's 1976 Annual Report (415) and the point was made that such screening not only aids disease diagnosis and treatment but also yields valuable scientific information. Incoming birds should be from a reputable source and placed in quarantine for at least two, and preferably four, weeks. During this time, in addition to observation and clinical examination, the laboratory tests outlined above can be carried out. Any bird that dies in quarantine *must* be submitted for a full pathological examination.

Post-mortem examination

This plays an important part in diagnosis and has contributed greatly to our understanding of diseases of birds of prey. As Keymer (252) pointed out, all those who keep raptors in captivity should be encouraged to submit carcasses for *post-mortem* examination; instructions for the despatch of these and other specimens, together with the relevant Post Office Regulations, are given in Appendices XIII and XIV. A dead bird should always be assumed to be infectious until proved otherwise. It must be removed promptly from the aviary or mews and placed in a clean plastic bag prior to examination. Occasionally it may be necessary to examine a raptor *post mortem* in connection with a legal case or insurance claim; under such circumstances it is particularly important that material is received as fresh as possible and that a comprehensive examination is carried out, with full documentation. Tissues should be retained in the deep freeze or fixed in formalin.

I originally described my techniques for *post-mortem* examination, in laymen's terms, in a paper in "The Falconer" (83)

The method differs little from that used for birds in any diagnostic laboratory and any reader who requires detailed information is referred to the sections in the book by Gordon (170) for descriptions of autopsy and other laboratory procedures in birds. Extra features, however, include, whenever possible, a whole-body radiograph of the bird in order to check for presence of lead shot, un-

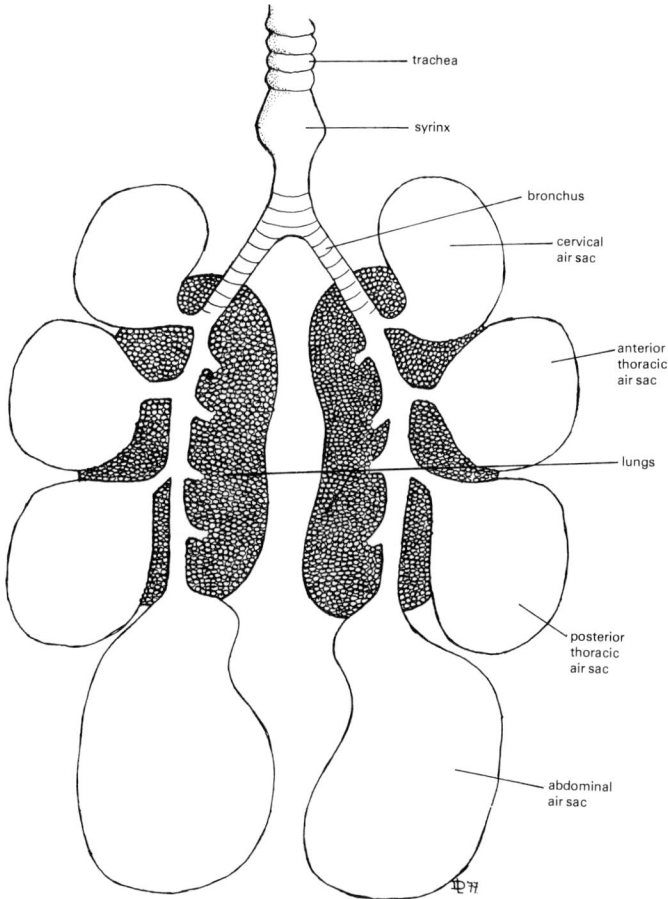

Fig. 5c   Basic structure of the avian respiratory tract

diagnosed fractures or skeletal disease. In addition, particularly careful attention should be paid to the exterior of the bird for evidence of skin, feather or foot lesions or the presence of ectoparasites. The bird should be weighed and in this respect it should be noted that there is weight loss following death, especially if there is delay before *post-mortem* examination. For example, a kestrel of weight 180 grammes at death may weigh only 155 g when examined 36 hours later. Whenever possible individual organ weights should also be recorded but this is time-consuming and not always feasible.

It is important that a record is kept of *post-mortem* findings and my own form is depicted in Appendix IV.

Having laid the bird on its back for *post-mortem* examination, a careful protocol should be followed. Feathers can be plucked from the breast or, if the body is required for taxidermy, the bird should be skinned. Once the sternum is lifted the main internal organs can be seen (see Figure 5a) but these will need to be displaced, removed and opened during the course of a full *post-mortem* examination. In addition, the pharynx should be dissected and both oesophagus and trachea opened fully. Depending upon the findings it may be necessary to dissect pathological lesions such as abscesses, adhesions or skeletal abnormalities.

It is advisable, whenever possible, to examine the brain although, as will be discussed in Chapter 8, *post-mortem* autolysis is rapid and subsequent histopathological examination may be hampered by fixation artefacts. If a nervous disease is suspected full examination of the nervous system is essential and this also is discussed in Chapter 8. If a bird has to be killed on humanitarian grounds it can, once unconscious, be perfused with formalin using either the carotid artery or the heart. This renders microbiology useless but very much improves fixation of the brain.

My own technique for brain examination is to remove the head and to skin the cranium. At this stage intraosseous haemorrhages may be seen in the skull. The skull is opened longitudinally using a scalpel blade (for small specimens) or a hack saw (for larger). Once an incision has been made, the skull can usually be split in half by inserting the points of a pair of scissors into the crack and opening them slowly. The skull and brain are then bisected; one half can be placed immediately in formalin for histopathology, the other dissected and examined. Both the brain and meninges must be carefully inspected and a low-power stereo-microscope is useful in this context. The brain should be sliced and each portion examined.

Post-mortem examination of the young bird differs little from that described above but radiography should be carried out in order to assess skeletal growth and it is important that the yolk sac is examined carefully. In addition, note should be taken of the presence or absence of the "egg tooth" on the beak and the size of the bursa of Fabricius should be recorded. There is also interest in the growth and differentiation of the brain in birds – differences were reported over twenty years ago between nidifugous and nidicolous birds (389) – and the brain of nestlings should, whenever possible, be weighed and dissected. This is one of the many fields in which the pathologist can provide data of value to his colleagues involved in avian biology and ethology.

Before a carcass is discarded note must be made of the tissues removed and the laboratory tests proposed. All too often one disposes of the dead bird and only later realises that valuable material was not removed. Unfortunately the method of preservation will influence the tests that can subsequently be performed. If in doubt it is wise to deep-freeze the carcass. Even if this is not possible, tissues (especially liver and brain) should be frozen for subsequent toxicological analysis.

The pathological examination of raptor eggs is a new field about which little is known. As such, it presents a challenge to all those involved in studies on diseases of birds of prey.

My own report form for eggs is reproduced in Appendix V. As can be seen, considerable emphasis is laid on description of the egg and adequate clinical history. The important external features are the size, shape and integrity of the egg. It should be measured, its shape recorded (or drawn) and any cracks or other external abnormalities noted. It is obviously of importance to ascertain whether the egg is fertile or not. If the egg *is* fertile, the age of the embryo at death should be assessed on the basis of its size. The embryo should be examined for evidence of physical abnormalities or infection. Bacteriological and mycological culture of the yolk sac, albumen and embryonic liver should be carried out. Histopathological examination of embryonic tissue may prove useful.

Infertile eggs must also be examined carefully. Some will be infected (contaminated) and culture should again be performed.

Whenever possible eggs should be "candled" before examination; this helps in subsequent correlation of pathological findings with clinical history.

Eggshells should be retained after examination. Their thickness should, if possible, be measured since eggshell thinning is a feature of chlorinated hydrocarbon toxicity and certain other pathological conditions. Failing this, measurements of length and width, coupled with weight, will provide equally useful data. There is also interest in the structure of avian eggshells and some interesting work on this subject has been published (47, 397); such investigators might welcome material from the avian pathologist. Egg contents can be preserved and deep-frozen for subsequent chemical analysis.

Post-mortem samples

Removal of specimens for laboratory investigations is usually straight-forward. In the case of external material the technique resembles that described for clinical samples. When dealing with internal tissues care must be taken not to contaminate material unnecessarily. For example, if the lung is to be examined bacteriologically it should be handled with clean forceps *before* the intestinal tract (which almost always harbours *E. coli*) is opened. Specific lesions may be swabbed or removed for further investigations. If a blood-borne infection is suspected a swab of heart blood should be taken; the heart should be removed and incised with sterile instruments before a fine nasopharyngeal swab is inserted into a ventricle. At the same time a blood smear can be taken.

The tissues chosen for histopathology will depend upon the lesions found and the degree of autolysis present in the carcass but whenever possible a full selection should be taken. Careful dissection of the anterior part of the kidney will usually permit kidney, adrenal and gonad to be included in one section. Two pieces of heart – a transverse and a longitudinal section (LS) – should be taken from larger specimens, together with a transverse section of the vessels if required. In the case of smaller hearts such examination may prove impossible and instead an LS of the heart alone must be taken.

The material to be taken for toxicological examination is entirely dependent upon the poison suspected and the tests to be performed. The sampling of feathers for mercury content was mentioned earlier. Liver, brain and body fat may be needed for organochlorine analysis. If there is any doubt over the tissues to be submitted it is best to deep-freeze the carcass, carefully wrapped in a plastic bag, until instructions from the chemist are received.

Laboratory investigation

Space does not permit detailed discussion of all laboratory techniques and therefore reference will be made to a number of relevant publications. Subsequent chapters will cover some procedures and these will not be discussed here in any detail. Where that is not the case, however, rather more information, together with examples of "normal" values, will be given in this chapter.

Although the main aim of laboratory investigations is to aid diagnosis and prognosis one must not forget how little information is as yet available on such data as haematology, clinical chemistry or even parasitology of birds of prey. Every effort should, therefore, be made to collect specimens for examination whenever possible and if necessary to submit them to an appropriate laboratory or authority. The results may not directly benefit the bird in question but will often yield useful scientific data.

Microbiological examination follows routine methods. It does not appear necessary to incubate cultures at temperatures higher than 37°C despite the higher body temperature of the bird. Aerobic and anaerobic culture should always be performed and the standard media used are blood agar plates, MacConkey agar plates, deoxycholate citrate agar (D.C.A.), selenite F and Robertson's cooked meat. Needham (312) described the use of these media with a variety of specimens taken from animals. For fungi, Sabouraud's agar should be used, with incubation at 37°C and 25°C for at least seven days. The attempted isolation of mycoplasmas should be in liquid medium following the technique described by Furr and colleagues (165). Bacteria are identified by standard techniques (115) although it is possible that some avian isolates may need special treatment. The differentiation of staphylococci is an example; the tests differ from those applied to isolates from man (311). Jeffrey Needham and I used this technique with avian isolates and in a subsequent publication (109), pointed out that the use of homologous (bird) plasma may be advantageous. A useful guide to the isolation and identification of avian pathogens is the book produced by the American Association of Avian Pathologists (208).

Microbiological techniques can also play a part in the maintenance of hygiene in mews and aviaries. Many organisms, such as *Staphylococcus aureus*, can be spread by air currents, and it is possible to monitor airborne contamination by employing bacteriological "settle plates" (312). This will be discussed again later in the book.

Once isolates of bacteria have been obtained from clinical or *post-mortem* lesions, they can be tested for sensitivity to antimicrobial agents. This is accomplished using standard agar plates and paper discs impregnated with the agents.

Parasitological examinations are again similar to those used in other species. In the case of a faecal sample it is often easier to prepare two direct smears and only perform a flotation test if parasites are seen. It is essential that a suitable sample is obtained and a useful guide to this, in a range of species, was given by Needham (313). Examination of the faecal sample may reveal features other than parasites; feather, fur and vegetable matter are common and excess numbers of erythrocytes and cellular debris may be seen.

Capillaria and other eggs may also be detected in scrapings from buccal cavity, crop or gut, in regurgitated food and in castings (pellets). The last named should always first be examined carefully for macroscopical abnormalities and then soaked in a small quantity of saline before parasitological or microbiological investigation.

Feather samples should be examined initially with a hand-lens or stereo-microscope; in either case the specimen should be viewed with both reflected and transmitted light. Following this, feathers can be soaked in 40% sodium hydroxide which renders them transparent and permits more careful examination for parasites or other abnormalities.

Blood for haematology should be submitted in the anticoagulant di-sodium ethylenediaminetetra-acetate (EDTA). My own technique is to measure packed cell volume (PCV), red cell count and haemoglobin. The techniques used, and preliminary results obtained, were outlined in earlier papers (92, 100). PCV (haematocrit) is measured using a standard micro-haematocrit centrifuge and red cells by the method described by Leonard (273). Natt and Herrick's solution is used for the red cell techniques. It is usually satisfactory but differentiation of cells may be difficult; use of dark ground illumination will make this easier. Many methods are available for haemoglobin estimation; in Kenya I used a conventional mammalian colorimeter method. Alternatively (and possibly preferably) techniques used in fish work can prove useful; an example was given in a review article by Hesser (204). A recent paper (379) reported the use of a semi-automatic system ("Coulter Counter": Coulter Electronics Ltd) for haematological measurements in chickens. The technique gave results comparable to those obtained by more conventional methods except in the case of haemoglobin and white cell counts.

My work in Kenya and subsequent investigations with British birds of prey have confirmed that in most species the PCV lies between 35 and 42% and the red cell count between 2 and 2·5 million per cubic millimetre (cu mm). Low PCV values are seen in debilitated and anaemic birds while elevated values indicate haemoconcentration, possibly on account of dehydration. They are often a feature in birds that have been transported. Elliott and colleagues (137) investigated white cell counts and gave a mean value of 24,000 cells per cu mm while Redig (351) presented some preliminary results on differential counts. Redig reported figures similar to those I have observed myself – approximately 50% lymphocytes, 41–42% heterophils, 0–1% eosinophils, 0–1% basophils and 2–6% monocytes. He also presented evidence of changes in the differential count in diseased birds and suggested that these could be used as an aid to diagnosis. Falconiform species have relatively large erythrocytes – up to $16 \times 8 \ \mu m$ – and while probably not of diagnostic importance, such measurements are worth recording for future reference; the possible significance of erythrocyte size was discussed in a recent paper by Palomeque and Planas (326). Balasch and colleagues (19) reported sedimentation rates for a number of birds of prey and it is possible that these too might prove useful in diagnosis. As was indicated earlier, there is increasing evidence that haematology can assist in diagnosis and prognosis, and all those working with birds of prey are urged to take and examine blood samples whenever possible.

Blood smears should be air dried, fixed with 100% methyl alcohol and stained with either Giemsa or Leishman stain. My own preference is Giemsa stain and this should be used at a strength of 10% at pH 7·2 for one hour; however, there is some evidence that Leishman shows eosinophilic granules and rods better. Careful examination, using oil immersion, is usually necessary to detect protozoa though microfilariae can be seen readily under low power. Smears can also be used for differential counts; for identifying the blood cells either the monograph by Lucas and Jamroz (281) or the chapter by Hodges (210) is recommended. If a bird is anaemic there are usually lowered PCV and/or haemoglobin levels, but another clue in some cases is an increase in erythrocytes with basophilic staining to their cytoplasm (290). Damaged white cells ("smudge" and "basket" cells) should be counted since not only will this ensure a more reliable differential count but it is also possible that increased numbers of such cells may be correlated with disease.

Blood for clinical chemistry must be submitted in an appropriate anticoagulant. Usually fluoride is best for glucose and lithium-heparin for other estimations. Total protein and uric acid can be estimated using plasma from the microhaematocrit. Clotted blood (serum) is preferable for calcium and other inorganic analyses. However, requirements vary from laboratory to laboratory and advice should always be sought before taking the samples.

It is also possible to employ chemically impregnated strips – as used extensively in veterinary practice – for certain tests, but I have some reservations about the accuracy of some of these when dealing with avian samples.

Although many of those working with raptors submit blood for clinical chemistry, this is an area where there is a particular dearth of information on "normal" values; as a result one relies heavily on data from poultry. The subject warrants more investigation. A similar situation applies to liver and kidney function tests although Redig (351) was able to report encouraging results for the former in red-tailed hawks, including one bird in which liver function had been impaired by treatment with carbon tetrachloride. Uric acid assay of blood may prove useful in assessment of kidney function: a suitable technique is that described by Bergmann and Dikstein (29).

Blood gas analysis is another procedure which may prove of use in future. The only reference I have been able to trace to the use of such a technique in birds of prey is that of Calder and Schmidt-Nielsen (66) who investigated panting and blood carbon dioxide levels in a number of species of bird including the turkey vulture. Results for this bird when it was resting at $22 - 25°C$ were blood pH 7·51 and pCO_2 27·5. During panting, at an air temperature of 44·5°C, these figures changed to 7·56 and 19·0 respectively.

For serological tests either clotted blood or serum is needed. My own technique for serum removal is to collect the blood in a tall narrow glass bottle, such as a "Universal" container, and to loosen the clot from around the edge with a sterile needle. The bottle is kept at room temperature for 24 hours to encourage contraction of the clot and the serum removed from the surface with a syringe and needle, if necessary after gentle centrifuging. Serological testing cannot be discussed here; suffice it to say that screening can play an important part in disease investigation and is likely to prove of increasing use in the future.

Material for histological examination should be fixed in at least ten times its own volume of 10% formalin, or, preferably, 10% neutral buffered formalin. The latter has the advantage that tissues can be stored in it for longer periods and there are less artefacts. This and other aspects are discussed in "Histological Laboratory Methods" (130), and other textbooks, to which reference should be made. Where applicable the specimen should be incised to permit penetration and in cases where there is much blood present a change of fixative after 24 hours is advisable. After fixation the material should be trimmed and processed. Decalcification is often necessary; for example, when investigating foot lesions it is far preferable to cut a transverse section of the whole digit, and to decalcify it before embedding, than to take the affected soft tissues only.

Paraffin sections are usually adequate although frozen sections may be necessary in emergency cases or where fat stains are required. The stain of choice is haematoxylin and eosin though others, especially Gram, P.A.S., Grocott and Ziehl-Neelsen may be necessary. There are no texts available on the normal histology or histopathology or birds of prey and the pathologist involved in such work must usually refer to standard poultry books, such as "Diseases of Poultry" (213) and "The Histology of the Fowl" (209). Other useful publications include those on comparative histology such as the books by Patt and Patt (329), Andrew and Hickman (2) or Leake (271).

For histology to be of maximum value, the tissues must be fixed promptly after death. Autolytic changes make interpretation exceedingly difficult; an example is pyknotic erythrocytic nuclei which can easily be mistaken for chronic inflammatory cells. Unfortunately, however, *post-mortem* change is often the norm rather than the exception, especially when a carcass is despatched by post. The avian pathologist will find the papers on sequential *post-mortem* changes in the chicken (*Gallus domesticus*) and mallard duck (*Anas platyrhynchos*) by Munger and McGavin (307, 308) and Morrow and Glover (303) respectively of help in deciphering such changes.

Histochemistry is proving of increasing value in veterinary medicine in a wide range of species, including poultry. Work on this subject in birds of prey is long overdue.

It is increasingly probable that the veterinary surgeon may be asked to examine semen samples from birds of prey. These will usually have been taken from the cloaca of the male following massage or natural copulation and should not contain urates or faeces. Semen samples should be kept cool (+4°C) but not frozen. If mixed with a diluent or saline the latter should be at the same temperature as the semen to reduce damage to spermatozoa. Various tests can be performed on semen; fixed samples can be stained and examined for abnormal spermatozoa or cells indicative of infection. Some variation in sperm size is normal and can be ignored. Fresh semen is used to assess motility and concentration of sperm. It must be remembered that the sperm concentration of some falcons is low compared with domestic birds (52). Other tests are used in mammals, amongst them enzyme analyses to monitor cellular damage following freezing, and it seems likely that these will ultimately play a role in raptor work. Bacteriological culture of semen may be carried out and this does not differ from other microbiological techniques.

Electron microscopy is likely to play an increasingly important role in diagnosis and research in future and the techniques used are similar to those in poultry. Consultation with the electron microscopist is important and he will give guidance on the type of fixative that should be used. In this context it should be noted that there is increasing interest in the use of one fixative for both light and electron microscopy – a mixture of formaldehyde and glutaraldehyde is an example – and a useful review article on this subject is by McDowell and Trump (284). My own experience of electron microscopy is restricted to the diagnosis of avian pox (86) and the examination of a variety of tissues from owls at the London Zoo in 1976. Diagnosis of pox is remarkably simple and is recommended whenever the disease is suspected; scrapings are lysed with distilled water and fluid placed on a grid and stained with phosphotungstic acid. Direct electron microscopy should reveal pox virus particles.

Toxicological examination cannot be discussed here. This is a specialised field and there are many publications on it. The laboratory will specify how it requires material to be submitted and it is vital that its instructions are followed. I must stress that a laboratory cannot look for "poisons" in general; it must be given some idea of the toxic agent suspected. It is, therefore, most important that a full clinical history is obtained, and appropriate pathology carried out, before tissues are submitted.

The use of experimental animals is necessary in some fields of raptor work. Rodents may, rarely, be used in the diagnosis of microbial disease or detection of toxins. More often embryonated eggs or chickens are employed for such work. Other birds may be of use in experimental studies – for example, at the time of writing, I am using starlings (*Sturnus vulgaris*) as models for bumblefoot. Raptors themselves have been used for toxicological research and it is probable that they will play a more important role in future. It is even possible that germ-free birds may be produced in due course. Experimental animals must be used humanely and, in Britain and certain other countries, the appropriate licences and/or certificates must be held.

Treatment

Although specific treatment will be discussed in subsequent chapters, basic points should be dealt with here. It should be noted that, in this book, the scientific names of drugs are used whenever possible. Reference is only made to tradenames when no suitable chemical name is available or when a particular preparation is being recommended. Dosages of drugs are given in Appendix IX.

As with other species, treatment can be either specific or non-specific. The latter is usually termed supportive or palliative.

Specific treatment will be discussed in considerable detail in subsequent chapters. Such treatment may be medical (by the use of drugs) or surgical. Many groups of drugs can be used safely and effectively in birds of prey, amongst them antibiotics, corticosteroids and anthelmintics. A list of agents is given in Appendix IX. There are, however, some contraindicated drugs and these also are listed.

Unfortunately, little work has been done on the metabolism of therapeutic agents in raptorial birds and one therefore relies largely upon clinical response to treatment and the data available from work with poultry. The latter are useful and have often provided a framework for the use of drugs in other birds but there are still many unanswered questions. Many of these relate to the specialised anatomy and physiology of the bird. For example, the bird's metabolic rate (and hence body temperature) is high and this will influence the absorption, metabolism and elimination of many agents. This feature is particularly noticeable in the case of injectable anaesthetics (e.g. CT 1341) where recovery is far quicker in the bird than the mammal. But it is possible that some drugs cannot function fully at the higher body temperature or that toxic metabolites may be formed. This also poses the problem of how frequently, and for how long, an agent should be given. For instance, in human medicine oral antibiotics are usually administered every 4 – 6 hours in order to maintain blood levels. In avian work, however, one tends to do so only once a day, despite the fact the bird has a higher metabolic rate. It is probable that the whole question of dosage needs reappraisal. The oral administration of antibiotics may, in any case, be a doubtful practice in birds. Fowler and Hussaini (151) discussed this aspect in poultry and referred to Williams Smith's (416) work in which he demonstrated only low serum levels of antibiotics following oral administration.

There is little doubt that the higher body temperature of birds may influence the fate and efficacy of drugs; indeed, even in mammals, the question of the effect of a fever on drug absorption has been investigated (399). On the other hand, research on reptiles has indicated that they tend to maintain themselves at a higher temperature when infected with bacteria and this has led to suggestions that the development of a fever may play a beneficial role in recovery of mammals from infection. This subject was discussed in an editorial in "The Lancet" (10); although birds were not specifically mentioned it is tempting to postulate that their higher body temperature may be advantageous.

When medication *is* to be given to birds of prey by mouth it must either be administered *per se* or secreted in food. As a general rule birds of prey drink very little and therefore incorporation of a drug "in the drinking water" is impracticable. Some falconers' birds will, especially if hooded, permit their beak to be opened and a tablet or capsule put in their mouth; I was particularly impressed with the ability of Arab falconers to do this when I was in Abu Dhabi. Alternatively the drug can be hidden in a piece of meat or inside a dead chick or mouse – although it is possible that absorption may be impaired in the latter case. Some liquid preparations can be injected into the prey while medical paediatric drops can sometimes be dropped into the bird's mouth while it is on the fist or if it is cast. Some of the latter preparations appear highly palatable and are readily taken by individual birds.

From time to time it may be necessary to medicate a raptor without handling it – birds in breeding aviaries and at hack are the prime example – and here there are often problems of diagnosis as well as treatment. In such cases the appropriate drug is usually best hidden in an item of food and this offered to the bird after 24 – 48 hours starvation.

If oral treatment has to be given forcibly the bird should be cast and the beak opened; the capsule should be pushed with a finger over the back of the tongue and down the oesophagus. Alternatively, for solutions and suspensions, a piece of rubber tubing (suitably lubricated) can be used as an oesophageal tube and passed down to the crop.

As a general rule oral medication should be given on an empty crop and stomach. However, from time to time a bird will regurgitate the drug under such circumstances in which case it should be given after a *small* meal of lean meat.

There is increased use of the injection route for the administration of drugs and clinical experience, with antibiotics in particular, suggests that this is likely to prove more efficacious than oral use. Falconers have traditionally been apprehensive about the use of injections and have recounted horrific stories of birds collapsing and dying after an injection. In other cases the hawk has not died but shown clinical signs of "cramp". Such effects are attributable, in my view, to the (now rare) administration of unsuitable drugs by this route – for example, procaine penicillin can result in tremors, incoordination and collapse. Nowadays there is far less concern about the use of the parenteral routes but the veterinary surgeon should still be careful to ensure that injections are given correctly, with the minimum of discomfort or tissue damage to the bird. As small a needle as possible should be used – if practicable, 25 or 26 gauge – and a small volume of drug. In the case of the latter, one must balance the need for a small volume with the dangers of inadvertent overdosage or local tissue damage if too concentrated a solution is used. Hygiene is important and the use of spirit to dampen the feathers helps visibility as well as (probably) reducing numbers of pathogenic organisms.

The important injection routes are intramuscular, intravenous and subcutaneous. Intraperitoneal injections can pose problems and should usually be reserved for euthanasia; if they are to be given the needle should enter through the midline midway between the sternum and the cloaca to reduce the risk of entering an airsac. For the intramuscular injection either the pectoral or leg (thigh) muscles should be used. I tend to favour the latter since the injections are often easier to give and do not present a hazard of impairing flight or of accidentally damaging delicate abdominal organs (see Figure 6). A hooded hawk on the fist can often be given a small intramuscular injection into the leg without restraint, so long as only a 25 or 26 guage needle is used. It is always advisable to withdraw the plunger

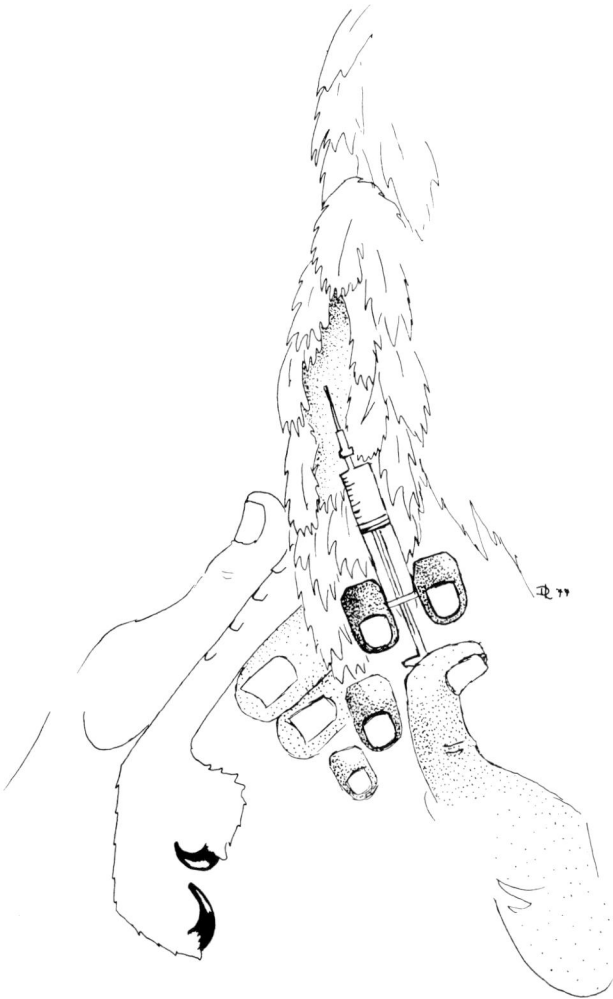

Fig. 6   Intramuscular injection in the leg. Note how one hand is used to extend the leg while the other holds the syringe

slightly before giving an intramuscular injection to help avoid inadvertently hitting a blood vessel.

Intravenous injections are best given into the brachial vein and instructions for locating this vein were given earlier in this chapter. It is important to ensure that air is not given intravenously although a few small bubbles appear to do no harm. In addition it must be remembered that, following removal of the needle, a sub-cutaneous haematoma will form; this can be minimised by applying pressure with a swab immediately. Blood under the skin will gradually break down (during which time the area will become green in colour) and it should be possible to use the vein again after 72 hours.

Subcutaneous injections are used primarily for vaccines and fluid replacement. Any area of exposed skin can be used but suitable sites are the nape and the skin overlying the medial surfaces of the legs. Moistening of the latter with alcohol will greatly facilitate the technique.

Non-specific therapy consists of nursing and the palliative treatment of wounds and clinical signs.

Nursing can be divided into four main areas, these being a) provision of warmth b) fluid balance c) feeding and d) minimum disturbance. Each will be discussed briefly.

Provision of warmth is vital whenever a bird of prey is being treated. Being homeothermic a raptor will attempt to maintain its body temperature and if the ambient temperature is low it will expend a considerable amount of energy in so doing. As a result the bird may become hypoglycaemic and die. In addition, however, a low temperature may act as a stressor and precipitate shock. Methods of keeping a bird warm range from bringing it indoors from an outside aviary to wrapping it in a towel or the provision of heating in the form of a "hospital cage" or a suitably wrapped hotwater bottle.

Heat loss can be significant during and after surgery and the maintenance of the bird's temperature at such time is crucial; this is discussed in Chapter 10.

Maintenance of fluid balance is important to counteract shock and should be considered particularly when a bird has suffered blood loss or shows clinical signs of diarrhoea or vomiting. The use of glucose-saline (5% glucose, 0·85% NaCl) is the simplest method of replacing fluid. Preferably it should be used orally but it can be administered subcutaneously at a dosage of up to 4% bodyweight. If used by injection it *must* be sterile. In order to improve renal function 2 – 4% lactated Ringer's solution can be given intravenously or subcutaneously (50). Other com-pounds can also be used in fluid replacement and many of these contain amino acids or other nutritives. An alternative technique is to use an oral electrolyte mixture – a technique which has been found of value in human cholera patients (310) and in calves with scours (197). At the time of writing I have not been able to carry out a full trial using such a technique in birds but initial results have been encouraging using the product "Ion-aid" (Syntex).

Unfortunately we know little about electrolytes and water balance in birds of prey with the exception of some experimental work – for example, on the red-tailed hawk by Johnson (236). It is of interest to note that the nasal glands of raptors appear to play only a minor role in electrolyte balance, in contrast to the situation in some other species of bird.

Feeding is important for the same reasons described earlier under provision of warmth. The sick raptor that does not feed will lose condition and a small bird, such as a sparrowhawk or merlin, may quickly reach a critical level at which it will die of starvation. If a bird refuses to feed voluntarily then it may need to be tempted or forcefed. Tempting a bird to feed needs patience and experience and can include ruses such as a change of diet, offering attractive morsels of fresh meat or viscera and taunting the bird with the food so that it opens its beak; the food can then be put inside and, with luck, will be swallowed.

Forcefeeding is not difficult. The bird's beak should be opened and a small moistened bolus of meat pushed over the tongue and down the oesophagus. It is always best to forcefeed "little and often"; any attempt to fill a sick bird's crop with food in one session is likely to result in regurgitation. Liquid food can be administered by oesophageal tube.

Minimum disturbance is an important adjunct to any treatment. A bird that is regularly disturbed by noise or movement will be stressed and may also damage itself in attempts to move. With diurnal species it is often wiser to keep the patient hooded, or in a closed box or dark cupboard, except when treatment is being carried out. Cardboard boxes are very useful.

Hand-in-hand with nursing is the first aid treatment of raptors. In a paper in "The Falconer" in 1971 (89) I discussed the provision of first aid and emergency treatment for the sick bird of prey. Many of these points have already been discussed or will be covered in a later chapter. Wounds should be cleaned, treated medically and, if necessary, sutured. Haemorrhage must be stopped by direct pressure or, in severe cases, by use of a tourniquet which must be released every 30 minutes. Often it is more important to nurse the bird, with supportive treatment, for the first 24 – 72 hours and to delay a definitive diagnosis until it has improved in condition.

The subject of nursing is complex and one that cannot be taught in a book. Many apparently hopeless cases recover because of dedicated care and attention by people who have the time and patience to devote themselves to the bird. Under this heading are many falconers, aviculturists and zoo personnel. Others include the staff of "wild bird hospitals" and similar establishments. These people are usually extremely proficient in the nursing care of wild birds and achieve impressive results in treatment. There is a tendency for some individuals to be sceptical of the work of wild bird hospitals but it has become increasingly clear to me that we have much to learn from them. Many a valuable bird could be saved if supportive treatment was improved and this will be emphasised often in succeeding chapters.

CHAPTER 4

Physical diseases

Many physical factors may cause disease or death in birds of prey. Of these trauma is the most important but others will also be discussed.

Trauma

Traumatic injuries are a very common cause of disability or death in raptors. Free-living birds may be shot, damaged by traps, struck by cars or hit electricity wires or windows; as a result many find their way into captivity as casualties. Falconers' birds can suffer a similar fate; they may also damage their wings or keel when bating on to a hard surface, especially if they are in poor condition. In zoological collections birds may hit or damage themselves on the wire fence; alternatively fighting may break out, with resultant injuries or death to a smaller or less aggressive individual. In breeding aviaries a number of physical mishaps can befall a raptor. Birds may strike a badly positioned perch or even become entangled in vegetation, such as ivy or honeysuckle, which is part of the "natural" flora of the enclosure. The latter can be a particular danger to birds which already have an injury, such as a healed wing fracture, and are thus less able to extricate themselves than are their healthy companions.

Predation can be a cause of injury or death and the "predators" involved can range from other raptors, such as the great horned owl in North America, to voracious social insects, such as safari ants (*Dorylus* sp.) in the tropics (Photo 3). Dogs and cats can injure birds of prey (although sometimes the role is reversed!) and humans can inflict similar damage intentionally or by accident. Falconers' birds may be injured or bitten by their quarry.

Damage can also be inflicted during capture and in transit. The cere and talons are particularly vulnerable and a severe case of cere damage, in a recently imported sparrowhawk, is shown in Photo 4. Such damage may lead to epithelial proliferation and the result can be a hypertrophied cere and partly or totally occluded nares – a condition somewhat similar to "brown hypertrophy of the cere" in psittacine birds (1). Obstruction of the nares leads to respiratory embarrassment and there is distension of the soft tissues around the eyes as the bird breathes. The nares can be widened surgically but often become obstructed again within a few weeks.

Injuries associated with transportation may be reduced by careful handling and packing and the use of well-designed cages and carrying boxes. Recent IATA Regulations have helped standardise containers for birds transported by air although, as Inskipp and Thomas reported in "Airborne Birds" (225) many bird

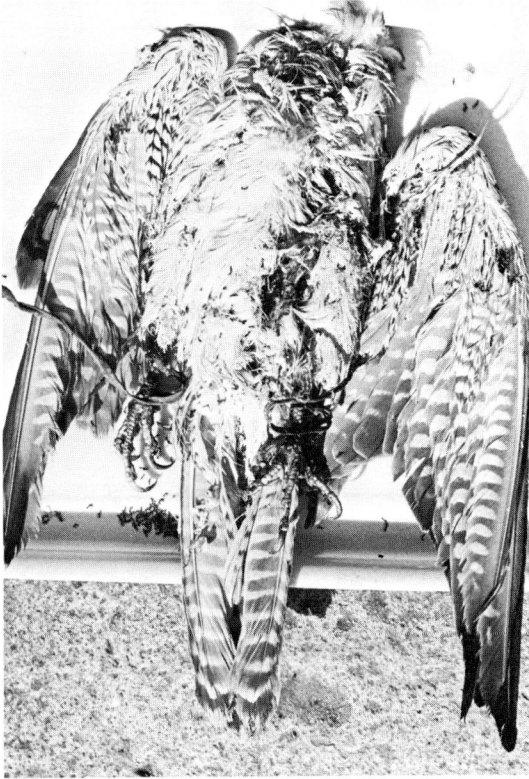

Photo 3.   A captive lanner killed by safari ants in Africa. Many ants are visible on the body and
plumage

exporters still do not adhere to them; examples were given of contraventions involving birds of prey. Not all aspects of the IATA Regulations will be accepted as desirable for raptors – for example the provision of perches – but in general they should be welcomed as a step forward. There is an excellent chapter on transport in Mavrogordato's book "A Falcon in the Field" (296) and reference should be made to it. Mavrogordato emphasised the advisability of not having perches nor absorbent material in a travelling box and recommended air-holes low down and a hole in the roof for the insertion of food. Like him I am a great believer in cardboard boxes for short journeys although I usually fold some newspaper on the floor and generally find that the bird does not damage it. For longer journeys, or as a permanent travelling container, a wooden box should be constructed.

Subdued light and hooding are useful aids to handling (see Chapter 3) and will reduce damage to the bird. Falconers' birds which are of nervous temperament need particularly careful management and the use of padded perches, such as a rubber tyre as a portable "cadge", will help reduce damage to wings.

The treatment of traumatic injuries in predatory birds is basically similar to that for other avian species but special care must be taken when restraining the

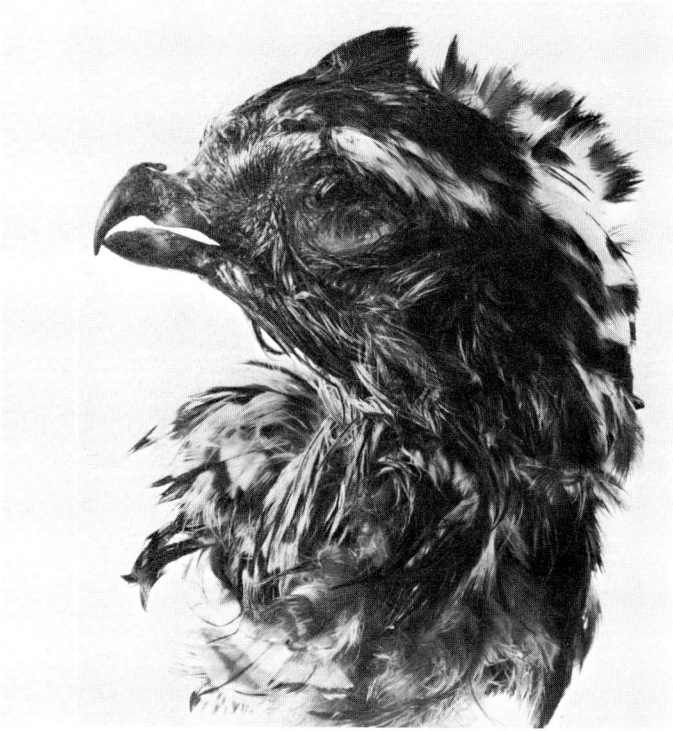

Photo 4.   Grossly damaged cere in a recently imported sparrowhawk

patient in order to reduce injury to it or the handler. Light anaesthesia may prove helpful. Fresh wounds must be cleaned and quaternary ammonium compounds are recommended for this purpose; gentian violet or tincture of iodine can be used for mild cuts and abrasions. The treatment of maggot-infested wounds is discussed in Chapter 6. Gunshot wounds pose no particular problems but radiography is important in ascertaining where shot is lodged and one must often give a guarded prognosis initially in view of the possibility of internal damage. Shot wounds should be cleaned but no effort made to remove the shot unless it is likely to hamper healing or, by virtue of its position (e.g. in the skull) produce specific clinical signs. If a talon is torn out it is usually best to dress the wound for two weeks as well as applying a disinfecting agent. Skin wounds can be sutured using nylon or silk for the skin and catgut for deeper tissues.

Injured birds should be kept warm, must be forcefed if necessary, and should receive fluids orally or by injection.

Occasionally an injured raptor shows subcutaneous emphysema; I have seen this in free-living birds and in young captive-bred falcons. The air in such cases appears to originate from a damaged air sac. It should be removed, aseptically, with a needle and syringe, repeating the procedure if necessary. The presence of green-coloured tissue around a wound is usually indicative of bruising – at least

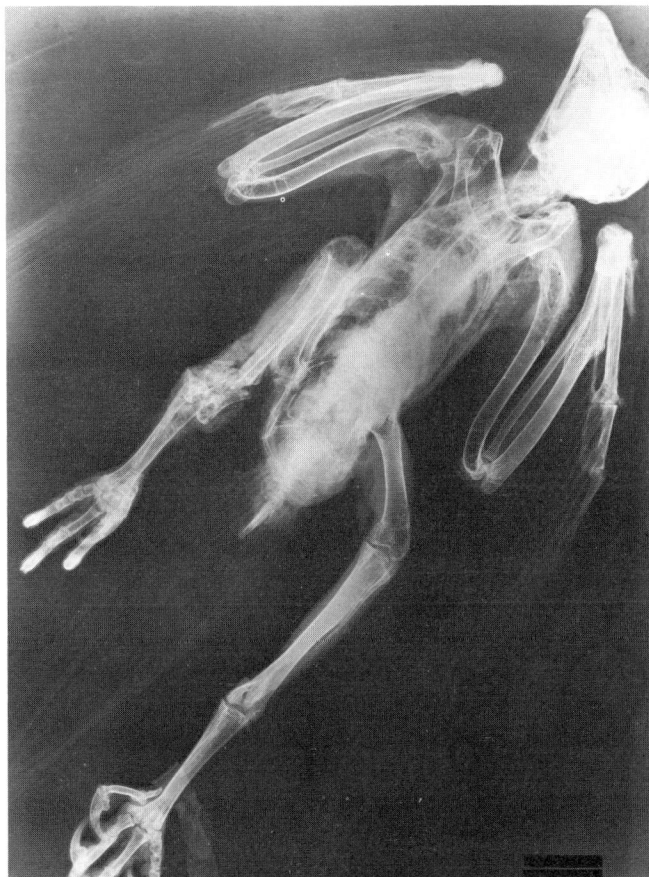

Photo 5. Radiograph of a saker showing impacted fracture (traumatic) of distal end of tibia

72 hours beforehand – but the possibility of infection (for example with a *Pseudomonas* sp.) must not be ignored.

Fractures and other orthopaedic conditions are common in raptors and considerable surgical assistance can be rendered to such cases. Most fractures follow trauma (Photo 5) but some may be due to a nutritional osteodystrophy (see later). In all cases, no attempt should be made to treat the injury surgically until the bird's fluid balance has been restored and the patient is in sufficiently good condition to withstand manipulations. Compound and complicated fractures should be treated symptomatically during this time by keeping the bird warm and quiet and by forcefeeding it if necessary. Simple support of the injured limb may be advisable for a few days. An X-ray examination is a valuable aid to diagnosis but even this may need to be delayed 36 hours in order to avoid unnecessary handling and stress to the bird at an early stage. For wing injuries, a ventro-dorsal radiograph, with the bird on its back, is usually satisfactory; for leg fractures, a lateral view is also recommended as a routine. In addition, it is always wise to radiograph the "normal" limb for comparison. The value of radiography in such work was emphasised in an earlier paper (108) when attention was drawn to the efficacy and safety of CT 1341 as an anaesthetic.

Whilst a number of cases of lameness or impaired use of the wing are attributable to a fracture or luxation, a percentage show no abnormalities on radiography and soft tissue damage must be assumed. In some instances there is history of an injury, for example a falconer's bird bating or being damaged by its quarry, and the clinical picture resembles a "sprain". The affected area is swollen, warm and painful. It usually heals spontaneously within 14 days and in my view treatment, other than rest, is of no value. Nerve damage also occurs from time to time, again usually following trauma. In some cases one can elicit pain on palpation but in others nothing can be detected and treatment must be palliative, with good feeding and rest in a suitable cage or room. It may be necessary to bind an affected wing to the body to prevent it from hanging. Such conditions usually recover spontaneously within three weeks. In the case of nerve damage to the legs, use of the limb or digit is impaired and there is usually flaccidity. Sometimes the foot "knuckles over" and the dorsal surfaces of the digits become abraded. There is sometimes, but not always, lack of sensation. My approach to such cases is to provide supportive treatment (for example, by protecting the digits or padding the perch) and to wait three weeks; if after this time there is no improvement I assume the condition is irreversible. Amputation may be necessary in some cases.

Another situation giving rise to lameness or incapacity of the feet is "surgery" of bumblefoot by laymen. A common sequel to this is damage to the nerves (or the tendons themselves) supplying the digital flexors; as a result the bird cannot flex the digit or digits. There is no treatment. The talon on a paralysed digit usually does not become worn and must be clipped frequently.

Fractures in birds of prey may be treated by external or internal fixation. Good results have been obtained by using the former for both leg and wing fractures with the exception of those of the humerus and femur. In the case of the compound fractures reduction is by traction and cleaning of the wound must be carried out. External fixation is done with splints or plaster of Paris bandage. Splints can be made of thick cardboard or plastic or, possibly best of all, strips cut from Zimmer orthopaedic splints; the latter are already padded and are easily moulded around a joint. For fixation of the radius or ulna the wing feathers may need to be cut away at their bases; the only exception is when they are growing ("in the blood") when cutting them will result in extensive haemorrhage. Alternatively it may be possible to secure a light splint to the wing by suturing it through the feathers or patagium (the membrane on the leading edge of the wing). The wing is usually strapped up or bound to the body and this technique alone, without splinting or plastering, may prove successful in the treatment of a simple fracture of radius or ulna. In order to bind a wing to the body a tubular elastic bandage can be used but it may be removed by the bird; care must also be taken to ensure that the bird is able to stand and that the cloaca is not occluded. Alternatively a one inch bandage can be used.

A disadvantage of external fixation is that one must check the bird carefully at regular intervals to confirm that the splinting is not causing tissue damage. There is also a danger that prolonged immobilisation of a limb may predispose to joint stiffness and possible impairment of use. Therefore the shorter the period of immobilisation the better.

Callus formation is rapid in birds and it may even be possible to release the free-living injured bird 14–21 days after fixation. In this context it is worthy of note that in 1855 Salvin and Brodrick (361) discussed the treatment of fractures in hawks and stated that a splint may be removed "after about three weeks' time . . . when the limb will be found straight and sound again".

Internal fixation is probably the most successful method of fracture repair in birds and good results by pinning, plating or wiring have been reported by many authors. The choice of technique depends upon a number of factors, especially the size of the bird, although Bigland (34) stressed that even small owls weighing only three ounces could be treated successfully by pinning. In a recent paper on experimental fracture healing in birds, Newton and Zeitlin (320) confirmed that intramedullary pinning was likely to give the most successful outcome for internal fixation. The use of such techniques in raptors is similar to that in other species (Photos 6a and b) and will not be discussed in detail. Every effort should be made to avoid damaging joints since this can result in arthritic changes; for example, when pinning the humerus the pin should be brought out at the shoulder and not at the elbow. It may even be considered wiser to insert a shorter pin into the medullary cavity and to supplement this by wiring, rather than risk joint damage. Mr B. H. Coles believes that it is more important to ensure joint movement than to obtain exact alignment of fractured bones. In an unpublished paper to the Avicultural Group of the British Small Animal Veterinary Association in 1977 he presented examples of fractures treated with such a combination of short pins and wires and reported that the majority healed well.

My friend Dr Patrick Redig of the University of Minnesota has made a particular study of the repair of fractures in birds of prey and at the 1977 Conference on Bird of Prey Management presented his results (351). He particularly drew attention to the different prognosis (in terms of complete recovery) for fractures, depending upon a) their position – for example, a proximal radial fracture carries a good prognosis if treated within five days while that for a distal facture of the same bone is only fair, and b) the bones involved – metacarpal fractures carry a poor prognosis whereas humeral fractures are usually excellent or good. In his paper Redig emphasised that surgical treatment of fractures *must* be carried out early (within five days) if optimum results are to be obtained. This in no way contradicts my own point that heroic surgery should not be embarked upon before the bird's condition has stabilised (101). An initial delay of 36 – 72 hours, during which time the bird is nursed, is invaluable; thereafter surgery should be undertaken promptly and the prognosis is usually good.

Fractures near the carpus are extremely difficult to treat surgically and arthritic changes, with resultant restriction of movement, are regrettably common. Usually all one can do is to apply external fixation. In contrast, fractures of the radius or ulna alone usually require only external support since the intact bone serves as a natural splint for the one which is damaged (Figures 7a, b and c). Humeral fractures should, in my opinion, always be treated by internal fixation since contraction of the strong muscles in this region usually results in severe overriding of the fractured portions. Although one usually approaches such fractures from the dor-

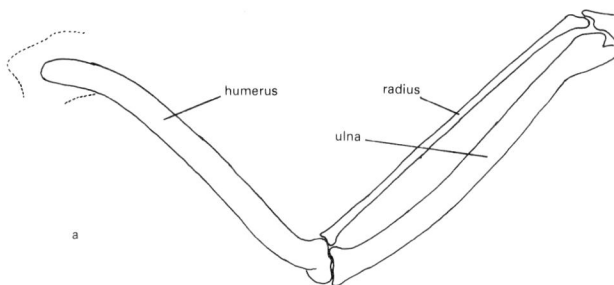

Normal humerus, radius and ulna

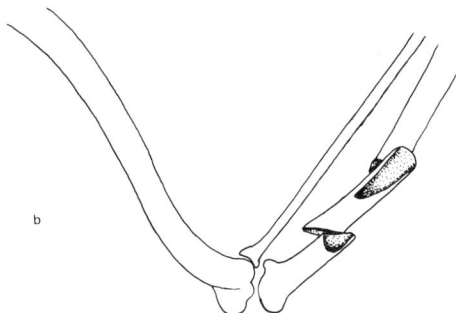

Comminuted fracture of ulna

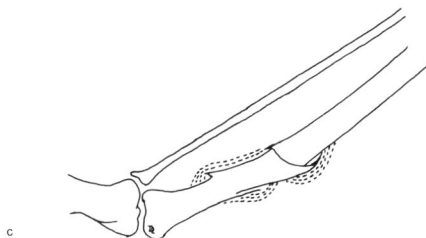

Callus formation resulting in healing of fractured ulna. Note how the intact radius serves as a natural splint

Figs 7 a, b and c

sal aspect of the wing, a ventral approach has the advantage of involving less plucking of feathers and tissue damage.

For falconry or release it is essential that a bird is able to use its feet or wings properly but in captive breeding establishments and zoological collections this may not be so important and therefore partial success in treatment may be acceptable. Indeed, in some cases, it may be considered best to amputate the distal portion of a limb, especially if a wing hangs down and becomes soiled or if a foot is only an encumbrance. Amputation is, in my opinion, often justifiable; birds treated thus can live for many years in captivity, appear to thrive and sometimes breed. One tawny eagle I treated in Tanzania has lived in a zoological collection for over ten years with only one foot. The amputation of a whole limb can often prove successful – an account of such an operation on a wing was given by Holt (215) but restriction of activity can result. The use of prosthetic limbs may prove of practical use, especially to aid mobility or copulation of valuable breeding birds. Such techniques are not new; the fitting of an artificial limb to a sea eagle was recorded in "The Times" of May 17th 1965 and as long ago as 1664 (140) John Evelyn, the diarist, recorded seeing in London a captive crane "having hadd one of his leggs broken, and cut off above the knee, had a wooden or boxen leg and thigh with a joint so accurately made that the creature could walke as if it had been natural"!

There should be no hesitation in amputating severely damaged digits or talons and even falconers' birds thrive surprisingly well with such a handicap. The procedure may also be necessary on account of frostbite (see later) or because a constriction on the leg (for example, injury by a trap or aviary netting) severely damages the tissues and results in a swollen insensitive foot which gradually develops dry gangrene.

As an alternative to amputation, the trailing tip of a wing may be remedied by surgical patagiectomy (358). This technique involves the removal of a piece of patagial membrane and is described in Chapter 10.

Two other orthopaedic conditions which occur frequently are dislocations (luxations) and arthritis. Captive hawks frequently dislocate a phalanx (Photo 7) and these cases are usually due to trauma, especially in the early stages of training or when the bird is first caged.

Dislocation of other joints, such as shoulder or elbow, may also occur. Some cases recover spontaneously but most require reduction, often together with immobilisation of the joint by plastering or bandaging. Reduction of a dislocation should be carried out within 72 hours; if there is delay irreversible damage may occur and arthritis can be the sequel. Luxation of the elbow (Figure 8) appears to be particularly difficult to treat successfully; in some cases wiring the bones helps keep them in place but the dislocation often recurs.

Arthritis is relatively common in birds of prey and may follow a traumatic injury or infection. Investigation of possible cases of arthritis should include tests of function. The joint must be fully flexed and extended and the angle of extension compared with the "normal" limb. The degree of freedom of movement of the joint is also important. Chronic arthritis may result in a thickened joint but often

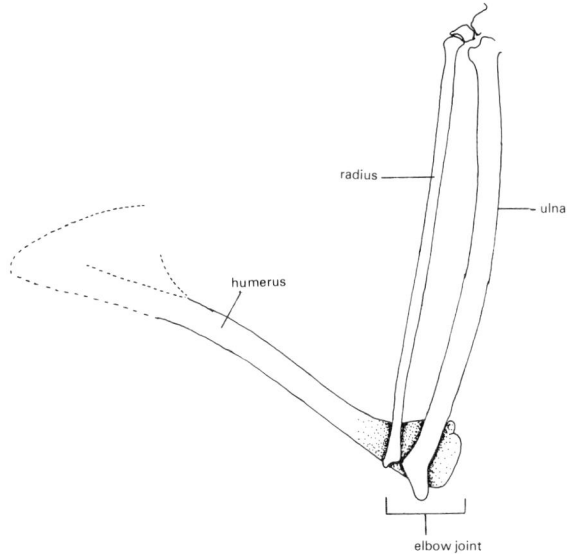

Fig. 8   Dislocation of the elbow joint. The radius and ulna are overriding the distal end of the humerus

no other abnormalities are visible. In acute cases, however, the swollen joint is usually also painful and warm to the touch. Pus can sometimes be aspirated but bacteriological culture may prove negative.

Early cases of arthritis appear to respond to appropriate antibiotics but when longstanding, for example following chronic "bumblefoot" (see Chapter 7), they are usually incurable. In one instance, a lagger, arthritis and ankylosis of the distal phalangeal joint had resulted in a "fixed digit" with the permanently erect talon an encumbrance to both bird and handler. The talon was amputated under halothane anaesthesia with good results and the bird was subsequently used successfully for falconry.

Other orthopaedic conditions which may be encountered from time to time include non-union of fractures with "false joint" formation and osteomyelitis (108). In neither case is the prognosis good and the latter may necessitate amputation. I have also encountered a case of bilateral degenerative disease of the heads of the humeri in a kestrel; clinically both wings drooped and if the bird fell on to its back it could not right itself. The aetiology is unknown.

When a bird is recovering from an injury exercise is important. Judicious design of an aviary, with perches at different heights, will help achieve this, as will "flying lessons" with the bird flown to a lure or tethered on a line. Many such techniques are used in the pre-release conditioning of casualty birds and reference can usefully be made to papers such as that by Snelling (380).

If captive or casualty birds are intended for release it is important to ensure that

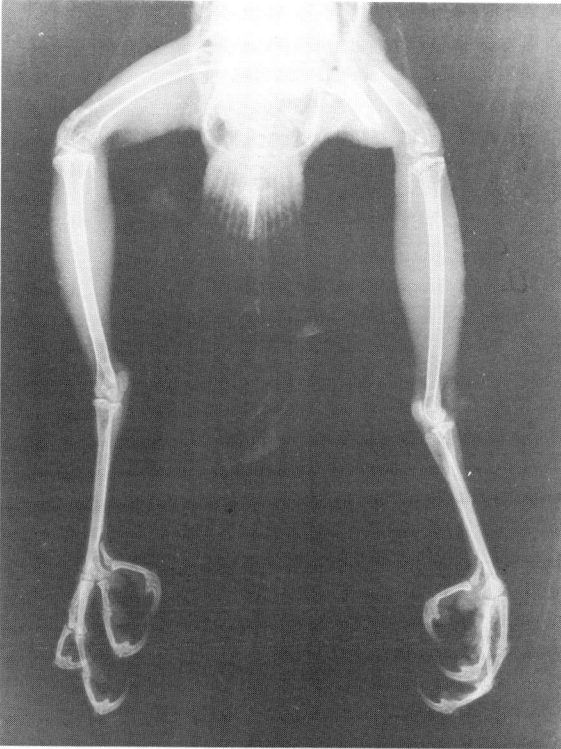

Photo 6a.   Radiograph of a merlin with a midshaft fracture of the left femur

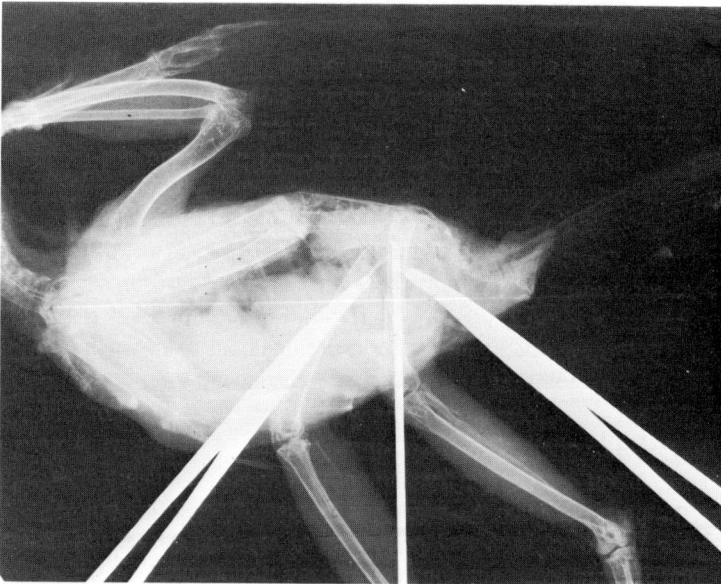

Photo 6b.   Surgery on the bird above. Intramedullary pinning is in progress

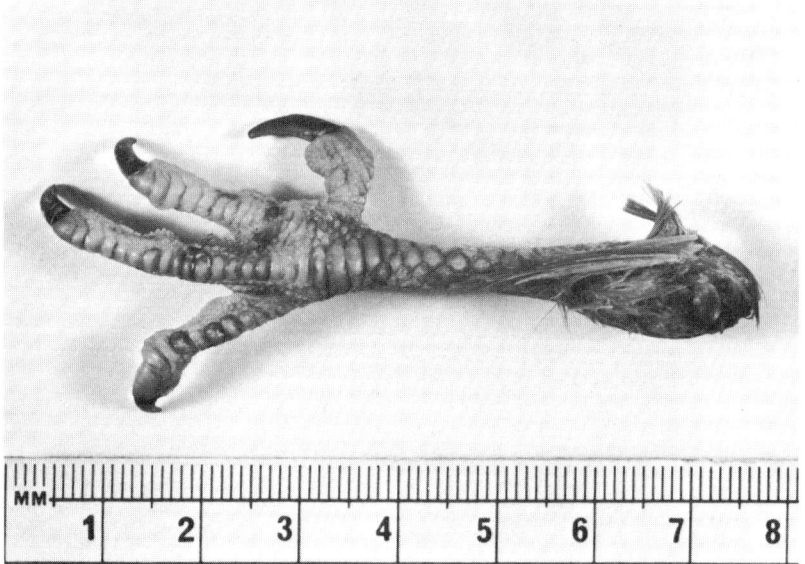

Photo 7.   Foot of a kestrel showing luxation of distal phalanx of lateral digit

a fracture or other skeletal injury has healed satisfactorily. My own approach has always been to insist that there is no impairment of function nor change in anatomy of a wing before a bird can be rehabilitated. This is not, however, the opinion of Mr B. H. Coles (quoted earlier) who has records of cases surviving (and in some cases breeding) in the wild following release with healed fractures where either the alignment was poor or the movement of joints impaired. Much, of course, depends upon the species and the locality into which it is released but Coles' belief is that most birds probably have "reserve powers" and are able to compensate for any relatively minor deficiency in wing (or leg) function. He substantiates this by reference to free-living birds (including some raptors) found with badly healed fractures which had apparently been able both to recover and, subsequently, to survive in the wild.

A number of anaesthetics may be used for the surgical repair of fractures and other orthopaedic procedures and these are discussed in more detail in Chapter 10. Halothane or methoxyflurane is particularly useful and systemic ketamine or metomidate can either be employed as a premedicant or may be sufficient on its own. Redig (351) recommended a ketamine-xylazine mixture.

Other physical factors

A number of other non-infectious factors may cause disease and death in raptors, amongst them excess cold and heat, burning, electrocution, and drowning.

The response of birds of prey to changes in temperature is of considerable ecological interest and a useful review is that by Mosher (304). In temperate climates birds are more likely to be exposed to low temperatures than high.

Frostbite has been reported in a number of species of bird (406). Affected birds show ischaemia and necrosis of digits which may later slough: some cases develop heart lesions. Frostbite is unlikely to occur in captive raptors unless exposed to very low temperatures although colleagues in North America tell me that they fairly often encounter cases. It is probable that species differ in their tolerance to cold; this has already been shown in snowy owls which have a lower critical temperature than other owls (365). It must also be remembered that a young raptor is usually less able to maintain its body temperature than is an adult and that certain drugs, particularly anaesthetics, will lower a bird's temperature and render it susceptible to pathological effects.

A drop in temperature *per se* need not prove dangerous to a bird of prey but it can serve as a stressor and may potentiate hypoglycaemia. Young (nestling) birds are particularly susceptible and may die following fairly non-specific signs of lethargy, fluffed-up plumage and reduction in food intake. An unacclimatised tropical bird can react adversely to low temperature and may develop respiratory disease as a sequel; this not infrequently occurs when lanners are imported in the Autumn from Nigeria. Karstad and Sileo (244) found gout, amyloidosis and heart lesions more prevalent in waterfowl in cold weather and it may be that a similar situation pertains in birds of prey. Some species, however, such as the snowy owl, which shows anatomical and physiological adaptations to cold, is likely to be more adversely affected by hot sunshine (see later) than a drop in temperature.

Any bird that has become chilled should be warmed gradually to a temperature of 35°C. It should be encouraged to feed and fluids must be administered. Frostbite damage needs topical treatment including, if necessary, amputation.

Although the importance of good ventilation has been emphasised elsewhere, it should not be forgotten that exposure to wind can be deleterious, especially to a falconer's bird on block or ring-perch. Birds show obvious dislike of a strong wind and I am in no doubt that exposure to it may predispose to disease – air sacculitis, for example. It will also result in heat loss and a subsequent increase in food consumption and this must be borne in mind when small birds, being kept for falconry, are exposed to such weather. Very often a slight change in management will help reduce the risk – for example, the provision of better shelter around a weathering ground.

A combination of wet and cold can rapidly prove fatal to a captive bird of prey. A falconer's bird in particular may become soaked if exposed on a perch in heavy rain or if it plunges into a pond or river during a flight. As a result the plumage becomes water-logged and the bird's insulation disappears. The bird appears hunched and stiff and may even show signs of inco-ordination. The cloacal temperature drops to 35° C or less. Treatment is entirely palliative; the bird should be warmed and the plumage dried with a towel, fan heater or hair drier. Under no circumstances should the bird be exposed to low temperature again until it has fully recovered – preferably not for 24 hours.

Although most birds of prey withstand high temperatures very well, they do not like excessive heat and try to avoid it. Overheating can occur in the tropics and, occasionally, in temperate climates. Birds being flown for falconry are particularly susceptible. A bird in confinement may become overheated on account of poor design of an aviary or because it comes into too close contact with an infra-red heater or light bulb in a "hospital cage". Another possible cause is if a bird is left in a car on a hot day without adequate ventilation or cooling. Eggs and nestlings can particularly easily become overheated and die if an aviary is poorly designed, especially if plastic or PVC sheeting is used.

An affected bird will pant, let its wings hang loosely and partly close its eyes. It will tend to seek a cool or sheltered place. In more severe cases there is prostration and a degree of hyperthermia detectable to the touch, dehydration may be apparent and the tongue and buccal mucous membranes are usually dry and discoloured (yellowish-brown) in appearance. Cutaneous erythema and other skin lesions may be present if burning has occurred.

Treatment of the affected bird must be prompt. It should be moved to a sheltered place and slowly cooled, if necessary using a cool damp cloth on the head, feet and underside of the wings. Fluids can be given and skin lesions should be treated topically. I have personally treated only a few cases of overheating. The one outside the tropics was a peregrine being flown at grouse in Scotland in 1975 which developed heat stress but responded to a cool environment and oral and parenteral glucose saline.

The response of birds of prey to hot environments was discussed by Mosher (304) who drew attention to the efficiency of panting as a method of heat dissipation so long as the bird can replace its lost water and maintain blood gas concentrations. Mosher also referred to the work of Bartholomew and Cade (21) who demonstrated a countercurrent system in the tarsus of American kestrels which presumably plays a part in withstanding high ambient temperatures. Calder and Schmidt-Nielsen (66) investigated panting and blood carbon dioxide levels in birds, amongst them a turkey vulture, and discussed the subject of heat stress.

Heat stress has been shown to cause eggshell thinning in poultry (343) and should perhaps be considered when birds in aviaries produce abnormally thin eggs.

Captive raptors may become burned or electrocuted, especially if they come into contact with electric heaters or, if being flown, powerlines. Often the only clinical signs visible are charred feathers but close examination will reveal skin burns of varying severity and haemorrhages. These lesions will be painful and the bird may show dehydration; shock is a common sequel. Treatment consists of nursing, especially the maintenance of body temperature and administration of fluids, and the topical treatment of the burns. Antibiotics and corticosteroids will help prevent infection and counteract shock.

Post-mortem examination of birds that have been burned or electrocuted will show internal lesions in addition to those described above. There may be free blood in the internal organs and this may be dark and unclotted in appearance. Petechial haemorrhages and discolouration are seen in muscles. In the case of electrocution the distribution of lesions depends upon the path the current took; careful dissection is necessary and the bird should be skinned.

An important step in the reduction of electrocution deaths in free-living birds, which will also apply to those flown by falconers, is the modification of design of power lines to minimise the chances of a bird electrocuting itself. Such work has mainly taken place in the United States, for example, in Idaho (314) where a captive (trained) eagle was used to study the problems.

Captive raptors occasionally drown, especially if in an aviary with an unsuitable waterbowl or if, due to some disability, they are unable to extricate themselves from it. In most cases the bird is dead before it is found – at *postmortem* examination the plumage is waterlogged (or matted, if it has dried) and there is fluid in lungs and air sacs. Petechial haemorrhages may be seen. In the unlikely event of a bird being found that is still alive, it should be treated by physically removing fluid from the respiratory tract – by holding it upside down, with beak open – and artificial respiration should be applied. The administration of oxygen may help. It is of interest to note that drowning has also been reported in free-living birds of prey (117), the authors suggesting, amongst other things, that the raptors might have been attracted to the water by potential prey species. This could be a hazard to falconers' birds.

I have no information on the effects of ionising radiation on birds of prey. However, it is reasonable to assume that excess exposure is undesirable and therefore use of radiography should be restricted whenever possible. It is of interest to note that in work on total body X-ray irradiation in the budgerigar (*Melopsittacus undulatus*) – one of the few publications not dealing with poultry – birds which died following irradiation were found to have a luxuriant growth of an *Aspergillus* sp. in the lungs (364).

CHAPTER 5

Infectious diseases

Under this heading I shall discuss those diseases of raptors caused by, or associated with, such infectious agents as viruses, chlamydiae, mycoplasmas, bacteria and fungi. Only the most common or potentially important conditions will be described in detail. Protozoan and metazoan parasites are covered in Chapter 6.

Several virus diseases have been reported from birds of prey, amongst them avian pox, Newcastle disease and hepatitis; these will be described later. It is probable that other viruses will be implicated in due course but isolation of these agents requires sophisticated equipment and many avian pathologists do not include virology as a routine part of clinical or *post-mortem* work. Nevertheless, every opportunity should be taken to submit material to appropriate laboratories for virological examination.

Chlamydiae have been reported from a number of birds of prey and the disease ornithosis, which can be transmissible to man, is known to affect members of both the Falconiformes and Strigiformes (250). I have not diagnosed it myself. Serological surveys would be of interest; a recent report from Oklahoma gave only negative results when 86 raptor samples were tested by the agar-gel precipitin test (262).

Mycoplasmas (Mycoplasmata) were only recently isolated for the first time from birds of prey (165) but their existence has long been suspected. Three isolates were from sick hawks (see later); one metabolised arginine and the other two glucose. Subsequent to that work we have isolated mycoplasmas from tracheal swabs of seven healthy peregrines at an establishment where there was a history of respiratory disease. One isolate hydrolysed arginine and the others glucose; they were all negative when typing was attempted using antisera against seven species of mycoplasma, amongst them poultry pathogens. The role of mycoplasms in raptor disease is still uncertain and more work is needed, including microbiological and serological surveys and experimental inoculation of birds.

Many species of bacteria are involved in raptor disease and considerable attention is paid to them later in this chapter. Bacteriological examination plays an important part in diagnosis and antibiotic sensitivity tests are desirable if therapy is to be successful. Much remains to be learned of the "normal" bacterial flora of raptors. Many organisms can be isolated from the feet, pharynx and cloaca of apparently healthy birds and it is possible that some such organisms may, under certain conditions, prove pathogenic. Some indication of the range of bacteria that has been associated with disease in non-domesticated birds was given by Fiennes (143) and although he referred little to birds of prey, his discussion and references are worth reading.

Relatively few fungi have been incriminated as a cause of disease in raptors. However, aspergillosis due to *Aspergillus fumigatus* is probably one of the commonest causes of death in captive birds and other species of fungi may also be involved in air sac and lung infection. Moniliasis has been reported in raptors (351); I also have isolated the fungus, particularly from the intestinal tract, on a number of occasions but have not considered it a factor in disease or death. Blastomycosis was reported from two birds of prey by Kaleta and Drüner (241); the infection involved the beak but no details were given. It is possible that other mycotic infections may occur from time to time, especially in skin infections. Keratinophilic fungi can often be isolated from the feathers of birds (345) but do not appear to be pathogenic.

It would be pertinent to mention that birds of prey may be a source of zoonoses; that is, diseases or infections transmissible to man, such as Newcastle disease and avian tuberculosis. In addition, birds can inflict wounds with their talons and beaks which may be infected with *Staphylococcus aureus* or other organisms, including *Clostridium tetani*. Occasionally, if a falconer or aviculturist becomes ill his doctor, or a hospital, may request information on the health of his birds on the grounds that a zoonosis might be involved. I have been asked for such assistance on a number of occasions but never has the bird been incriminated. Moreover, I have been unable to trace any evidence that birds of prey cause the allergic disease "bird-fancier's lung" in man. It seems probable, therefore, that raptors are only very rarely involved in human disease.

Hygiene is of great importance and I drew attention to the hazards of a build-up of infectious agents in the second edition of "A Hawk for the Bush" (94). In that chapter I suggested some rules to reduce the risk of infection, all of which hinged upon simple hygiene. I do not intend to discuss hygiene and disinfection in detail in this book; information is available in textbooks on veterinary medicine, especially those dealing with poultry diseases, and in published papers elsewhere.

However, a few general points will be made. It is usually impossible to sterilise a raptor's surroundings, with the possible exception of small items such as water containers, and the aim should therefore be to reduce the number of organisms by destroying and/or diluting them. A surface must be clean before it is disinfected. Hot water alone is a remarkably good disinfectant and scrubbing with soap and hot water is strongly recommended. If a chemical disinfectant *is* to be used, it should be chosen carefully; some guidelines were given in a paper published in the "International Zoo Yearbook" (104) and examples are listed in Appendix IX. Probably the safest disinfectant is a surface-acting compound, such as cetrimide, but the efficacy of such chemicals against viruses is doubtful and they may be inactivated by soap. Phenol compounds and formalin are both effective against bacteria but only the latter has any virucidal activity. Following adequate exposure of a surface to a phenol or formalin the disinfectant must be washed off. Washing soda is cheap and effective against viruses but rinsing is again necessary. In Britain there are "Approved Disinfectants" for use against certain pathogens of farm animals, including poultry, and details of these can be obtained from the

Ministry of Agriculture, Fisheries and Food. Fumigation of a mews or enclosed quarters, using formaldehyde and potassium permanganate, can be an effective way of reducing the numbers of organisms in a building but must be carried out effectively.

It is virtually impossible to disinfect adequately an enclosure that contains vegetation. Hurrell (224) suggested that exposure to rain and sun reduces the numbers of pathogens and this is probably so. Nevertheless, breeding aviaries should be examined in the Autumn and such items as feeding platforms and water containers cleaned. Replaceable materials, such as logs and bark, can be removed and burned. If such an enclosure becomes infected (for example with avian tuberculosis organisms) the only long-term solution is probably to remove the birds and leave the aviary to "rest"; removal of the vegetation and, if possible, the top few inches of soil will probably help.

The management of a large collection of captive birds of prey necessitates an appropriate health programme and one important aspect of this is maintenance of hygiene. Much of this is routine and will not be discussed here. A number of techniques can be employed to monitor ventilation while the use of bacteriological settle plates, as mentioned in Chapter 3, will help in assessing the contamination of the building. The different numbers of bacterial and fungal colonies which grow on each plate give an indication of the relative contamination (Photo 8). For example, when investigating respiratory disease of hawks in one falconer's mews I obtained a count of 1160 colonies in one ("dirty") corner, 56 in a "clean" area and only 4 in the owner's domestic living room. Results such as these need careful analysis but often give a guide as to where changes in management or design might be advantageous.

In the succeeding part of this chapter the more important infectious diseases will be discussed. In many cases they will be grouped together under a clinical heading, such as "Respiratory conditions", regardless of the aetiological agent involved. Some organisms, however, will be listed separately and not related to specific pathogenesis or clinical signs. Certain infections are included in Chapter 11.

Infections of the integument and superficial tissues

Infectious conditions of the feet ("bumblefoot") are discussed in Chapter 7. However, many other infections of superficial tissues may also be encountered.

The beak and talons are particularly susceptible to traumatic damage but may also become infected. Secondary bacterial infections of the cere and digits may follow injury and a variety of organisms are isolated, including *Staphylococcus aureus, Escherichia coli* and *Proteus* spp. Falconers often speak of "fungus" infections of these sites but I have not confirmed such diagnoses other than a single isolation of *Mucor hiemalis* from sloughed material from the talons of a golden eagle. Although this fungus is usually a saprophyte, it is possible that it was involved in the condition; unfortunately histology was not possible but the bird recovered after topical antifungal therapy. Local infections of the cere may result

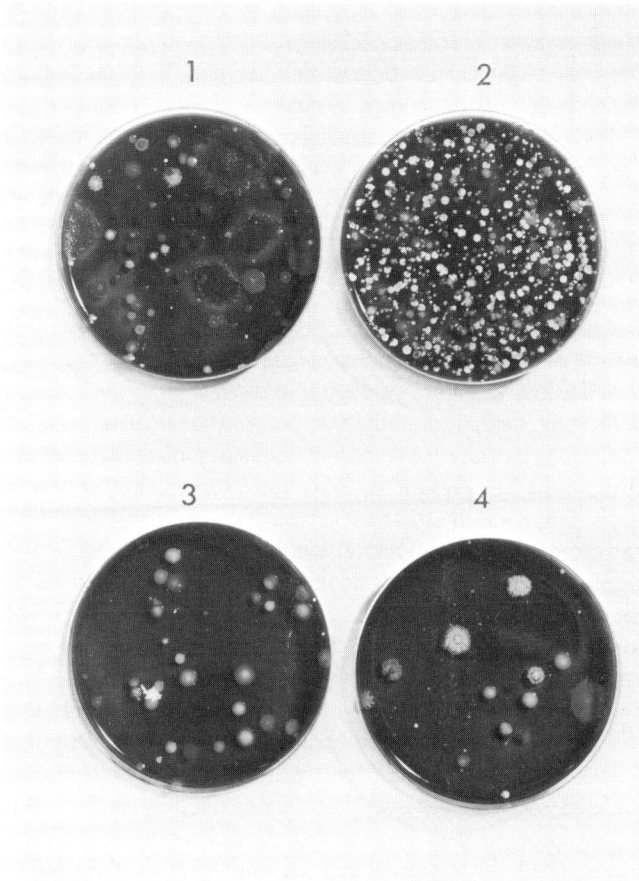

Photo 8.   Bacteriological "settle plates" placed for 30 minutes in different aviaries and then incubated for 18 hours. The number of colonies on each plate gives an indication of the relative contamination

in partial obstruction of the nares, with clinical signs of noisy respiration. The nares should be cleaned with a small swab soaked in cetrimide and local antibiotic applied daily for a week.

Skin infections are relatively uncommon in birds of prey but may occur following injuries. In such cases a variety of bacteria can usually be isolated. Treatment is often successful using a disinfectant, such as cetrimide, rather than sulphonamides or antibiotics.

Skin granulomas are seen from time to time and are commonly associated with *S. aureus* although sometimes no organisms can be isolated. Surgical excision and/or antibiotics should be employed in treatment. In a paper on cutaneous diseases of wild birds Blackmore and Keymer (43) described tumour-like masses on one wing of a kestrel; these proved to be due to tuberculosis. Similar tuberculous lesions were reported in a barn owl by Bucke and Mawdesley-Thomas (60) and I have seen them in two buzzards. Infection with a *Mycobacterium* sp. should therefore always be considered in differential diagnosis of cutaneous lesions and a Ziehl-Neelsen stain of the tissue carried out.

Conjunctivitis and keratoconjunctivitis may occur from time to time, again often following trauma. Bacteria are usually involved; frequent isolates are *S. aureus* and *E. coli*. Arnall and Keymer (15) reported *Mycoplasma* infections of the eyes of birds of prey but gave no details. If treatment is not prompt, excoriation of surrounding skin and purulent dermatitis may occur and this feature was reported in 1619 by Bert (32) who described a "hot humour that runneth out of the eye, and scaldeth all the feathers from that part under the eye, and maketh it bare". Bert went on to describe clinical signs of "wiping of the eye against the wing" and this is often a feature of such infections.

Antibiotic therapy, using an ophthalmic preparation, is usually satisfactory and I often also administer vitamin A in case a deficiency is involved. If severe ulceration and photophobia are present suturing the eyelids together will help prevent further damage. Generalised ophthalmitis may respond to parenteral antibiotics but often the sequel is a non-functional eye and/or enucleation.

Otitis externa has been seen occasionally; it may progress to otitis media and otitis interna. Clinically, cases of otitis externa show damp feathers in the region of the auditory meatus. If the inner ear is involved the bird's head may be held on one side. Treatment should be with systemic antibiotics.

Bursitis can occur on both the wing and the leg. "Blain", which has long been recognised by falconers, is probably bursitis of the carpus and I have seen a number of cases of this condition. The "watery blister" on the joint frequently becomes damaged so that fluid seeps out giving the feathers a wet appearance. The condition probably follows trauma; two cases I examined were in birds which had repeatedly struck their wings against the walls of the mews. The lesion can be drained, taking sterile precautions, and antibiotic applied topically. If the fluid is cloudy, suggestive of infection, a suitable intramuscular antibiotic should be used, preferably following culture. One of my cases developed myiasis (maggot infestation) but made a complete recovery following topical application of an antibiotic and insecticidal product ("Negasunt": Bayer). Writing in 1855 Salvin and Brodrick (361) discussed the treatment of blain and mentioned that "it is very difficult to cure, and . . . if of long standing, will generally produce a stiff joint". Such arthritic complications are still often seen if treatment is delayed or antibiotics are not used. Another sequel, which can also follow other infections or traumatic insults to the end of the wing, is that the part of the wing distal to the carpus may be sloughed.

I have only seen one case of bursitis on the leg – a buzzard which suddenly, and inexplicably, developed a soft, painful, well circumscribed swelling over its patella. The lesion showed up well radiographically. It was drained under CT 1341 anaesthesia but subsequently became infected; it was later operated upon and its wall was cauterised. It recurred after several months and the bird finally contracted aspergillosis and a cloacal calculus.

Bursitis may be confused with acute arthritis which is discussed in Chapter 4.

Cloacitis occurs from time to time in raptors and it is frequently associated with calculus formation; this aspect is discussed in Chapter 11. Cloacitis *per se* can occur, however, and is commonly associated with excoriation and inflammation of the skin round the vent and soiling of the area with urates. Clinical signs vary but usually the bird shows discomfort when defaecating and may ruffle its feathers and attempt to peck at the cloacal region. Diagnosis is based on visual inspection and examination; the presence of cloacal calculi should be excluded by palpation or radiography. *E. coli* appears to be the usual cause of the infection but bacteriological culture is always advisable; I have isolated *S. aureus* from one case and this necessitated cloxacillin treatment. Oxytetracycline *per cloacam*, parenterally or orally, is frequently effective in treatment when *E. coli* is involved. The administration of oral liquid paraffin will ease discomfort and local treatment of the vent area is advisable. Following recovery the mutes may appear unusual in that faecal and urate portions are mixed; this I attribute to damage to the cloacal chamber.

A variety of other organisms can be isolated from the cloaca of healthy birds – for example *Proteus* spp. and *Streptococcus* spp. – but their role, if any, in disease is not known.

It is possible that cloacitis may become more prevalent following the use of instruments, such as specula, during artificial insemination. Care must be taken whenever such aids are used and they should be disinfected between birds.

Respiratory conditions

Respiratory diseases have long been recognised in captive birds of prey (32, 269). They can be manifested by a mild localised rhinitis, sinusitis, pneumonia, air sacculitis or a generalised aspergillosis. In the series of cases discussed in the first edition of this book respiratory infections, including aspergillosis, were responsible for 62 out of 208 deaths. "Stress" factors seem to play an important role in the onset of respiratory diseases; they often follow a change of environment (especially in recently imported birds), other infections, or traumatic injuries. It is also possible that a vitamin deficiency, particularly vitamin A, can predispose to respiratory infections. Pathological examination plays an important role in investigation and if a bird dies or has to be killed it should be submitted for full *post-mortem* examination in order to ascertain which of the many respiratory conditions is involved. It should be noted, however, that some raptors which die following respiratory signs show only marked pulmonary congestion *post mortem* and no significant organisms can be isolated; the diagnosis in such cases is obscure.

Rhinitis is known to falconers as "cold" or "snurt". It is characterised by unilateral or bilateral nasal discharge, sneezing and, sometimes, anorexia. Affected birds should be kept warm and unless a secondary infection supersedes will usually recover spontaneously. Some cases appear to become chronic; the nares are blocked and there may be intermittent bouts of noisy respiration and sneezing.

The nares should be cleaned with a small human nasopharyngeal swab dampened in saline and the bird kept under careful observation. This syndrome may possibly be associated with sinusitis and air sacculitis (see later).

Sinusitis in falconiform birds is not at all uncommon. It has been reported by other authors (385) and I have personally treated several cases, particularly in the Autumn and Winter. However, it appears to be rare in owls.

Affected birds are often anorectic, may show a nasal discharge and usually have a swollen face, especially around the eyes (Figure 9). Other conditions of the

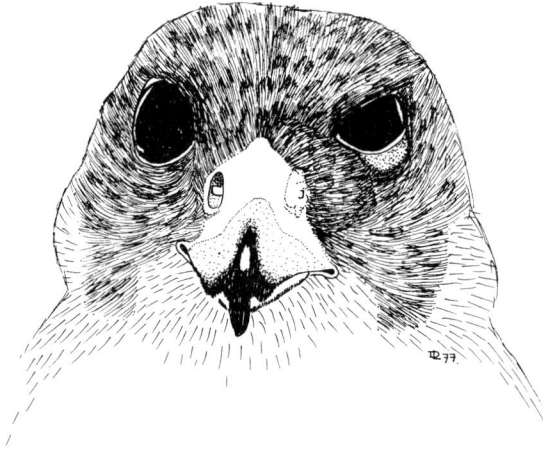

Fig. 9   Sinusitis in a falcon. The bird's left eye is slightly closed, the nostril is blocked and there is swelling of the face below the eye

head should be considered in differential diagnosis – for example, bee sting and inflammatory lesions of the buccal cavity. There is considerable overlap between sinusitis and rhinitis on the one hand and sinusitis and air sacculitis on the other and it is quite possible that all three conditions are closely related.

Success in treatment of sinusitis has been achieved with spiramycin or lincomycin, often together with betamethasone, but it is important that these are administered intramuscularly rather than orally. In some cases the causal organisms are probably not completely killed, since the condition recurs. On other occasions the characteristic facial swellings disappear but the bird may continue to show respiratory signs and blocked nares. Surgical removal of pus can prove valuable in particularly resilient cases, particularly if accompanied by systemic antibiotic therapy. The operative technique recommended is similar to that used in poultry (366). The earliest report I have been able to trace of surgically draining sinuses in raptors is that of Campbell, in Canada, who reported in 1934 (68) that he had "operated on several eagles and vultures for mycotic sinusitis, removing the fungus growth that collects and painting the cavities with iodin". I have little doubt that the "fungus growth" was straightforward sinusitis and not mycotic in origin.

Occasionally a subcutaneous soft tissue swelling of the head region may be seen following sinusitis. Such swellings contain caseous pus and may be pedunculated. They appear to arise as a result of extension of infection from the sinus and can be removed surgically.

The casual organisms in sinusitis are not known but, using the analogy of poultry, it is tempting to incriminate a *Mycoplasma* sp.; the rapid clinical response to spiramycin in some cases might support this. Although usually only single birds are affected, in Kenya I was consulted (by telephone only!) concerning an "epizootic" which killed seven birds of prey (95), suggesting either a common source of infection or transmission from one bird to another.

Birds with pneumonia usually show signs of dyspnoea, especially on exertion. Most cases are probably bacterial in origin although there seems little doubt that predisposing factors include chilling and transportation. Organisms isolated from cases at *post-mortem* examination have included *E. coli*, *S. aureus* and a *Pasteurella* sp. Affected birds usually respond to a 7–10 day course of antibiotics, especially chlortetracycline. As with so many avian diseases careful nursing, particularly warmth, fluids and feeding by hand, can be an invaluable aid to recovery.

Greenwood (177) described bronchitis as a rare condition of hawks: this too will respond to appropriate antibiotic therapy. It must be distinguished from syngamiasis and physical obstructions of the upper respiratory tract, both of which can produce similar clinical signs.

Air sacculitis of hawks is a condition which I have recognised for some years but which was not described elsewhere for a considerable period, other than mycotic air sacculitis associated with *Aspergillus fumigatus* (385) and inflammatory lesions of the air sacs due to *Serratospiculum* worms. In the past three years, however, others have reported a similar clinical syndrome and Redig (351) associated it with *E. coli* infection. My own early cases were in the cold Autumn of 1968 when many birds of prey were being imported into Britain from tropical countries; a number of these showed a clinical disease which, on *post-mortem* examination, proved to be an air sac infection.

Clinical signs of air sacculitis may be slight but affected birds are usually anorectic and often regurgitate food. Respiratory signs are variable. Regurgitation usually occurs within five minutes of ingestion but may be delayed up to an hour. The respiratory rate is often accelerated (up to 60 per minute) but dyspnoea is often not apparent unless the bird is either exerted or *in extremis*. Radiological examination of chronic cases may reveal a narrowing and opacity of the air sacs (Photo 9a).

The lesions seen at autopsy are a thickening of the air sac walls (Photo 9b) and, often, the serosae. Usually some yellowish debris is present on the air sac walls. On histological examination the air sacs are inflamed and often adherent to other tissues (Photo 9c).

When cultured the debris from the air sacs often yields *Escherichia coli* while, as was reported in the first edition, in three *post-mortem* cases a glucose-

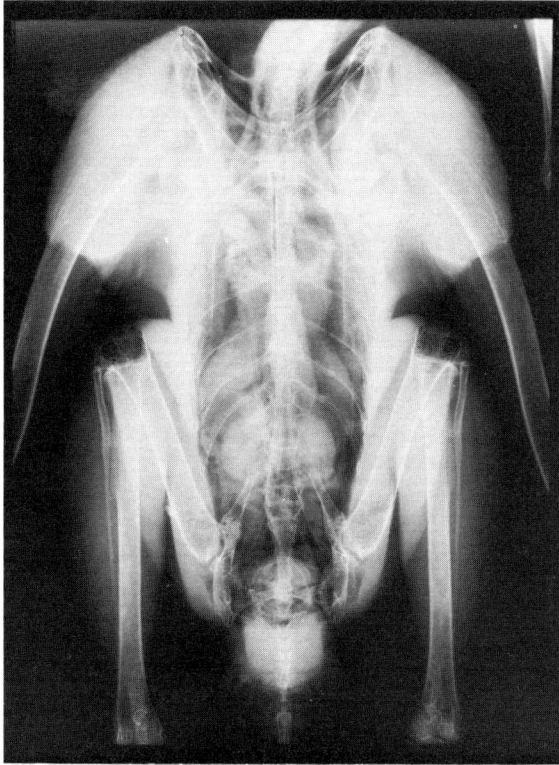

Photo 9a.   Air sacculitis: radiography of a hawkeagle showing opacity and narrowing of the air sacs

fermenting *Mycoplasma* was isolated but not processed any further. Mycoplasmas have also been identified from hawks with clinical signs of respiratory disease (165). However, as was mentioned earlier, there is as yet no proof that these organisms are responsible for disease and it is possible that they are part of the normal flora of the respiratory tract.

Treatment of cases of air sacculitis with tylosin or spiramycin has been based on the assumption that the condition might resemble that in poultry and the clinical response to these drugs has been most encouraging. In one instance, reported in the first edition, there was an epizootic at a commercial establishment and nearly a dozen birds died. Following a diagnosis of air sacculitis at autopsy, a course of tylosin by injection was given to all sick birds and no further deaths occurred. Similar results have been obtained on many subsequent occasions and the rapid alleviation of clinical signs with such therapy is a useful diagnostic aid.

I personally believe that air sac infection may also be a feature of other respiratory diseases in birds of prey, including rhinitis and sinusitis; clinical examination of some such cases would certainly suggest so. Birds which have recovered from such infections often seem prone to further respiratory disease. In

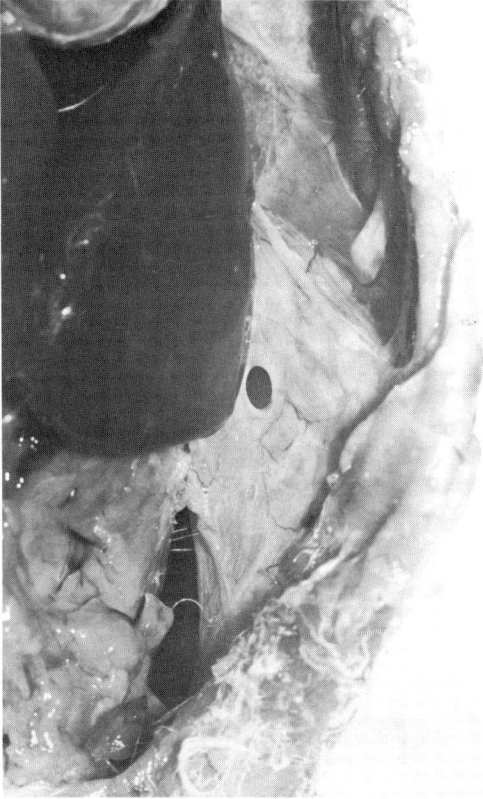

Photo 9b.   Air sacculitis: *post-mortem* examination showing a thickened air sac wall in which a hole has been made with scissors. In the top left-hand corner is the liver and the apex of the heart is just visible

some instances, even after apparently recovering from air sacculitis, a bird will show slight persistent dysnoea or tachypnoea and the soft tissues anterior to the eye may become distended as the bird breathes. The latter is a useful clinical feature that is quickly noted by falconers. I have observed it in sakers in the Middle East, some of them with a previous history of respiratory disease as well as in other falconiform species in Britain. Although the old falconers' terms "kecks", "croaks" and "pantas" probably cover a variety of respiratory conditions, I suspect that Bert's description of "a Hawke that bloweth, and is short or thicke-winded" referred to a chronic case of air sacculitis.

Aspergillosis has been recognised in birds of prey for many years. The earliest reference I have found to it was a communication to the Pathological Society of London (119). The subject was a captive peregrine falcon and the description of the lesions is sufficiently accurate and similar to those seen today to be worth repeating:

> "The pericardium was studded with small round elevated tubercles; and the spleen and liver were also tuberculated. The peritoneum, in some places, was covered with

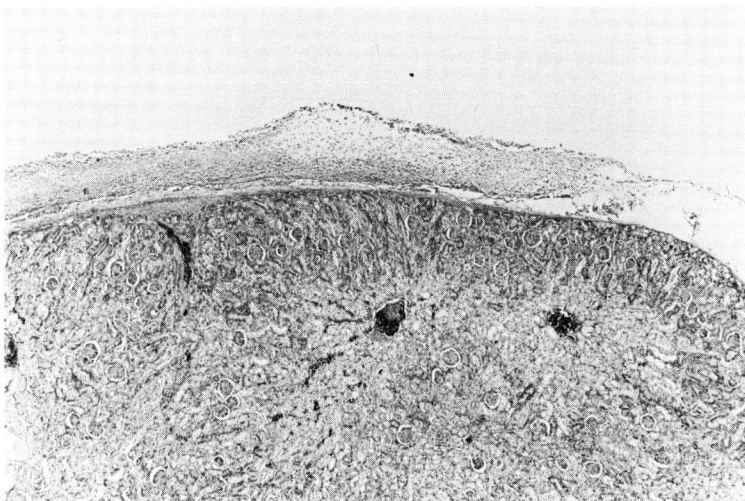

Photo 9c.   Air sacculitis: low power photomicrograph of kidney showing grossly inflamed air sac wall adherent to its capsule

patches of thick lymph of old standing, which had a mouldy appearance; and on microscopical examination the sporules of mould were very apparent".

Aspergillosis is generally believed to be the commonest cause of death in captive raptors in Britain (84, 249) and Dr Patrick Redig confirms that this is the case, in his experience, in the United States. The disease appears to be less common in owls than diurnal birds of prey, although this is not necessarily the case; for example, in 1935, Hamerton described two cases in eagle owls at the London Zoo (192).

Medical authors have described *Aspergillus fumigatus* as "opportunistic" and the same situation appears to apply in avian work, since aspergillosis is usually a sequel to some other factor, especially low condition or intercurrent disease. It is also a common cause of death in recently imported birds; in a letter to Mr J. G. Mavrogordato in 1940, now in my possession, the Pathologist at the London Zoo, Colonel A. E. Hamerton drew attention to this when he wrote "it is a comparatively rare disease among hawks at the Zoo and only occurs amongst new arrivals that have been kept in unsuitable conditions . . .". There is also increasing evidence that long-standing deficiencies, especially of vitamins A and B1, are involved in predisposition to aspergillosis (162). As with domesticated birds (184) it seems probable that a spore-laden environment will enhance the chances of the disease developing and for this reason falconers and aviculturists are well advised to avoid musty hay lofts and other poorly ventilated buildings for their birds. The use of bacteriological settle plates will help to monitor the air-borne contamination of an enclosure, as outlined earlier. There is no evidence that aspergillosis can be transmitted from one bird to another; more than one affected bird on the same premises is probably indicative of an infected environment. Work on passerine birds has shown that the majority of nests harbour *A. fumigatus* and, often, other fungi (12) and this should be borne in mind when cleaning and disinfecting breeding quarters at the end of the season.

The onset of aspergillosis is often insidious, with loss of weight and lethargy common early signs. Dyspnoea is often only observed when the lungs are involved or the bird is subjected to exercise; *post-mortem* cases with extensive fungal lesions in all air sacs have been seen when no respiratory signs were evident in life. Some birds may appear relatively unaffected when at rest, on a perch, but can develop severe dyspnoea and cyanosis when cast on their back for examination. Many cases are chronic, with extensive fungal lesions – one goshawk examined *post mortem* had an aspergilloma forming a complete cast of the left abdominal air sac. Others appear more acute, with active lesions in the lungs as well as air sacs. Occasionally *post-mortem* examination of a raptor reveals small granuloma-like lesions on the air sacs which, when examined histologically, are found to contain fungal hyphae but death is due to some other cause such as trauma. Such instances suggest that *Aspergillus* lesions may not prove fatal but become "walled-off" – possibly to initiate an infection later?

Diagnosis of aspergillosis is not easy. A serological test has been used in humans (279) and in domestic mammals (111, 112, 268) and has recently been applied with some degree of success to birds of prey (351). The test is qualitative rather than quantitative; a positive result is assumed to indicate an active case. Intradermal tests have been investigated in penguins and other birds (16) but I have been unable to trace similar work in birds of prey.

Radiography may be of value in diagnosis, for example as described by Ward and colleagues (410) but in my experience only when lesions are fairly extensive. Both lateral and ventro-dorsal views should be taken. Usually distinct nodular lesions are seen and there may be a reduction in size of the air sacs. Opacity of the air sac fields is more likely to be indicative of air sacculitis or large numbers of *Serratospiculum* worms. Microbiology is of only limited value in diagnosis. Tracheal swabs and air sac aspirates may yield *Aspergillus fumigatus* on culture, but the fungus can also often be isolated from unaffected birds. Redig reported the use of "air sac lavage" to diagnose the disease in experimentally infected turkeys (*Meleagris gallopavo*) and suggested it might be used in raptors (351).

Usually aspergillosis is diagnosed *post mortem*. Affected birds are thin and there are nodular yellow lesions in the air sacs and other internal organs. Distinct fungal growth is often visible in lung lesions. On histological examination septate fungal hyphae are seen in the affected tissues (Photo 10); the stains of choice are P.A.S. or Grocott.

Treatment also poses problems. In few "successful" cases has the disease been definitely diagnosed. Fuller and colleagues (164) used amphotericin B by both the intravenous and aerosol routes and this was also recommended, without any apparent personal success, by Ward and colleagues (410). I have had reports of good results with pimaricin while Beebe and Webster (24) recorded one apparent recovery after nystatin therapy. Success with amphotericin B inhalation therapy, coupled with hygiene, has been claimed in work with cormorants (*Phalacrocorax*

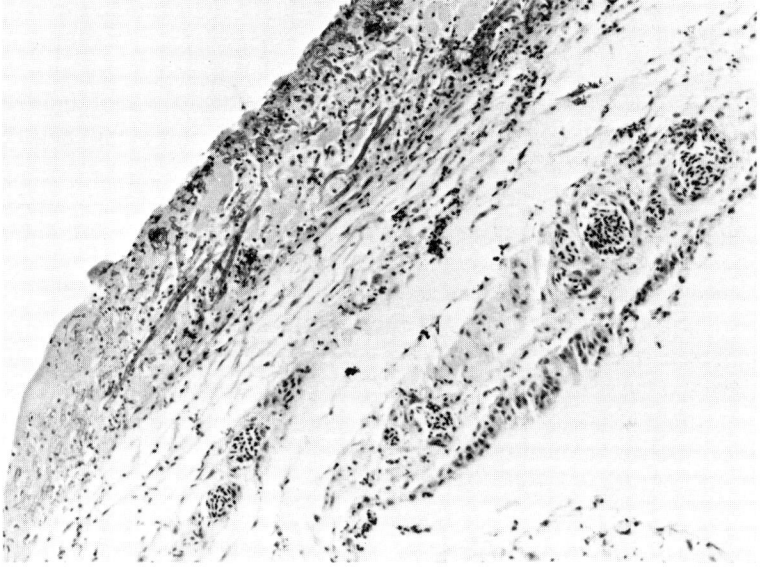

Photo 10.   Low power photomicrograph of air sac wall of an African fish eagle showing inflammatory reaction and *Aspergillus* hyphae

auritus) but there was no control group of birds (33). In humans emetine hydrochloride by intramuscular injection has proved successful in small numbers of human patients (234) and might usefully be tried in birds of prey.

My own attempts at therapy have included aerosols and injections into the air sacs of amphotericin B, nystatin, fentichlor and pimaricin, all apparently unsuccessfully, but these failures may have been attributable to the progressed state of the lesions at the time of treatment. Intratracheal administration of amphotericin B and chloramphenicol produced a marked clinical response in a golden eagle but the bird later died and it was not possible to evaluate the treatment fully on account of marked autolysis. Similar administration of the antifungal drug pimaricin was carried out (on one occasion only) in an African fish eagle. There was no obvious improvement but in this case the bird had a concurrent tuberculosis infection (242). An important point is to avoid corticosteroids in cases where aspergillosis is suspected since there is evidence from both mammalian and avian work that immunosuppression can result in active infection (396).

Although *A. fumigatus* is the usual isolate in cases of mycotic air sacculitis and pneumonia, occasionally other *Aspergillus* spp. may be involved. *Aspergillus niger* has been associated with pneumonia and oxalosis in a great horned owl (420). A *Mucor* sp. was isolated from a case of air sacculitis in a kestrel by Kaleta and Drüner (241). *Geotrichum candidum* was recently identified by the Commonwealth Mycological Institute from a buzzard in which the gross and histopathological lesions were identical to those in *A. fumigatus* infection.

Prevention of aspergillosis is based upon ensuring that birds are in good condition and not exposed to excess numbers of spores. An aerosol of nystatin has been recommended as a prophylactic measure in cagebirds (56) and Ward and colleagues (410) suggested similar adminstration of amphotericin B to prevent the disease in "susceptible species of raptors". I personally am not in favour of the prophylactic use of antifungal drugs. Vaccination would be of inestimable value and is a field in which research might prove fruitful. In 1972 encouraging work was reported in London on vaccination of mice (91) but no subsequent studies appear to have been done.

Gastro-intestinal conditions

In this section a number of conditions of the gastro-intestinal tract will be discussed, including some that are not due to infectious agents. Nevertheless, they are included here since they must be considered in differential diagnosis.

Many different bacteria may be isolated from the alimentary tract of apparently healthy raptors. In the case of the lower intestine, or a "clean" faecal sample, the usual isolates are *E. coli* and *Proteus* spp. Many other organisms can be cultured from the pharynx including *S. aureus, Bacillus* spp. and *Corynebacterium* spp. The role of these is unknown but it is not unreasonable to assume that they might adopt a pathogenic role under certain circumstances. Stomatitis is discussed in the next chapter, under trichomoniasis, but it should be noted that this condition can also be due to bacteria.

Enteritis is common in birds of prey. I have diagnosed it at *post-mortem* examination on many occasions, in some cases associated with gastritis, and often the aetiology is obscure. Affected birds show discoloured (dark) mutes which are often foetid; in addition there may be regurgitation of food. Occasionally fresh blood is seen in the mutes and while this is probably a manifestation of intestinal damage it should be noted that haemorrhagic enteritis has been described as a sign of "shock" in birds (144). Often in enteritis the mutes are voided with less force than is usual though it should be noted that this can also be a feature of other debilitating diseases.

Laboratory examination of mutes and regurgitated material from cases of enteritis/gastritis may suggest that a parasite is involved, for example *Capillaria* worms. Alternatively, in severe cases of enteritis, ascarid worms may be "flushed out" by the passage of ingesta and mislead the owner or veterinary surgeon into thinking that they are the cause. Often, however, the only significant laboratory finding is a profuse pure growth of *E. coli*. It is my belief that these bacteria can be the cause of enteritis/gastritis and both clinical and *post-mortem* observations support this. For example, an African goshawk developed enteritis shortly after being moved to a new (colder) locality and only oxytetracycline sensitive *E. coli* could be isolated from faeces; it recovered rapidly after oxytetracycline therapy. A peregrine examined *post mortem* showed enteritis together with hyperaemia and oedema of the proventriculus and gizzard; a profuse growth of *E. coli* was isolated in pure culture from the affected areas and no parasites were found. These and many other cases help substantiate the role of *E. coli* in specific gastrointestinal conditions. Clinical diagnosis of *E. coli* infection must be based upon the isolation of *E. coli* (usually β-haemolytic) in pure culture from mutes and upper alimentary tract and clinical signs of alimentary disease. Treatment consists of antibiotic therapy and nursing, including fluid replacement and small meals at frequent intervals.

E. coli can also be involved in other infections. Brisbin and Wagner (55) described an outbreak of "coli bacillosis" in a captive collection of American kestrels which was treated successfully with oral furazolidone.

A secretary bird I examined in Kenya died of acute pancreatitis from which only *E. coli* could be isolated and I have obtained the same isolate from cases of pneumonia, pericarditis and nephritis. Hamerton (194) isolated *E. coli* from a case of purulent pericarditis and Fiennes (144) from a hepatic abscess, both in falconiform birds. The role of the organism in septicaemia is discussed later.

Falconers sometimes speak of their hawk having a "chill". The condition is not a clearcut clinical entity but commonly follows a stress factor, such as a drop in temperature or heavy rain. The affected bird flies poorly, often shows a reduced appetite and may be hunched or "fluffed-up" in appearance. Occasionally it regurgitates or may pass loose faeces. There is usually spontaneous recovery within 48 hours – my advice is to bring the bird indoors and keep it warm. My own view is that such "chills" are possibly due to a low grade *E. coli* infection or perhaps an upset of the normal bacterial flora. *E. coli* has been isolated from the faeces of some such cases – which is not unusual – and also, in profusion, from pharyngeal swabs.

E. coli can pose problems when it is isolated from organs at *post-mortem* examination. It is a normal part of the gut flora and if examination of a carcass is delayed the organisms can be detected in the liver, kidneys and lungs. Isolation in pure culture from the heart blood is, in my view, more significant although caution must still be taken in incriminating the organism as the cause of death. Interpretation of the role of *E. coli* depends upon a number of factors, particularly the clinical history, gross *post-mortem* findings, and degree of autolysis of the carcass. One must also take into consideration whether the organism was isolated in pure culture and how profuse or scanty was the growth. In some cases histopathological examination will help support or refute a diagnosis of *E. coli* infection.

"Inflammation of the crop" has been recognised in falconers' birds for many centuries. It is characterised by regurgitation of food a short time after swallowing. Most of the 19th and 20th century authors discussed it in some detail but Mavrogordato, in the first edition of "A Hawk for the Bush" (295), reported having never seen the condition. In my view "inflammation of the crop" may be due to bacterial or parasitic oesophagitis, gastritis or certain other non-alimentary disorders, particularly air sacculitis.

A number of cases recover without specific treatment; others appear to respond to oral tetracyclines plus careful feeding with fluids or, as Woodford (422) suggested, protein hydrolysate. Greenwood (177) discussed crop infections in young birds and described clinical signs of immediate regurgitation and flicking of food. He recommended treatment by infusion of antibiotic into the crop. The response to antibiotics in such cases would suggest a bacterial aetiology. I have often observed discrete, raised lesions of the crop in birds at *post-mortem* examination which appear to be small abscesses and presumably bacterial in origin. Some or these show cocci or bacilli in sections. The only bacteria that I have isolated from swabs of regurgitated food from affected birds are *E. coli* and other member members of the Enterobacteriaceae and it is again probable that these may be involved. On one falconer's premises cases of regurgitation occurred on a number of occasions in trained hawks. Some cases showed clinical signs of air sacculitis and appeared to respond to tylosin. When throat swabs were taken after an outbreak a number of bacteria were isolated, amongst them *S. aureus* and a *Corynebacterium* sp. The significance of these organisms is uncertain but it is possible that they played a part in the syndrome.

Oesophageal capillariasis is discussed in Chapter 6; it is probably one important cause of "inflammation of the crop".

Regurgitation of food is also a common clinical sign in birds suffering from other diseases, especially air sacculitis, and, in some cases, aspergillosis. Such birds may show crop lesions at *post-mortem* examination but these are usually only areas of hyperaemia or inflammation which are secondary to the repeated regurgitation of food. In my view the primary cause of the regurgitation is inflammation of the air sacs (particularly the interclavicular?) and serosal surfaces.

Regurgitation in birds of prey need not be pathological. Most normally regurgitate indigestible material (such as bone and fur) as a "casting" or "pellet" and the observant owner will get some guide as to the health of his bird by examining this pellet. In a healthy hawk, it is well-formed and once voided, dries quickly; in a sick bird it is misshapen, wet and may contain undigested food. Persistently misshapen pellets occur in some hawks and are sometimes associated with difficulty in casting; a lesion of the stomach or crop may be responsible. In other birds the production of pellets is intermittent – a bird will, for example, cast every 2–3 days instead of at its usual 24 hourly intervals. Although delay in casting can be a sign of disease some such birds appear quite healthy and the pellets they produce are normal. The reason for this is unknown; much work is needed on the "meal to pellet interval" (MPI) as emphasised by Duke and colleagues (134).

Occasionally a bird may vomit due to "motion sickness". This was described by de Bastyai (126) and I have known other cases, including a kestrel which, when transported hooded in a car, would vomit unless allowed to face the front of the vehicle! Other birds may regurgitate when cast, injected or given certain drugs.

There is little information on disease of the gall bladder in birds of prey although scattered reports exist – for example, cholecystitis in a Javan fish owl at the London Zoo (192). An enlarged gall bladder is commonly seen in birds which have died of inanition or been chilled.

Peritonitis and septicaemia

Birds of prey may develop peritonitis or septicaemia and often these follow trauma, such as fractures or shot wounds. *E. coli* is commonly the cause but I have isolated other organisms from such cases including a *Pseudomonas* sp. and *Staphylococcus aureus*.

Birds with peritonitis usually die quickly, with few clinical signs other than anorexia and depression. Occasionally the bird shows diarrhoea and regurgitation for 24 hours before death. Treatment with antibiotics does not, in my experience, appear to be of any value.

Diagnosis of a septicaemia is also not always easy. Clinically affected birds show severe lethargy and pyrexia may be detectable. Bacteria can be cultured from the blood or, at *post-mortem* examination, from the heart. The failure to isolate organisms from the heart blood of cases which show a typical septicaemia at autopsy is often attributable to the administration of antibiotics before death. Prompt use of an appropriate antibiotic may prove effective in treating a bird with a blood-borne infection and for this purpose the intravenous route is recommended.

Tuberculosis

Avian tuberculosis is frequently diagnosed in birds of prey (Photos 11a and b). It primarily involves the liver and intestinal tract although interesting atypical cases have included an African fish eagle with concurrent aspergillosis (242) and a (free-living) buzzard with a large cystic tuberculous lesion on its leg (81). In view of these cases, and those reported by others elsewhere (43, 60) an acid fast infection should always be borne in mind when dealing with an unusual case. Culture of the causal organisms may take a long time but a direct smear of the lesion, if stained with Ziehl-Neelsen stain, may help diagnosis.

More typical cases of tuberculosis in birds of prey show clinical signs of a chronic loss of weight over several weeks. The appetite usually remains good but water may be drunk to excess. There are few other clinical signs although some birds show a tendency to close their eyes as if sleeping. Occasional cases show intermittent diarrhoea.

Clinical diagnosis of tuberculosis is not easy. A tuberculin test was recommended by Stehle (385) in Germany but has never proved successful in my hands, even in proved cases of tuberculosis. The staining of a faecal smear with Ziehl-Neelsen stain has been useful in some cases, though care must be taken not to mistake small numbers of saprophytic acid-fast organisms for pathogens. However, some positive cases do not appear to pass bacteria in the faeces. Additional aids to diagnosis are radiography and laparotomy and these are likely to prove of increasing value in the future. A number of my tuberculosis cases have shown an enlarged liver and narrow air sacs on radiography. I have examined one suspect case by laparotomy, under general anaesthesia – using this technique the enlarged liver, studded with tubercles, was readily visible. Haematology can also

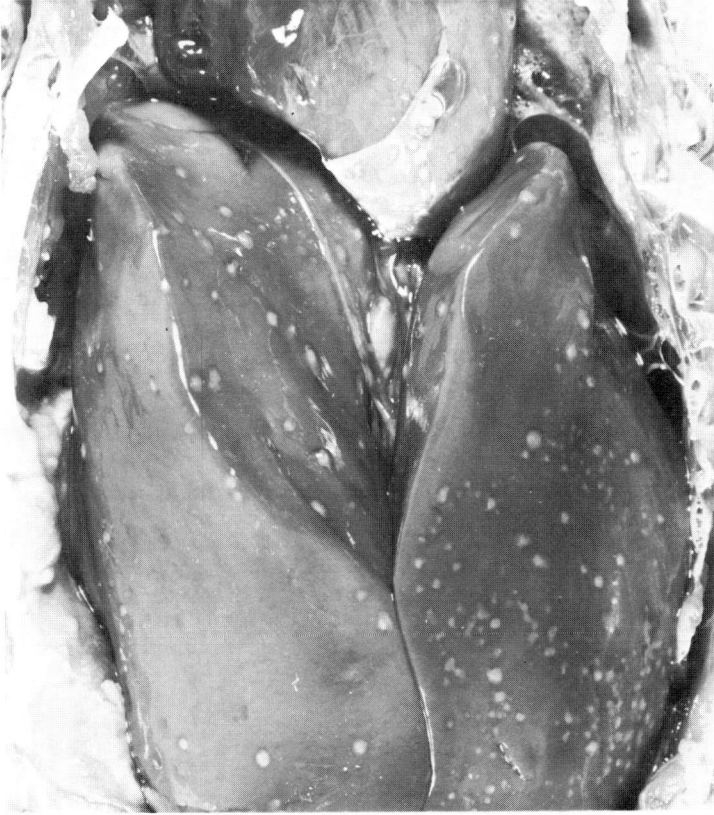

Photo 11a.   Freshly opened carcass of a goshawk to show liver lesions due to avian tuberculosis

aid diagnosis; many of my cases have shown low PCV and haemoglobin levels.

In my view raptors with tuberculosis should not be treated but destroyed. Others, however, have recommended chemotherapy; for example, Greenwood (177) advocated the use of rifampicin and reported two instances where treatment appeared to be successful. A definitive diagnosis of tuberculosis could not, however, be made in the birds involved.

Prevention of tuberculosis is not easy though care should be taken to check any birds for internal lesions of the disease before offering them as food. In the case of wood pigeons (*Columba palumbus*) the tendency for infected birds to have a darker plumage may be a useful clue (283). Vaccination would be of great benefit and was discussed in an earlier paper (99) but is unfortunately not yet feasible in raptors. Host resistance is probably an important feature; Kenward (247) reported that a goshawk ate at least one pigeon in which tuberculosis was diagnosed without contracting the disease.

In view of the resistant nature of the Mycobacteria all steps should be taken to prevent their being introduced to a collection. Free-living birds are probably the

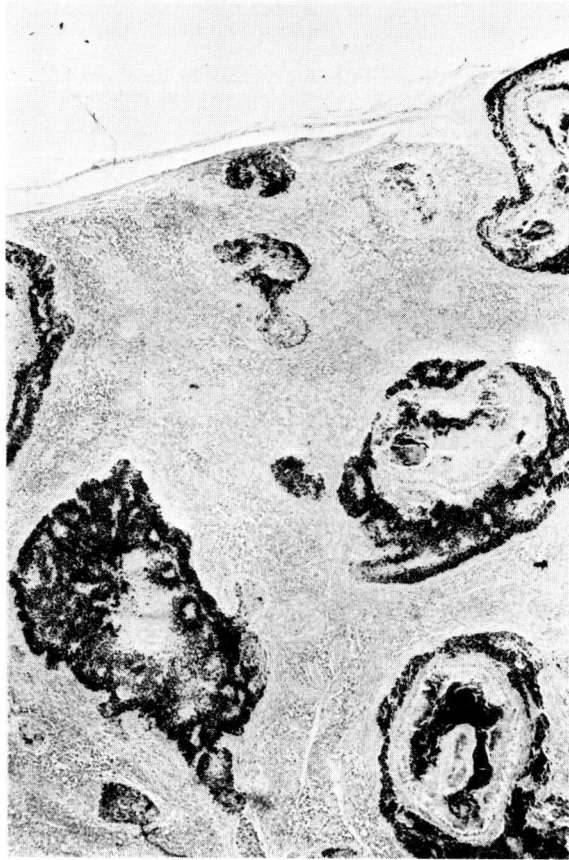

Photo 11b.   Low power photomicrograph of portion of spleen of a saker stained with Ziehl-Neelsen and showing foci of (dark) acid-fast organisms

main hazard but other species may harbour the organism including the hedgehog, *Erinaceus europaeus* (294). Once a case has been diagnosed thorough disinfection with phenol or formalin is recommended. The possibility of human infection must also be borne in mind; Marks and Birn (289) reported ten such cases in Britain and others have been recorded subsequently from a number of countries.

Other bacterial infections

Keymer (249) listed anthrax, erysipelas, listeriosis, pasteurellosis and salmonellosis as bacterial diseases that could be contracted from infected food.

I have diagnosed pasteurellosis in a free-living tawny owl and also isolated a *Pasteurella* sp. from cases of pneumonia in a number of species. Probably the infection is not uncommon and possibly it can be contracted by means other than ingestion of infected food. Subacute pasteurellosis was reported in a captive goshawk by Woodford and Glasier (423) and in a peregrine by Bougerol (51). My friend Paul Jacklin had a jack (male) merlin which died of acute pasteurellosis in 1955, the *post-mortem* examination being carried out by Mr. W. E. Parish.

Anthrax is relatively rare in captive birds although there are a few reports; for example, Hamerton (196) reported two fatal cases in eagles fed infected meat at the London Zoo. The disease must, therefore, be taken seriously and care taken to ensure that infected food is not given to captive birds. Any mammal that dies unexpectedly should be checked for anthrax. The situation in the wild is of interest since raptors, especially vultures, seem rarely affected clinically but possibly play a significant role in the dissemination of the organism. Studies on this aspect have usually involved the use of captive experimental birds (45, 398); Dr. David Houston and I used a white-backed vulture in our work in Kenya (219).

I have been unable to trace any records of erysipelas infection in captive falconiform birds although there are a few reports of it in free-living or casualty individuals (249, 351). However, there are at least three records of the disease in captive owls and therefore this infection, which like the others being discussed under this heading is a zoonosis, must be considered in diagnosis. The series of cases described by Blackmore and Gallagher (42) included a little owl and this bird, in common with most of the others affected, showed no specific signs of disease. This point emphasises that many of the generalised bacterial infections do not produce typical clinical signs and a definitive diagnosis in such cases must usually be based on pathology and microbiology.

Listeriosis does not appear to be an important condition in either captive or free-living birds of prey; however, in view of the difficulty in culturing the organism, cases may have been missed. Keymer (249) could locate only one record of a case in a captive bird.

There are relatively few records of salmonellosis in captive birds of prey despite the numbers of suspect wild birds and mammals that must be fed to them. Keymer (249) listed the publications describing either clinical salmonellosis or the carriage of *Salmonella* spp. I have encountered no cases of salmonellosis in raptors, nor have I ever cultured a *Salmonella* sp. from their faeces despite routine microbiological examination of large numbers of birds in both Britain and East Africa. An *Arizona* sp. (Serotype Pc 196/Minn 98) was cultured from the intestine of one of my cases, an African goshawk; this was an interesting finding in view of the known pathogenicity of this genus to domestic turkeys but it was not considered responsible for the goshawk's death.

Although pseudotuberculosis, caused by *Yersinia pseudotuberculosis,* is a relatively common and important disease in cage and aviary birds (143) it does not appear to be so prevalent in birds of prey. I have never encountered a case. It is possible that some cases have been misdiagnosed since "typical" caseous lesions on the gut, liver and spleen are often a feature of tuberculosis and aspergillosis. In the letter to Mr. J. G. Mavrogordato to which I referred earlier, Colonel A. E. Hamerton drew attention to this confusion when he wrote "I think by pseudotuberculosis you probably mean *Mycosis* – a disease of the air sacs which produces lesions resembling those of tuberculosis".

Clostridial enterotoxaemia, caused by toxins of *Clostridium* spp., has been reported on a few occasions in individual birds of prey. For example, Köhler and Baumgart (264) recorded fatal cases in three captive hawks due to the feeding of meat contaminated with *Clostridium perfringens* Type A. Affected birds may be incoordinated and show diarrhoea and haemorrhages. Routine pathology and toxicology often fail to detect any case of death in such cases and diagnosis must be based on clinical history unless facilities permit the toxins to be demonstrated. Specific antitoxins would almost certainly be effective in treatment but are usually not available; antibiotics and adsorbents should be tried.

While certain vultures appear resistant to the toxins of *Clostridium botulinum* Types A, B and C by both oral and injectable routes (243) this is not true of all birds of prey. Botulism has been reported from a variety of free-living birds (276) but is probably unlikely to present a significant threat to captive raptors. However, the feeding of infected maggots could possibly pose a hazard to small species kept for aviculture, as reported from the London Zoo (378).

Virus infections

Newcastle disease
Newcastle disease has been described in the past from a number of birds of prey; for example, Keymer and Dawson (254) recorded it in a free-living kestrel and in three young captive barn owls. Clinical signs were minimal. Serological surveys have also shown evidence of infection; for example, a positive titre in the serum of a red-tailed hawk in a survey by Kocan and colleagues (262) and in 28 out of 432 samples from birds of prey in Germany by Kaleta and Drüner (241). I have not consistently been in a position to carry out virological investigations on raptors. In a small number of cases in Kenya attempts to isolate Newcastle disease virus by egg inoculation were all unsuccessful. Nor did serological (haemagglutination inhibition) tests on a number of birds give any positive results. More recently I have submitted material from several birds to Dr. H. P. Chu at Cambridge but again with negative results.

Recent legislation in Britain (the Importation of Captive Birds Order 1976) prohibited the importation of birds into Britain unless under licence and this legislation was aimed at protecting poultry from exotic strains of Newcastle disease and other infections. Some falconers remain sceptical of the claim that birds of prey may pose a threat of Newcastle disease but there is increasing evidence that this is the case. In addition to Keymer and Dawson's paper mentioned earlier, there are other reports of the isolation of Newcastle disease virus from raptors. Pierson and Pfow (340) reported eight cases of the disease in "Shaheen hawks" (presumably shahins) and seven out of the eight died. There were no clinical signs suggestive of the disease but the virus could be isolated in the laboratory. Another paper, by Chu and colleagues (73) described studies in Britain. Newcastle disease virus was isolated from 11 out of 14 birds of prey that died in captivity between 1971–74. In each case the virus isolated was of the velogenic (highly fatal) type.

Some of the birds showed clinical signs of innappetance, head twisting and incoordination but in the majority the only common feature was death. Experimental inoculation of birds by Winteroll (419) resulted in clinical signs of convulsions and paralysis and significant histological lesions were described.

It would seem wise, therefore, to look upon Newcastle disease as a potential hazard to captive predatory birds. There is no specific therapy and the aim should be to prevent entry and establishment of infection. I have used inactivated (betapropiolactone) vaccine in several captive East African species with no ill effects and would suggest its use in the face of an outbreak, although, as discussed elsewhere (99) I have reservations about the protection it confers. Attenuated vaccines may be preferable; Chu and others (73) reported the safe use of live Hitchner B1 vaccine and Winteroll (419) successfully protected falconiform and strigiform species with both LaSota and Galivac live vaccines. Winteroll's birds resisted experimental infection but the antibody titres obtained were low.

There are steps other than vaccination that can be taken to help prevent or exclude Newcastle disease. The use of poultry as food for birds of prey can be hazardous and, as a general rule, contact between raptors and other species of bird should be avoided. In the case of aviaries, free-living wild birds may prove a threat – not only of Newcastle disease but also of other avian pathogens. A recent report suggests that house mice (*Mus musculus*) may also, occasionally, be hosts of Newcastle disease (235).

Avian pox

Pox has been recorded in captive birds of prey on a number of occasions including cases in peregrines imported into Britain (86, 180) and a red-tailed hawk in America (188).

The disease produces classical clinical pock lesions, especially around the eyes and beak and on the feet (Photos 12a and b). The pocks are slightly raised plaques which are brownish in colour. Occasionally they may be seen on the mucous membranes. Affected birds usually retain their appetite and appear in good health although extensive scabbing may result in closure of the eyes and inability to feed. In addition, the lesions may be pruritic and secondary infection can follow scratching by the bird's feet or beak.

Diagnosis of pox infection can usually be made on the basis of the clinical signs. Confirmation can be by direct electron microscopy of scab material (86) or histological examination, using Lendrum's (phloxine-tartrazine) stain, of a skin biopsy when characteristic ballooning of epithelial cells and intra-cytoplasmic inclusion bodies are seen. Treatment is non-specific and may include the use of antibiotics to control bacterial infection and vitamin A to aid healing. Prevention of the disease depends upon the exclusion of the virus from collections; recently imported birds are a particular threat and the statutory quarantine period for incoming birds in Britain and other countries may help to reduce this risk. Hygiene will minimise the risk of the (relatively resistant) virus being spread mechanically and control of biting insects is also desirable. Prophylactic vaccination is likely to prove of benefit in the future; in the United Arab Emirates Dr Abdul Qayyum has

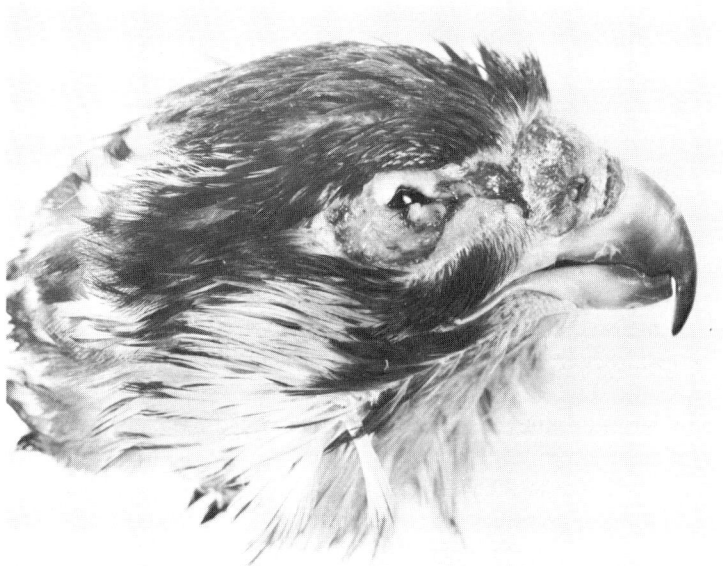

(a)

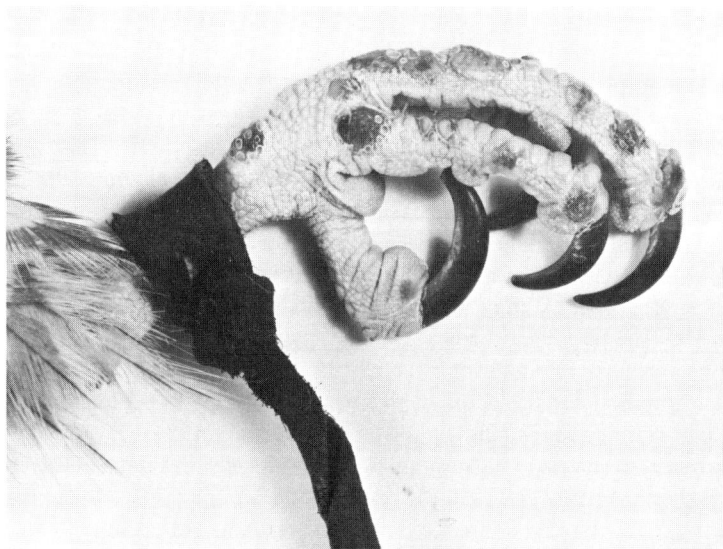

(b)

Photo 12a.   Pox infection in a peregrine showing scabs on the cere and eyelids.
b.   Foot of the same bird as above. There are conspicuous brown scabs on the feet

safely used an attenuated pigeon pox vaccine in hawks and this appears to be giving protection.

Other viral infections

A viral hepatitis (hepatosplenitis) has been described in owls in the United States (176) and Europe (62) and there is a very similar disease in falconiform birds in North America (174). The disease has not, however, been reported in any bird of prey in Britain. The causal agents are usually referred to as owl herpesvirus (OHV) and falcon herpesvirus (FHV) respectively. A useful review of the host spectrum of OHV was given in a paper by Burtscher and Sibalin (63); it is interesting to note that both the tawny owl and barn owl proved resistant to a massive experimental infection.

The disease is usually peracute and often fatal. In subacute cases clinical signs are restricted to lethargy, anorexia and diarrhoea. At *post-mortem* examination the liver and spleen are swollen and owls may show pharyngeal and intestinal lesions. On histopathological examination there are characteristic lesions of necrosis in the liver and intra-nuclear inclusion bodies may be seen. A detailed description of lesions and diagnostic techniques was given by Peckham (333) in the book "Isolation and Identification of Avian Pathogens". The diagnosis can be confirmed by inoculation of fertile eggs, tissue culture or susceptible birds. Both OHV and FHV are pathogenic for owls, ring-necked doves (*Streptopelia* sp.) and kestrels (European and American) and, additionally, FHV for other species of falcon. An alternative approach to diagnosis is direct electron microscopy of tissues (261, 375). With the help of colleagues I used an electron microscope to investigate deaths in owls at the London Zoo in 1976; we could detect no virus particles, and as will be mentioned later in the book, the owls were subsequently found to be poisoned.

There is no specific treatment for viral hepatitis; affected birds should be isolated or, possibly, killed to reduce the risk of spread. Vaccination against viral hepatitis could be of great value and as I discussed in an earlier paper (99) might be feasible in due course.

Hepatitis is a potential hazard to captive birds of prey in Britain and it is to be hoped that recent restrictions on importation of birds will prevent its entry. However, Greenwood (179) suggested that selective import controls on prairie falcons and European eagle owls might be desirable until more is known about the ability of recovered birds to carry the virus.

I have not encountered cases of Marek's disease or leucosis in raptors but Woodford and Glasier (423) recorded the former in three sparrowhawks while Halliwell (187) described lesions indicative of the disease in a great horned owl and Jennings (233) in a little owl. Another report has recently appeared of lesions indistinguishable from Marek's disease in a free-living tawny owl (18) but as the author pointed out, in none of the reports listed has virus been isolated. In a virological and serological survey of zoo birds in the United States (72) ten raptors were examined but all were negative for Marek's disease as were the other non-galliform species. Some positive birds were identified in a survey of 432 sera in Germany by Kaleta and Drüner (241) but these were described as "isolated cases". Marek's should probably, under present circumstances, be looked upon as a disease of little practical relevance to captive raptors but this is not to suggest that the situation may not change with more intensive systems of management. Under such circumstances vaccination could prove useful.

A disease of goshawks which clinically resembles Marek's is described in Chapter 8; it is probably unrelated. Other neoplasms are discussed in Chapter 11.

Rabies antibodies were detected in 15 out of 65 (23·1%) predatory birds in a survey in the United States (172) and the authors of that paper reviewed the literature on avian rabies. They listed examples of experimentally induced rabies in owls, hawks and falcons but stressed that natural transmission was rare except when a bird was exposed to a rabid mammal. The same authors (240) later reported the development of antibody titres in a great horned owl fed a rabid skunk (*Spilogale putorius*). The owl suppressed the infection until corticosteroids were administered when a maximum antibody titre was attained; there were no definite clinical signs other than possible slight irritability and reluctance of the bird to sit on its perch. The authors concluded that carnivorous birds might conceivably initiate a rabies infection. This work is of little relevance to captive birds of prey but does suggest that, in countries where rabies is enzootic, care should be taken not to feed rabid carcasses to birds.

There seems little doubt that more viral infections and diseases of birds of prey are likely to be recognised in future. One has only to glance at the long list of viruses that can infect galliform birds to appreciate the advances made in our understanding of avian virology in the past 20 years. It seems reasonable to suppose that search for similar agents in falconiform and strigiform species is likely to prove fruitful. Work on free-living passerine birds has shown that many harbour arboviruses and similar investigations in birds of prey should be considered. Louping ill virus has been isolated from red grouse (*Lagopus scoticus*) in Scotland (355) and in view of the fact that falconers' birds are often flown at grouse, search for the virus would be of interest. Workers in Germany (241) have isolated chicken embryo lethal orphan virus (CELOV) and respiratory enteric orphan virus (REOV) from birds of prey but the role of these is unknown. It is particularly important that serological surveys for viruses are performed; in a recent study (262) a positive titre to type-A influenza was reported in a red-tailed hawk but no titres to either Eastern equine encephalitis or Western equine encephalitis. In Kaleta and Drüner's survey antibodies were detected to a number of viruses, amongst them Newcastle disease, CELOV and REOV. Similar studies are needed elsewhere.

Increasingly captive raptors are being maintained under "intensive" conditions and, as with poultry, it may be that such changes of management will result in an increase in significance of viral infections. Already birds die from time to time from what appears to be an infectious disease but no bacteria can be isolated. Although previous therapy with antibiotics may be responsible in some cases, it seems probable that viruses (or, perhaps, mycoplasmas or chlamydiae) might be involved. For example, in a previous paper (104) I reported unexplained deaths in fledgling (captive bred) kestrels which *post mortem* showed grossly enlarged spleens, strongly suggestive of a viral or chlamydial infection, but from which neither Newcastle disease or chlamydiae could be isolated. Constant surveillance is undoubtedly needed.

CHAPTER 6

Parasites

Parasites of many species are associated with captive birds of prey and some may cause disease.

In this chapter only the metazoan (many celled) and protozoan (single celled) parasites will be discussed; the microorganisms – all of which are, strictly speaking, parasites – are covered in Chapter 5.

The main groups of parasites of birds of prey are as follows:

Ectoparasites
Ticks and mites (Acarina)
Fleas (Siphonaptera)
Hippoboscids and other flies (Diptera: Pupipara and others)
Biting lice (Mallophaga)

Endoparasites
Roundworms (Nematoda)
Tapeworms (Cestoda)
Flukes (Trematoda)
Acanthocephala
Protozoa

These and certain other parasites will be discussed under the two main headings and emphasis will be laid on those of practical clinical importance. A list of those parasites found or identified by myself is given in Appendix VIII: this is not intended to be comprehensive but gives some indication of the species likely to be encountered during the course of routine clinical or *post-mortem* work. It is particularly hoped that it will encourage the reader to submit parasites for identification.

The majority of parasites of raptors are transmitted from bird to bird, in some cases via an intermediate host (or hosts). Close contact between birds is likely to favour a build-up of parasites, especially if it is coupled with poor hygiene. The role of food in the spread of parasites is discussed in Chapter 9.

Ectoparasites

Ticks are occasionally found on birds of prey in the tropics, especially on the cere and around the eyes; they are aesthetically undesirable and suck blood but are seldom important clinically except, possibly, as vectors or piroplasms (*Babesia* spp.). If left alone they will, after engorging themselves on blood, drop off but they are best removed with forceps, preferably after painting with alcohol, and making sure not to leave the mouthparts embedded in the tissue. Recently taken birds of

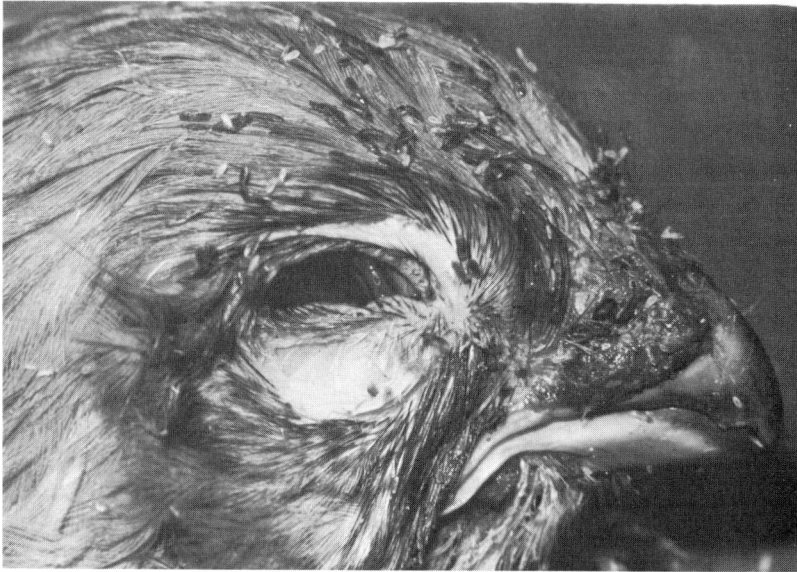

Photo 13.   Heavy louse infestation on the head of a kestrel

prey may have heavy tick burdens and larvae, nymphs or adult ticks may be involved. One such case, a newly imported lanner, was reported by Parsons (328). The bird had a massive infestation of larval ticks (*Argas* sp.), approximately 300 being counted. The areas of attachment (under the thighs) showed gross lesions of excoriation, haemorrhage and necrosis and these were confirmed histologically. It is of interest to note that the bird also had a heavy louse burden, damage to beak, cere and feet, and stomatitis (probably trichomoniasis). In the wild state certain ticks can be responsible for irritation or even disease in humans and this may be a possibility with recently captured raptors. An example of the former was recorded by Hoogstraal and colleagues (216) who described allergic reactions, pyrexia and skin lesions in personnel who ventured into a cormorant and osprey breeding area in Abu Dhabi. Both species of bird were infested with a species of tick and it was postulated that an arbovirus might be transmitted by its bite.

Mites cause trouble more frequently than ticks. The most important ones are probably the red mite (*Dermanyssus gallinae*) and Northern mite (*Ornithonyssus sylviarum*). The former lives in the building but attacks birds at night causing irritability, skin lesions and, possibly, anaemia. It may be difficult to detect unless the mews or aviary is examined with a torch at night; the parasites may then be seen. I have never found red mites on a bird of prey and have only incriminated them as the cause of disease on the basis of clinical signs and the presence of the parasites in the vicinity. *O. sylviarum* infestation is much easier to diagnose. It lives on the host and also sucks blood; as Salvin and Brodrick (361) stated in "Falconry in the British Isles":

". . . it is a species of *Acarus,* and makes its first appearance in the nares of the Hawk, burrowing in these parts, as also into the eyelids".

Trained hawks often become infected from affected prey, especially rooks (*Corvus frugilegus*).

Both these species of mite can be killed with insecticides but great care should be taken in view of the apparent high susceptibility of predatory birds to chlorinated hydrocarbons (51, 80). Following removal of the bird the accommodation can be dusted with 2% malathion or fumigated with formaldehyde and potassium permanganate and either of these techniques will help eliminate red mites.

In the case of *O. sylviarum,* a pythrethrum, derris or piperonyl butoxide product can be used to dust the bird but none of these is completely effective. Alternatively the bird can be sprayed with a 0·15% solution of trichlorphon which will kill the mites readily. This product was investigated in Kenya (97) and was found to be safe in 13 birds of ten species.

Despite careful examination of the skin and feather lesions, I have never found the mite *Cnemidocoptes* on a bird of prey but Dr. David Blackmore told me that he encountered a cnemidocoptic infection of the legs of a snowy owl, and Bougerol (51) recorded a *Cnemidocoptes* sp. on accipiters but gave no details. A number of feather mites may infest birds but care must be taken not to confuse them with those non-parasitic species which damage dropped feathers. Mumcuoglu and Müller (305) recorded the death of a free-living eagle owl from aspergillosis and a *Pseudomonas aeruginosa* infection and it is interesting to note that these authors suggested that feather mite damage predisposed to the dual infection.

Fleas are generally rare on captive birds of prey other than as temporary visitors derived from the prey or, occasionally, on nestlings. A possible exception is the stickfast flea *Echidnophaga gallinacea,* a tropical species, which attaches itself to the skin of the host. I found large numbers of this flea on the feet of a free-living (casualty) black-shouldered kite in Kenya, suggesting that it could be of significance in captivity. A number of species of flea are found in the nests of both falconiform and strigiform birds; examples of British species were listed by Smit (377). It is possible that fleas may assume increasing importance in establishments where captive breeding is carried out. Control of these parasites is not easy since the life cycle is completed off the host; nesting material and casting, which may harbour ova, larvae or pupae, should be removed and burned.

Hippoboscids are common on birds of prey but are rarely seen; they may crawl or fly off during anaesthesia or restraint. They appear to be harmless but suck blood, and, as Keymer (248) pointed out, they may possibly transmit *Haemoproteus* and other protozoal parasites. They can be removed manually (if one is quick!) or the bird can be treated with insecticides as outlined earlier for other parasites.

Other flies may also cause tissue damage or even death. Examples are *Lucilia* and *Calliphora* spp. Such flies lay their eggs in wounds and the larvae which hatch feed on dead (and in some cases living) tissues; this is termed myiasis. It has been reported in free-living raptors but is probably a particular problem in captive birds, especially when they have open wounds or large areas of damaged tissue. Flies tend to prove troublesome in hot weather; under such conditions wounds must be examined carefully – at least once a day – and the prophylactic use of a *safe* insecticidal product may be desirable.

Treatment of myiasis consists of the cleaning of the wounds, preferably by irrigation with warm water containing soap or a quaternary ammonium disinfectant. Necrotic tissue should be removed and a suitable insecticidal/antibiotic product applied. Some reports of myiasis in free-living birds have suggested that the larvae of certain species of fly feed for only a short time and then fall back into the nest (207) – but it is not clear whether this applies to raptors. Nevertheless, if myiasis should occur in young birds in breeding aviaries it would seem reasonable to check (and possibly burn) nesting material.

Mosquitoes of the Family Culicidae will feed on birds of prey and can probably transmit avian pox. Unexplained swellings on the head may be attributable to such bites. They usually resolve spontaneously. Attacks by a biting fly *Prosimulium* sp. have been reported as a common cause of death in young red-tailed hawks in rainy seasons in California (59) but I have been unable to trace any references to the role of this, or other species, in captive birds.

Bees (*Apis mellifera*) are not, strictly, parasites and could probably be covered under a number of other headings in this book. They are insects in the Order Hymenoptera. I know of at least two birds of prey that died following bee stings – one almost immediately, the other after several days. I have no records of wasp stings but in 1969 Mr. R. B. Comyn told me of a kestrel which died suddenly and unexpectedly and at *post-mortem* examination the only finding was a queen wasp (*Vespa* sp.) in the stomach.

Biting lice are common on captive birds of prey. They can cause damage to feathers and irritation. They often increase in numbers when raptors are sick, possibly because such birds do not preen properly (Photo 13). Lice also multiply, or become more apparent, in recently imported birds of prey. Treatment with insecticides must again be carried out with care; pyrethrum powder or flowers of sulphur are relatively safe and, if given on several occasions, effective. Trichlorphon (see earlier) has been shown to be effective against poultry lice and, in view of its apparent safety, is recommended. Some success has been achieved by manual removal of the larger species of lice (e.g. *Craspedorhynchus* spp.) and, in small birds, by use of a plastic bag containing cotton wool soaked in ether or chloroform; the bird is placed into the bag, with its head outside, for about five minutes. The lice are anaesthetised or killed and drop off into the bag.

Removal of "nits" (eggs) is best achieved manually by pulling, or cutting off, the affected feathers and if this is done regularly it can help reduce numbers of lice considerably.

Although traditionally biting lice have been associated with feeding on feather and skin debris and not blood, a recent report (370) described the transmission of a heartworm parasite of waterfowl by a biting louse which regularly fed on blood. It is possible, though unlikely, that a similar situation may apply in raptors.

Endoparasites

The endoparasites of particular importance in raptors are flukes (trematodes), roundworms (nematodes), tapeworms (cestodes) and protozoa. Some examples of the eggs and immature stages of certain of these parasites are shown in Figure 10. It should be noted that these figures are somewhat diagrammatic and are intended to aid identification.

Flukes are mainly found in the intestinal tract. In my opinion they are rarely pathogenic. However, Dedrick (127) reported a fatal disease characterised by low condition and diarrhoea associated with flukes in a captive prairie falcon, and Greenwood (177) described severe enteritis in infected birds imported from the Far East. Fluke eggs are commonly seen in faecal samples and their numbers fluc-

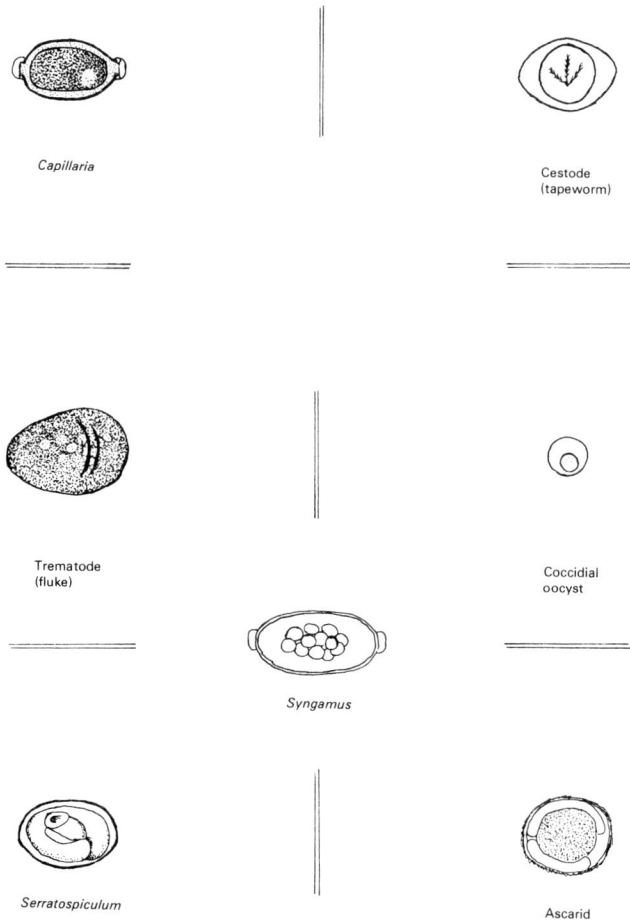

Fig. 10   Examples of eggs and immature stages of endoparasites

tuate from day to day. No treatment is usually required; when it is necessary rafoxanide can be tried (177). Fortunately there is little chance of tropical flukes completing their life cycle in this country, since suitable intermediate hosts are unlikely to be present, but the same cannot be said for temperate species and care should be taken under aviary conditions.

Tapeworms are of less clinical importance than roundworms. They are usually diagnosed when proglottides or eggs are seen in the faeces; large numbers appear to be correlated with poor condition. Treatment with appropriate drugs usually results in the parasites' being regurgitated or voided in the faeces. Care should be taken, however, as some birds react adversely to the medication and may vomit. At the time of writing I am investigating the use of mebendazole in birds of prey; it is hoped that this drug, which kills both cestodes and nematodes, will ultimately prove both safe and effective in raptors. Its successful use against *Syngamus trachea* in turkeys has already been reported (392).

Roundworm infestation in hawks may or may not cause clinical signs, depending largely upon the species and number of parasite, their locality and the health of the host. Intestinal ascarids, for instance, cause little trouble in small numbers in a healthy host but are probably pathogenic in large numbers. Two genera of ascarids, *Ascaridia* and *Porrocaecum* spp., are not uncommon in birds (both captive and free-living) which have died of inanition; in such cases the worms may block the lumen of the intestine and tens of thousands of eggs per gramme are present in the faeces. *Capillaria* worms are, similarly, often harmless, even in quite large numbers, but may on occasion cause clinical capillariasis. The affected bird is anorectic and has blood-tinged or, more commonly, dark chocolate-brown faeces; death follows rapidly unless fluid therapy is instituted. At *post-mortem* examination *Capillaria* worms are often difficult to find unless the material is very fresh but they and large numbers of eggs are usually visible in smears or histological sections of the gut. The carcass is usually anaemic and dehydrated and there are often tags of fresh blood in the intestinal tract. Occasionally I have encountered rather more chronic cases, characterised by illness of several weeks duration with diarrhoea, anorexia and weight loss the main clinical signs. The carcass is again anaemic and *Capillaria* worms are found in the intestinal tract.

Recently imported birds often exhibit high *Capillaria* egg counts (up to 30,000 eggs per gramme) which drop following acclimatisation and I discussed this syndrome in some detail in the second edition of "A Hawk for the Bush" (94). I do not advocate treatment initially; rather the bird should be allowed first to improve in condition.

Capillaria contorta infestations of the upper alimentary tract can cause disease of varying severity (85, 394), and this I believe to be one cause of the condition described by earlier falconers as "inflammation of the crop" (see Chapter 5) as well as sometimes being a differential diagnosis for trichomoniasis. Affected birds show white necrotic exudate or a diphtheritic membrane in the buccal cavity and, in some cases, pharynx, oesophagus and crop. A scraping of this material will, if examined under the microscope, show characteristic *Capillaria* eggs. In birds which die there is usually a severely inflamed upper alimentary tract on the surface of which adult worms can be demonstrated. On histological examination worms are seen in the mucosa and there is usually associated oedema and varying degrees of inflammatory reaction. Clinical oesophageal capillariasis does not appear to be as common in the Strigiformes as the Falconiformes though *C. contorta* worms are often seen in the buccal cavity of owls and can usually be removed with forceps. The worms and eggs may also occasionally be detected in sections of the buccal cavity or pharynx of apparently healthy birds of prey of both orders during histological examination.

Methyridine, levamisole or tetramisole can be used to treat *Capillaria* worms but it may be necessary to repeat the drug, at least once, after 7–10 days.

Two groups of nematode are relatively common in the respiratory tract of hawks; *Syngamus trachea* in the trachea and *Serratospiculum* spp. in the air sacs (Photo 14). A *Cyathastoma* sp. was found in the air sacs of one goshawk I examined and Bougerol (51) recorded six adult *Ascaridia* in the lung of a peregrine.

Syngamus can cause mild gurgling sounds or severe dyspnoea but I have not personally seen the latter. Usually there are only one or two worms present and

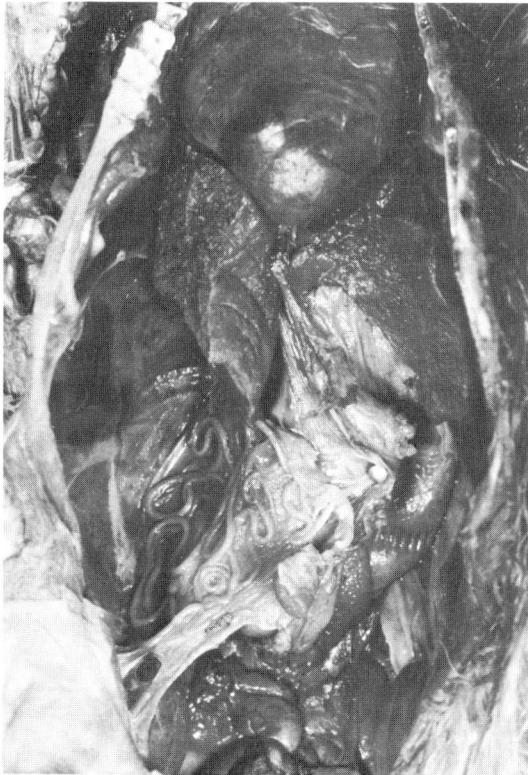

Photo 14.   Freshly opened carcass of lanner showing a *Serratospiculum* worm coiled in abdominal air sac

these can be seen in the trachea when a bird is examined clinically or *post mortem*.

Serratospiculum is commonly encountered in large numbers in the air sacs of falcons. The earliest reference to it that I have been able to trace is a communication to the Pathological Society of London by a Dr. Crisp, in 1854 (119). He described several "filaria" which were "embedded in the cellular tissue at the root of the great vessels; one of these worms was six inches in length".

Although there is usually considerable inflammatory reaction, including squamous metaplasia, around *Serratospiculum* worms I do not usually consider them pathogenic. Certainly I have never personally encountered clinical or *post-mortem* cases where I felt that the worms played any part in the disease and Greenwood (179) expressed a similar view. Some colleagues are doubtful of this claim, however, and pathogenicity has been attributed to *S. amaculata* in prairie falcons in North America (35, 409, 260). In the cases described by Bigland and colleagues (35), embryonated ova were found in the lymphatics of the lung and hepatic veins of the liver and living larvae in a chronic lesion involving the proventriculus. Ward and Fairchild (409) described disease in a peregrine and a prairie falcon which, on rather flimsy evidence, they diagnosed as serratospiculiasis. The affected birds showed clinical signs of regurgitation and there were plaque-like lesions in the mouth in which typical *Serratospiculum* eggs could be seen. Use of thiabendazole appeared to produce clinical improvement. Kocan and Gordon (260) hinted that air sacculitis (see Chapter 5) might be associated with the presence of these worms but this cannot be the cause in all instances since air sacculitis has been diagnosed in birds which were shown, at *post-mortem* examination, to harbour no air sac parasites. *Serratospiculum* worms and eggs are not uncommonly seen in association with lesions of aspergillosis (for example in Dr. Crisp's case) and it is tempting to link the two but I personally think that predisposition to *Aspergillus* infection by worm infestation is the exception rather than the rule.

The eggs of both *Syngamus* and *Serratospiculum* may be seen in the faeces and are characteristic in appearance; those of *Serratospiculum* are embryonated. It appears that *Serratospiculum* is essentially a parasite of the tropics and sub-tropics although it is worthy of note that Jefferies and Prestt (230) observed it in peregrines found dead in Britain; they did not ascertain whether the peregrines were native or escaped birds.

Syngamus may be treated successfully with thiabendazole. As was mentioned earlier, mebendazole has proved effective in turkeys when administered in the food for three days (curative) or 14 days (prophylactic) (392). If a *Syngamus* worm is situated near the glottis it can sometimes be removed with forceps. I do not treat *Serratospiculum* since I fear that dead parasites may do more damage in the air sacs than live ones, but Scott (368) reported an apparently good clinical response to oral tetramisole and Ward and Fairchild's cases appeared to improve following the use of thiabendazole.

In many collections birds are treated regularly for intestinal parasites. Some falconers worm their hawks at the end of the moult – that is, once a year – and this is a useful routine. My own view is that if administration of an anthelmintic can be carried out without too much difficulty this should be done every three months. I do not advocate the regular use of other anti-parasitic drugs unless there is evidence of infection. Piperazine and thiabendazole can be used but neither drug is particularly effective against *Capillaria* spp.; methyridine, levamisole or tetramisole is more suitable in such cases. Predatory birds will usually take oral anthelmintics if they are crushed in a piece of meat, or, in the case of large hawks, placed inside a dead mouse which can be swallowed whole. A parasitological examination a few days later should help ascertain whether treatment has been successful. However, it must be remembered that strict hygiene will go a long way towards the control of parasites and this must always be practised.

Routine faecal examinations (at 2–3 month intervals) are a useful indicator and some people rely on them as a guide to when anthelmintic treatment is needed. Recently imported hawks should always have faeces examined but I do not recommend treatment in their first week of captivity unless clinical signs are present. It is also wise to check faeces of all birds which are to be put in an aviary for breeding since parasites can easily multiply in these natural, yet intensive, surroundings and it is useful to know which parasites one is likely to be introducing into the enclosure. At the Hawk Trust aviaries all incoming birds are injected with levamisole while in a special quarantine enclosure. If faecal samples show that worm eggs are still present the treatment is repeated.

A word should be said about worm egg counts. Although in the past I always reported the numbers of "eggs per gramme" found in mute samples I have now ceased to do so. There are many factors involved and I do not believe that a worm egg count does more than give a *very rough* indication of the parasite infestation. This hypothesis has been borne out often when I have repeated parasitological examinations on raptors and obtained different counts from samples taken at only 48 or 72 hour-intervals.

Nor can one assume that a particular worm egg count is an indicator of pathogenicity. Earlier I mentioned the very high *Capillaria* egg counts seen in recently imported hawks which clinically appeared healthy. This should be contrasted with the findings in a peregrine which died of severe oesophageal capillariasis. The crop, which was inflamed and eroded, contained many adult *Capillaria* worms. In a smear taken from the crop 218 *Capillaria* eggs were seen; comparable samples from the mid intestine showed nine eggs and from the rectum only two eggs. Previous faecal samples from this bird had shown either low egg counts (below 500 eggs per gramme) or, on occasion, no eggs at all. This case illustrates that, at least in the case of *Capillaria contorta* in the crop, the faecal egg count means little.

My conclusions over egg counts are that:

(a) the finding of eggs in a faecal sample demonstrates the presence of the parasite and very little else.
(b) repeated faecal examinations over a few days, or pooled samples, will give more reliable results than one specimen.
(c) although note should be taken of the actual egg count, little reliance should be

placed upon a single result in terms of estimating the parasite burden. The results must be carefully assessed, taking into consideration the bird's history, its overall health and the findings in previous or subsequent faecal examinations.

I have only ever found microfilariae in one bird of prey, a red-chested owlet, and this also harboured protozoal parasites (93). Microfilariae have been recorded elsewhere, for example in birds that died in the London Zoo (195, 356), but their significance is uncertain.

Acanthocephalan parasites are found in birds of prey from time to time and may possibly cause disease; Keymer (249) discussed this but reported that he had no experience of the parasites in raptors. I have found Acanthocephala in two species of bird but in neither case was there any evidence of pathogenicity.

A number of blood protozoa have been recorded from birds of prey (413) but, as with other avian species, few detailed studies or investigations are documented. As will be mentioned later, there is little information on the role of such parasites in disease.

In the first edition I listed the blood protozoa identified from birds of prey in my series of clinical and *post-mortem* cases, and a number of parasites, including *Haemoproteus* spp., *Leucocytozoon* spp., and a *Trypanosoma* sp. (Photos 15a and b) were reported. Since then my colleague Michael Peirce and I have surveyed blood smears from both British and East African species and added to, or expanded, that list.

In a survey of 70 birds of prey in Britain 15 (21·4%) showed haematozoa parasites (334). It is of interest to note that several of these parasites, including a haemogregarine in a captive bred snowy owl, were detected during the course of routine screening. In the case of our survey of haematozoa of East African raptors (335) ten out of 52 birds (19·2%) were found to harbour one or more parasites. Kocan and colleagues (262) recently surveyed 86 Oklahoma raptors for haematozoa and found them in 29 out of 36 (80·5%) of strigiforms and 24 out of 50 (48·0%) of falconiforms. These figures, which are considerably higher than our own, are similar to those reported in Colorado by Stabler and Holt (383).

Transmission of blood protozoa is usually by biting arthropods, such as hippoboscids, mosquitoes and mites, but again there is little information available regarding those species parasitising birds of prey. A report by Wolfson (421) of the successful infection of canaries (*Serinus canarius*) with *Plasmodium oti* is of interest in that it may indicate interspecies transmission. However, Garnham (166) suggested that *P. oti* is probably a synonym or subspecies of *P. hexamerium*. Several species of *Plasmodium* are known to infect a broad spectrum of avian hosts from different Orders.

Khan (255) carried out extensive observations on the life-cycle of *Leucocytozoon ziemanni* in saw-whet owls and its development in simuliid vectors. The leucocytozoids of the Falconiformes have recently been discussed by Greiner and Kocan (181).

The lack of information on the role of blood parasites in disease has been mentioned and Keymer (249) went so far as to say that "Nothing is known regarding

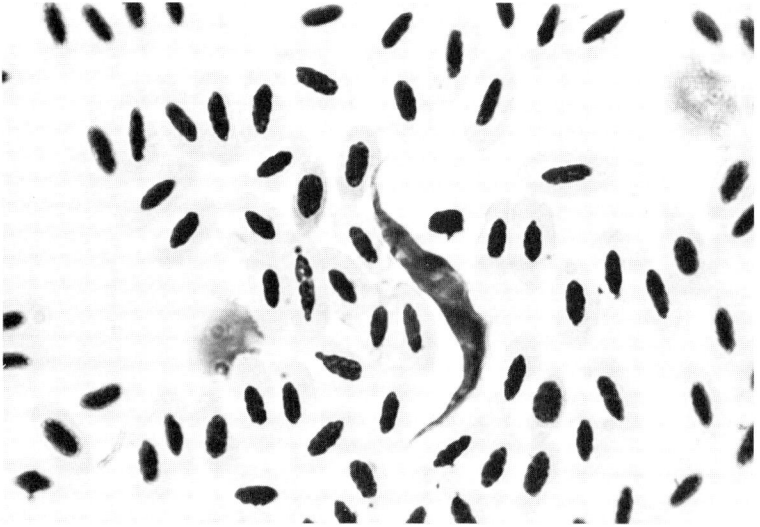

a

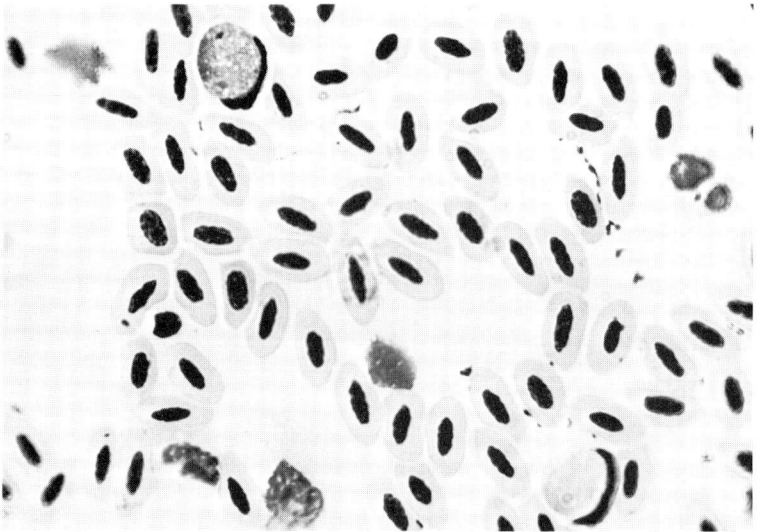

b

Photo 15a.   Blood smear of a peregrine stained with Giemsa and showing a *Trypanosoma* sp.
b.   Blood smear from the same bird showing a *Leucocytozoon* sp. The parasite in the top of the picture is a macrogametocyte, in the bottom a microgametocyte

the pathogenicity of most blood protozoa to birds of prey". This emphasises the need for more investigations and those who regularly examine raptors are urged to take blood smears for examination. There are also few data on the pathology of blood parasites in birds although Keymer (248) referred to work where lesions such as splenic enlargement were observed in passerine and psittacine birds infected with *Plasmodium, Haemoproteus* and *Leucocytozoon* spp.

Some scattered information on pathogenicity is available. In 1918 Wasielewski and Wülker (412) recorded acute pathogenicity of a *Haemoproteus* sp. in young kestrels followed by relapse of a more chronic type in older birds. They stressed, however, that clinical signs are not often seen and that death can rarely be attributed to this parasite. It is of interest to note that they also suggested that the kestrel was the most suitable species for studies on the lifecycle of *Haemoproteus*.

More recently Kingston and colleagues (257) reported clinical signs of loss of stamina and listlessness in a female gyrfalcon which had been bred in captivity at Cornell in the United States. Blood smears revealed red cells heavily (16%) infected with *Plasmodium relictum* and a further 12–14% of the cells showed signs of immaturity suggestive of anaemia. Treatment (see later) proved successful and reduced the parasitaemia to less than 0·01%. In their article Kingston *et al* described their report as the second of *Plasmodium* in the gyrfalcon, referring to a bird that died of a "fulminating malaria" due to *P. relictum* in 1956.

In my cases there has been no evidence of pathogenicity. A saker with a chronic paralysis of the wings was infected with a *Haemoproteus* sp. but there were no lesions at *post-mortem* examination to suggest that the parasite was in any way responsible. A rise in parasite numbers in the blood may be associated with stress, as suggested by Peirce and Mead (336) who reported a high parasitaemia of *Haemoproteus tinnunculus* in an injured hobby; this is another reason for recommending that, whenever possible, smears are examined from birds undergoing treatment and the parasites seen are both identified and counted.

In the event of clinical disease being associated with protozoan blood parasites a number of drugs are likely to prove efficacious in treatment. As long ago as 1937 Coatney and West (76) described the successful (and safe) use of quinacrine hydrochloride in treating a *Leucocytozoon* infection in two species of raptor. Kingston *et al* (257) treated their gyrfalcon with chloroquine phosphate by mouth over a three day period and reported clinical improvement within 24 hours.

Flagellate organisms have long been associated with birds of prey – in a review of *Giardia* spp. from birds in 1925 Hegner (202) drew attention to a isolate "from the blood" of a black-shouldered kite as early as 1911. However, it is *Trichomonas gallinae* that is the most significant and well documented insofar as the health of birds of prey is concerned and it is disease due to this organism that is known to falconers as "frounce".

Trichomoniasis due to *T. gallinae* is basically a stomatitis but the early signs may be only mild – the "flicking away" of food or difficulty in swallowing. On clinical examination one may see yellow caseous material in and around the mouth. Later the bird loses its appetite and may become dehydrated. Eventually the lesions can involve the ears, pharynx, larynx, respiratory tract, and other organs. Occasionally mouth lesions are associated with a foetid smell.

Definitive diagnosis is not difficult so long as therapy has not started. A moist swab of the exudate should, if expressed into warm isotonic saline, reveal motile flagellate organisms with undulating membranes.

I have never diagnosed trichomoniasis at *post-mortem* examination and have had little experience of it clinically but the reason for this dearth of cases is almost certainly because most falconers recognise "fronce" and at the slightest sign of any mouth lesion administer a suitable drug. Dimetridazole or the medical preparation metronidazole are probably the most effective and safe. Caution should be taken if the older preparation 2-amino-5-nitrothiazole is used since toxic side effects, such as nervous signs, can follow its use. Judged from reports of falconers and a small number of veterinary colleagues treatment with appropriate drugs is usually effective.

I have not been able to trace any records of trichomoniasis in raptors in zoological collections; this may be due to the fact that the parasite is often acquired by feeding on freshly killed pigeons and the latter are probably less likely to be fed to a zoological specimen. Clinical cases of trichomoniasis have been reported almost entirely from the Falconiformes although the isolation (and, indeed, culture) of a *Trichomonas* sp. was recorded from an unnamed owl by Tanabe as long ago as 1925 (390) and there are recent records of trichomoniasis in a tawny owl (6) and barred owl (351). Perhaps more owls should be examined for these parasites.

The danger of trichomoniasis is another reason for ensuring that care is taken when pigeons are used for food. At one time it was assumed that a healthy pigeon posed no threat but it is now realised that even healthy individuals can harbour *T. gallinae*. A useful precaution, which seems to be successful, is to freeze and thaw pigeons before using them as food; this appears to kill or incapacitate the parasites. Nevertheless, one must bear in mind that *T. gallinae* can probably also be transmitted directly from one bird to another, as reported in an American kestrel by Stone and Janes (387).

In addition to cases in Europe and North America trichomoniasis has been reported in recently imported birds such as lanners from Nigeria (328), and, in my own experience, in falconers' birds in the Middle East and Pakistan. Such cases appear to respond to appropriate antiprotozoal treatment. Stomatitis is also not uncommon in young captive bred falcons in Britain; I have not examined any such cases myself but the condition appears to respond to dimetridazole therapy, suggesting that it is, indeed, trichomoniasis.

Other conditions may simulate "fronce", in particular oesophageal capillariasis (85, 394) and various types of stomatitis. Stehle (385) listed eight possible causes of stomatitis (German "diphtherie") in hawks including vitamin A deficiency, pox and fungal infections. Physical factors may also occasionally be involved; Fox (155) described tongue lesions in two Australasian harriers which he attributed to a band of animal tissue, probably tendon, which constricted the base of the tongue. It is important, therefore, to ensure that any cases of stomatitis are examined clinically and swabs or scrapings taken for examination and/or culture before treatment is instigated. The aetiology of some cases is obscure, however, and these can be particularly troublesome since the lesion is frequently proliferative or associated with a build-up of necrotic debris. There may be no response to antiprotozoal or antibiotic drugs and treatment must be palliative, with removal of desquamated material and application of a mild antiseptic such as gentian violet. In chronic cases, especially where there is an ulcerative lesion, I have found daily spraying with 10% sodium chloride solution of value. More research is needed into these non-specific cases of stomatitis and their treatment.

Chronic granulomatous lesions of the buccal cavity occur occasionally. I have seen such cases in goshawks and they were recently reported in two free-living kestrels (18). My approach to these lesions in captive birds is to remove them surgically; blood loss is usually considerable and cautery is useful.

A number of species of coccidia have been reported from both the Falconiformes and Strigiformes: these were described and discussed by Pellérdy (337). Keymer (251) stated that "there is no proof" that coccidia are pathogenic to birds of prey: I cannot entirely agree with this but I do accept that in many avian species coccidiosis is misdiagnosed on the basis of finding oocysts in faeces. This is particularly true of falconers' birds where, for many years, diagnoses of coccidiosis were made with alarming regularity, particularly by veterinary surgeons and laboratories more acquainted with poultry. In this context it should be remembered that, as with other parasites, the finding of oocysts in a raptor's mutes may merely indicate that the prey was infected and the parasite is being passed through the bird's intestinal tract. It is important to note that coccidia are very host specific and therefore a bird of prey fed upon a chicken infected with coccidiosis will *not* contract the disease. However, prey items may act as an intermediate host – the vole *Microtus arvalis* for a coccidian of the kestrel, for example (69).

A definitive diagnosis of coccidiosis cannot be made on clinical grounds alone, even if signs of dysentery or diarrhoea are accompanied by the finding of many thousands of coccidial oocysts in the mutes. To confirm the diagnosis one needs to examine a portion of intestinal tract histologically and this can only be done in a dead bird.

I have confirmed clinical coccidiosis in only four birds of prey; in each of these the intestinal tract was either examined histologically or scrapings of severely damaged mucosa showed many coccidia. Two of those cases were recently imported birds and another a young bird bred in captivity, suggesting that the disease may be important in nestlings or at times of stress. Again my figures may be deceptive since coccidiosis is another condition readily suspected by falconers and treatment of possible cases is usually quickly carried out with oral sulphadimidine. I have detected oocysts in the mutes of otherwise healthy birds on many occasions.

I do not usually recommend treatment for coccidia unless clinical signs of diarrhoea or dysentery are present. It is preferable to control re-infection by hygiene and to ensure that the bird remains in good condition. When treatment is deemed necessary oral sulphonamides prove remarkably effective, especially if combined with fluid therapy.

Such response to treatment does not, of course, prove conclusively that the bird was suffering from coccidiosis since the sulphonamides will also control certain bacteria, including *E. coli*. Nevertheless, the fact that in some such cases a recurrence of clinical signs is seen, coupled with the reappearance of oocysts in mutes, when treatment is restricted to a three day course, adds weight to my argument that coccidiosis *is* a clinical entity in raptors. My own regime for treatment in such cases is as in poultry – three days of treatment, followed by two days without and finally another three days of treatment. It should be noted, however, that small numbers of oocysts sometimes continue to be detected even after such therapy.

CHAPTER 7

Foot conditions

Various conditions may affect the feet or legs of birds of prey, especially those kept for falconry, and the subject is discussed in a separate chapter in view of its practical importance. Although many conditions are infectious there seems little doubt that in most cases there is a predisposing factor such as trauma.

Traumatic injuries of the legs are not uncommon. A condition that is frequently seen is a swelling of the "ankle" (metatarso-phalangeal) region associated with excess bating. This occurs particularly in goshawks and sparrowhawks and is probably entirely traumatic in origin. The provision of better fitting jesses of softer leather is recommended, together with changes in management in order to reduce trauma.

Poorly fitted jesses may also result in infection: the skin of the leg becomes abraded and fails to heal due to continuous chronic irritation by the jesses (Figure 11). Bacteria may enter and a dermatitis result. The offending jesses should be removed and the bird released in a suitable large room or aviary. Treatment of the wound with a sulphonamide powder or tincture of iodine is advisable and, in severe cases, a course of antibiotic may be considered desirable. Similar infections may result when birds are trapped and birds in collections may damage their feet

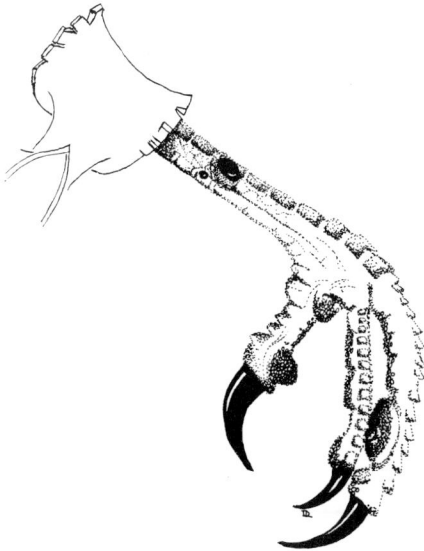

Fig. 11   Jess damage on the metatarsus. There is also an early bumblefoot lesion on one digit

97

or legs on the wire of the cage. Another cause of such lesions can be closed rings on the legs of captive-bred birds; such rings rarely cause problems on their own but can be traumatic when a jess is also applied to the leg.

Other infectious lesions of the legs which occur in birds of prey are described in Chapter 4. Arthritis and osteitis are not uncommon; they will be discussed later in connection with bumblefoot but it must be remembered that they can occur independently. Metabolic and other generalised diseases which may produce leg or foot lesions – for example, articular gout – are discussed in Chapter 11.

Bumblefoot

Inflammatory conditions of the foot are one of the most important clinical problems in captive hawks and will be discussed in detail. In falconry literature they were recognised and recorded as long ago as the 17th century (32, 269), while the Arabs, who have practised the sport for centuries, list them as one of the most significant diseases of their trained falcons. In recent years there have been several publications in falconry journals on their clinical features, prevention and cure. A useful paper in this respect was that by Halliwell (186) who presented a review of foot conditions seen in falconers' birds in America including discussion of their aetiology. In Germany the term "dicken Hände" is used for foot diseases and in a paper by Kösters (265) the relevance of this description and the importance of healthy feet to a falconer's bird were emphasised.

Foot conditions have also been recorded in birds in zoological collections (192). They are, however, mainly seen in the Falconiformes. I have seen cases in owls myself and North American friends tell me that the condition is particularly prevalent in snowy owls.

The terminology of foot conditions in birds of prey is confused; falconers refer to both "corns" and "bumblefoot" (301) but the distinction is often not clear. In this book a variety of lesions is referred to as "bumblefoot" but only in certain cases is the clinical picture identical to that described for classical "bumblefoot" in chickens (25, 372). My own approach is to consider each case of foot disease as a separate entity. The classification given later is a useful guide but no two cases are identical and the surest approach to treatment is to carry out as full an investigation as possible and to commence therapy early before chronic changes occur.

Some general points should be covered before the different types of bumblefoot are discussed in detail.

It is important to understand the anatomy of a raptor's feet before debating upon the cause, treatment and prevention of bumblefoot. The foot is protected by a thick layer of stratified squamous epithelium over which lies a layer of keratin. On the plantar surface there are hard papillae which assist in grasping. Underlying tissues consist of connective tissue, muscle, bone, nerves and blood vessels. In the succeeding few pages I shall describe the different types of bumblefoot and shall discuss their natural history. In all, however, the pathology is related to damage of the epithelium and, in some cases, the entry of pathogenic organisms.

The tendency for foot lesions to become infected is interesting since birds are generally fairly resistant to infection of wounds, whether natural or surgical. I suspect that the lower skin temperature of the feet may be contributory and it is possible that the digits may have a relatively poor blood supply. There is also, of course, the important point that the feet are more likely to become contaminated by bacteria than other parts of the body although this does not necessarily explain why *Staphylococcus aureus* (which is uncommon in raptor faeces) is so often the predominant organism rather than enteric bacteria such as *E. coli* or *Proteus* spp.

It is possible that the source of the infection may be organisms which live on the surface of the feet themselves and routine swabbing of the feet of healthy raptors has shown that many species of bacteria can be isolated. Often these are indicative of faecal contamination – *E. coli* and *Proteus* are common isolates – while the occasional culture (anaerobically) of *Clostridium tetani* would suggest that soil may have contaminated the area. More often, however, the bacteria cultured are staphylococci and it is these that are most commonly involved in foot infections. In one survey (109) 10·8% of 37 birds of 12 species yielded *S. aureus* and 62·1% *S. epidermidis*. We have also isolated *S. aureus* from throat swabs of apparently healthy birds suggesting that this site too may serve as a focus of infection. Bacteriology plays an important part in the diagnosis and treatment of bumblefoot and, together with antibiotic sensitivity tests, is advisable whenever a case is being investigated. An important point here is to remember that anaerobic culture may yield organisms not detected aerobically; my colleague Jeffrey Needham and I have occasionally even cultured *S. aureus* in cooked meat when routine aerobic cultures have proved negative.

Histology also plays a significant part in the investigation of bumblefoot and could perhaps be used more extensively. If surgery, however minor, is carried out the material that has been removed should not only be cultured bacteriologically but also examined histologically. Such examination will help ascertain whether bacteria are still present – pockets of *S. aureus* in particular are frequently seen – and will also enable the degree of fibrosis and other reaction to be assessed. Biopsy of foot lesions can also prove useful, especially when they are proliferative, and histology should again be performed. Bumblefoot rarely kills a bird directly but any foot lesion seen at *post-mortem* examination should also be examined.

At the time of writing I am carrying out an investigation into the histological changes that occur in *S. aureus* infection of the foot, using natural cases in raptors and experimental material from starlings (*Sturnus vulgaris*). It is hoped that the results will yield useful information, of clinical relevance to raptors, and thus aid prognosis and treatment.

I have particularly emphasised the role of microbiology and histopathology in the investigation of bumblefoot since I believe that they are not always utilised to the full. However, it must be remembered that these and other laboratory techniques should only be used to back up clinical observations. Careful examination of foot lesions is vital, if necessary under light anaesthesia, and in many cases radiography is desirable.

Prevention of the different types of bumblefoot will be discussed later but a general point should be made here. There are three main aspects of preventing foot lesions, these being reduction of trauma to the foot, hygiene and ensuring that the bird is in healthy condition on an adequate diet. Vaccination might play a part in prevention but, so far as I am aware, no work has been done on this subject other than studies on the immunising properties of staphylococcal toxins in mammals (149). This is another aspect which could be investigated using an experimental "model" in starlings or other species.

Treatment of bumblefoot may be managemental, medical or surgical and is often a combination of all three. These aspects are discussed in detail later.

Types of bumblefoot

1 Type 1 bumblefoot

Here there is a mild localised lesion, often of only one digit. The lesion may be proliferative (a raised "corn") or degenerative with a flattening and thinning of the epithelium or, in some cases, ulceration (Photo 16). Both types may progress to a scab. Such cases are often benign and frequently no organisms may be cultured or seen in histological sections, They are commonly associated with poorly designed

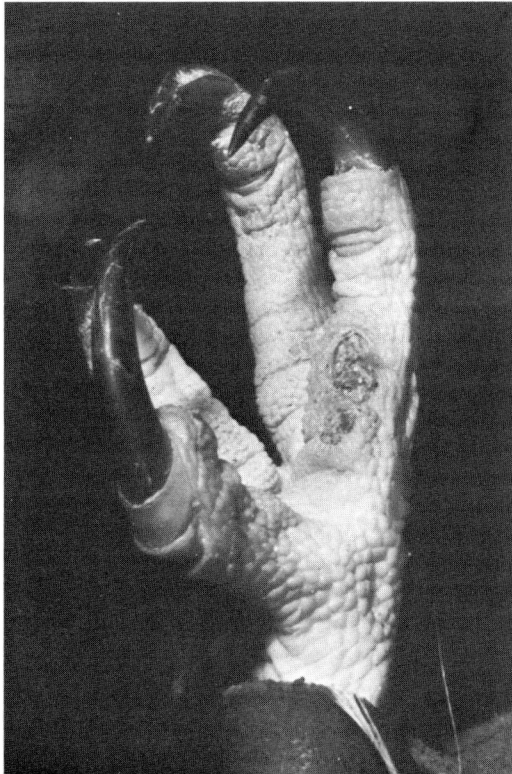

Photo 16.   Type 1 bumblefoot showing early ulcerative lesion of digit (black-shouldered kite)

perches or abrasive surfaces and changing these will often result in spontaneous recovery though proliferative lesions may never disappear completely (see later). Although a change of perch will usually result in improvement, sometimes the converse may apply and the lesions deteriorate.

Very occasionally foot lesions actually develop following what appears to be only a minor modification to a perching surface. For example, a 13 year old peregrine, which had never previously suffered a foot infection, developed bumblefoot within three weeks of a change of perching surface from a stone block with a convex top to one with a flat top. No other factors could be incriminated. This bird finally needed surgery for Type 2 bumblefoot.

Clinical signs associated with Type 1 bumblefoot vary. Some cases may show a tendency to favour one leg: alternatively the affected foot may be slightly swollen or warm to the touch. Sometimes the lesions can be seen without any accompanying clinical signs.

Ulcerated lesions should be treated with local cetrimide or antibiotic while a light dressing will, if left in place by the bird, discourage the entry of infection.

Some proliferative lesions may be benign papillomata, possibly of viral aetiology. These can be removed surgically. The majority, however, are composed of thickened epithelium and scab which overly a small focus of infection. Such cases often respond to a suitable antibiotic (see later) or, as Salvin and Brodrick described in "Falconry in the British Isles" in 1855 (361) ". . . the contents may be easily removed by merely cutting down upon them with a sharp knife, and squeezing the matter out".

The presence of a scab on a foot or digit may indicate a Type 1 bumblefoot lesion, but often is a sign that infection is, or has been, present. In this respect scabs may represent an intermediary between Type 1 and Type 2 bumblefoot. It is therefore important to ascertain whether they are traumatic or infectious in origin and to take appropriate action before the condition deteriorates.

2 Type 2 bumblefoot

This is more extensive (Photos 17 and 18) and is almost invariably associated with pathogenic bacteria; essentially there is an acute inflammatory lesion although histological examination usually shows the presence of chronic reaction, such as fibrous tissue and mononuclear cells, as well as abscessation.

Some cases result from a deterioration or infection of Type 1 bumblefoot but others appear to arise spontaneously. A sharp talon (in the case of falcons, usually the hind one) can easily pierce the sole of the foot and introduce infection (Figure 12). Some birds tend to "clench" their feet as a part of normal behaviour and the majority will do so during recovery from anaesthesia or restraint. I can find no evidence that the provision of "perches which are too slender" causes the ball of the foot to be pierced by the talons, as stated by Keymer (251). Poorly designed perches may predispose to traumatic injuries, however, and sharp edges in particular may be responsible for the establishment of a foot infection.

Some cases of Type 2 bumblefoot are attributable to infection following the entry of a foreign body. A common cause in tropical areas, and occasionally in

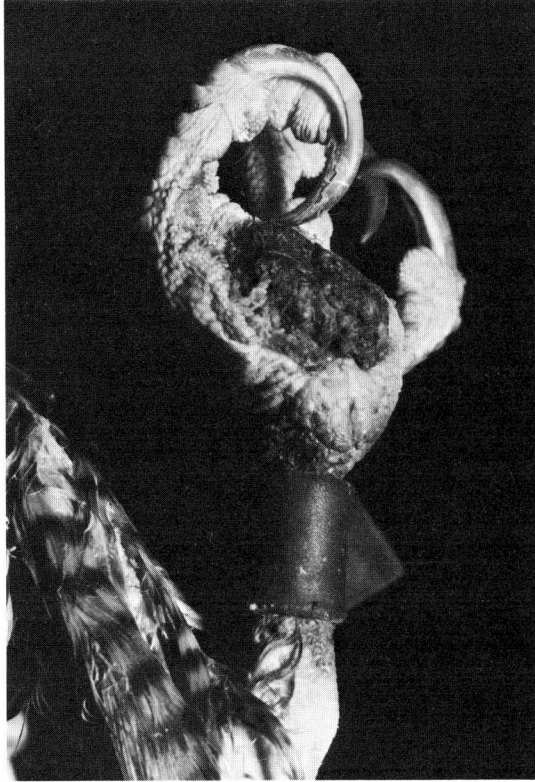

Photo 17.   Severe Type 2 bumblefoot showing scab on plantar surface (peregrine)

temperate, is a sharp thorn entering the sole of digit. The area becomes swollen, hot and painful but often there is little or no overlying scab. The thorn may be visible, as is a splinter in a human finger, and should be removed. Local antiseptic or antibiotic will usually control the infection. Recently imported hawks sometimes show infected foot lesions, especially of the digits, which are probably attributable to trapping or wire netting damage. In addition, if the heavier birds are kept on concrete they may abrade their feet and infection can enter, as described in tawny and steppe eagles in a paper earlier (102); a change of floor surface will accelerate healing.

The characteristic clinical features of this type of swelling (usually of the sole but sometimes of only one digit) are heat and pain. There is usually scab overlying the swollen area. Affected birds often lie down or stand in their waterbath in order to reduce the pain. The swollen tissues usually contain pus which may either be caseous in appearance or a clear serous exudate. Culture of the pus will normally reveal bacteria and in early cases these are often coagulase positive *S. aureus* but other organisms have been isolated, including *Streptococcus pyogenes* from the hind digit of an African fish eagle and a *Corynebacterium* sp. from a Wahlberg's

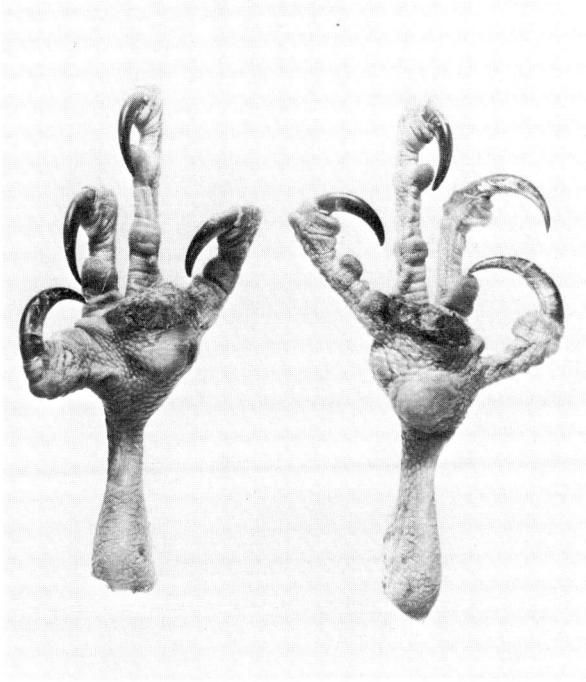

Photo 18.   Type 2 bumblefoot progressing to Type 3. Note scab on plantar surface and active infection ("pointing") on foot on right (peregrine)

eagle. The presence of *E. coli* is probably an indication of subsequent infection with faecal organisms, and in my experience can make treatment difficult (see later). Moore and Ronniger (301) suggested that *E. coli* in one of their cases might have originated from dog (*Canis familiaris*) faeces which contaminated the lawn where the hawk sat but it seems to me more probable that the organism comes from the bird's own faeces. Other organisms may establish themselves as a result of unhygienic surgery or following extensive antibiotic therapy; examples include *Pseudomonas* spp. which are notoriously difficult to kill. I have attempted to isolate mycoplasmas from foot lesions on a few occasions but this has never proved successful. I have seen yeasts in direct smears but never cultured them. Kösters (265) warned against the longterm use of antibiotics to treat bumblefoot on the grounds that "a fungus infection can develop" but no evidence was given to support this theory.

Histological examination of material removed surgically from Type 2 bumblefoot cases has confirmed that staphylococci are often present in large

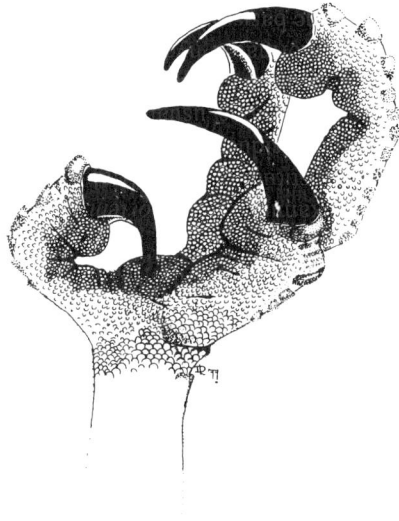

Fig. 12   Foot of a falcon showing the ease with which the hind talon can pierce the sole and introduce infection

numbers in the scab, as well as the underlying soft tissues. Histologically the scab in such cases closely resembles the human clavus ("corn") in that there is an area of excessive hyperkeratinisation which exerts considerable pressure (and hence damage) on the underlying tissues. It is therefore not surprising that such cases often recur.

Type 2 bumblefoot is treated initially with an appropriate antibiotic following a sensitivity test. Early treatment is important. Experimental work on the acute inflammatory response in poultry has shown that fibroplasia begins to occur as early as 3–5 days after tissue damage (309) and my own feeling is that chemotherapy is far less likely to prove successful once fibrosis is extensive.

Cloxacillin and lincomycin are particularly valuable in the treatment of *S. aureus* infections but other drugs, including oxytetracycline, have also been used successfully. At the time of writing I have started to use flucloxacillin which has the advantage of being better absorbed from the intestinal tract than cloxacillin while equally effective against penicillin-resistant staphylococci (388). Andrew Greenwood has used clindamycin or gentamicin (given twice daily by injection) often coupled with a steroid applied topically in dimethyl sulphoxide (DMSO). I have no experience of either of these antibiotics in birds of prey and I try to avoid using aminoglycosides but evidence from the human field (70) suggests that gentamicin is likely to prove highly successful in the treatment of staphylococcal infections. Staphylococcal osteomyelitis in poultry has been satisfactorily treated with oral sulphadiazine and trimethoprim (237) and such combinations should, perhaps, be investigated.

In cases where there is a mixed infection, especially if *E. coli* is involved, a mixture of ampicillin and cloxacillin is valuable. On occasions I have also prescribed a small dose of betamethasone, with apparently good results. All these drugs are best given by intramuscular injection. Response to antibiotic treatment is usually fairly rapid – a reduction in swelling within five days – but on some occasions a delay of 14–21 days may occur.

I also administer vitamin A routinely (orally or by injection) since a number of people have suggested an association between bumblefoot and nutritional deficiencies, especially vitamin A. This theory could be correct in view of the evidence from work on bumblefoot in poultry, for example by Jaksch (229) but it should be noted that foot diseases are not uncommon in hawks fed on day-old chicks, which are a rich source of the vitamin. On the other hand, the only severe case of bumblefoot in both feet which I have encountered in an owl was a young bird which also showed swollen eyelids and ocular lesions suggestive of a vitamin A deficiency.

Therapy of the condition must be accompanied by husbandry measures. The possible role of the perching surface was mentioned earlier. There is considerable dispute amongst falconers as to whether hard or soft surfaces on block perches predispose to bumblefoot but one point that seems certain is that once a bird has Type 2 bumblefoot then it should have a padded perch in order to reduce trauma and pain to the feet. In some cases a change from a block to a padded ring perch alone will result in improvement and even recovery. An affected bird should also be given every opportunity to rest the foot by lying down, should be fed well (on a mixed diet) and must not be flown. There is no doubt that a captive bird stands for longer each day than it would in the wild and this may predispose to foot conditions but flying a bird to the fist or lure when it has Type 2 or 3 bumblefoot will only exacerbate the condition. Heavy inactive birds, especially eagles, gyrs and sakers, seem particularly prone to bumblefoot and it is probable that in such cases the prolonged pressure on the feet is deleterious and permits damage to the epithelium through which bacteria may enter. The fact that cases of both Type 1 and Type 2 bumblefoot will sometimes heal spontaneously if the bird is released or given the freedom of a large aviary adds support to this theory.

Hygiene is probably also important in order to reduce further bacterial infection of the lesion. In particular the perches on which the bird stands should be cleaned and disinfected. I have cultured many species of potentially pathogenic bacteria from such perches and also from falconers' gloves and attempts to clean the latter are advisable. Particularly ancient gloves and other equipment should be destroyed! As was mentioned early, *S. aureus* can be cultured from the feet of healthy birds and it is possible that it may be acquired from human carriers, as Jeffrey Needham and I postulated in 1976 (109); personal hygiene is therefore also advisable.

It has been shown in poultry (128) that certain antibiotics, administered orally, will suppress skin populations of *S. aureus*. I do not suggest that antibiotics should be used routinely in such an empirical way in birds of prey (nor, indeed, in their owners!) but prophylactic use might be deemed necessary in an individual bird that regularly contracts bumblefoot. Whenever possible, however, more basic control measures, such as improved management, should be implemented.

Prevention of Type 2 bumblefoot is not easy but one useful precaution is to cut the talons of all birds when they first come into captivity or when handling is necessary. Such a procedure is not new; as Kösters (265) pointed out, it was often done to falconers' birds in the Middle Ages. In addition, it is important to ensure that injuries to the feet are treated early to prevent infection; daily cleaning with cetrimide is recommended. Well designed perches which avoid sharp edges and rough surfaces are probably a useful preventive measure whilst attention to the general health of the bird, including regular examination of the feet, can enable early recognition of lesions.

If chemotherapy fails or is only partly successful, surgery of Type 2 bumblefoot is necessitated and this will be discussed later.

3 *Type 3 bumblefoot*

This is essentially chronic and almost invariably follows Type 2. There is often still some infection present but this has usually been walled off by fibrous tissue to produce one or several pus-filled sacs. In severe long-standing cases the locomotory system may be affected, with damaged tendons and arthritis of the phalanges (Photos 19a and b) or tibio-tarsal joint. It is important that such cases

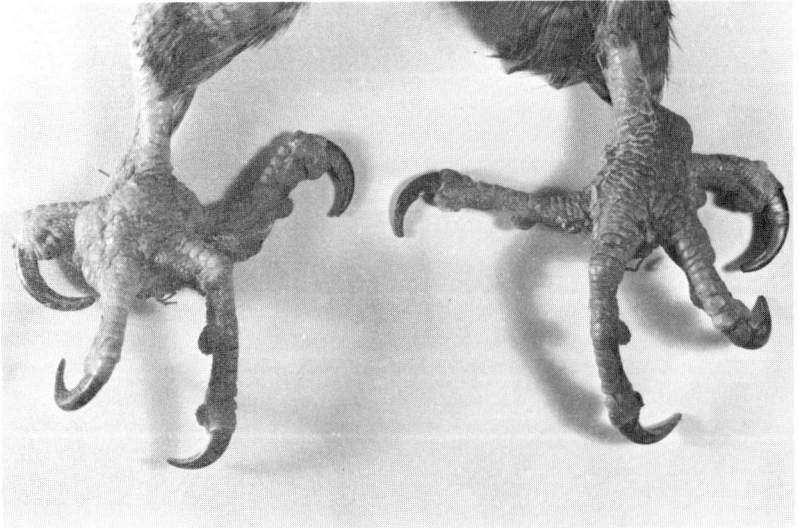

Photo 19a.   Type 3 (chronic) bumblefoot showing distortion of digits

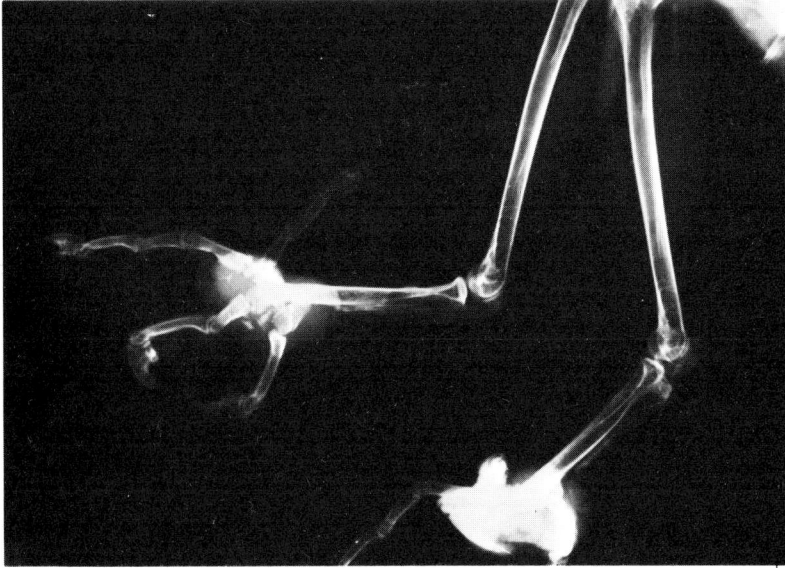

Photo 19b.   Radiograph of case previous showing arthritis and soft tissue reaction (peregrine)

are radiographed in order to assess the degree of bone involvement. Arthritic changes are usually destructive and can extend into the shafts of long bones.

Chronic cases of bumblefoot are often only hot and painful intermittently but the bird is usually unable to use the foot (or feet) satisfactorily.

Treatment of Type 3 bumblefoot with drugs is rarely successful, partly because systemic drugs are unable to reach the affected parts and also on account of irreversible damage to the tissues. Antibiotics will often produce an initial response but the swelling returns within a few days of cessation of treatment. Local preparations are often recommended for this and Type 2 bumblefoot but their value in severe cases is doubtful. I have used staphylococcus toxoid systemically but with no apparent success; an autogenous vaccine might be more successful. The use of radiotherapy (employing X-rays and five doses of 150 rads) was reported from Canada (39): there was some initial success but David Bird subsequently told me that the birds thus treated had shown remissions later. In most cases of Type 3 bumblefoot, therefore, the only course of action is either surgery or euthanasia.

Surgery

A surgical approach to foot infections was first recommended by Latham (269) who wrote – in 1615:

"You must have your Hawke well and easily cast, and with a sharp knife search and pare out the pinne, or core ..... the which if it have not planted it selfe too deep amongst the sinews, whereby to annoy and hurt them, it will easily be amended . . . . . and so dresse it thrice in the week, and withall let her sit very soft and warme, and this will cure her out of all doubt".

This is a magnificent description and cannot be improved upon to any great extent; the reader who prefers a more scientific dissertation is referred to the description of Dr. K. W. Kost's technique in "A Manual of Falconry" (422). My only quarrel with Kost's procedure is that anaesthesia was not recommended; nowadays anaesthetics are far safer and should always be used. I have treated many cases surgically, all of them intractable cases of Type 2 or Type 3 bumblefoot.

Prior to surgery, radiographs should be taken to assess whether or not there is bone involvement; the presence of arthritis or osteitis will drastically reduce the chances of success. The operative technique is carried out with the bird on its back (Photo 20a). The rationale of surgery is to open the affected area (Photo

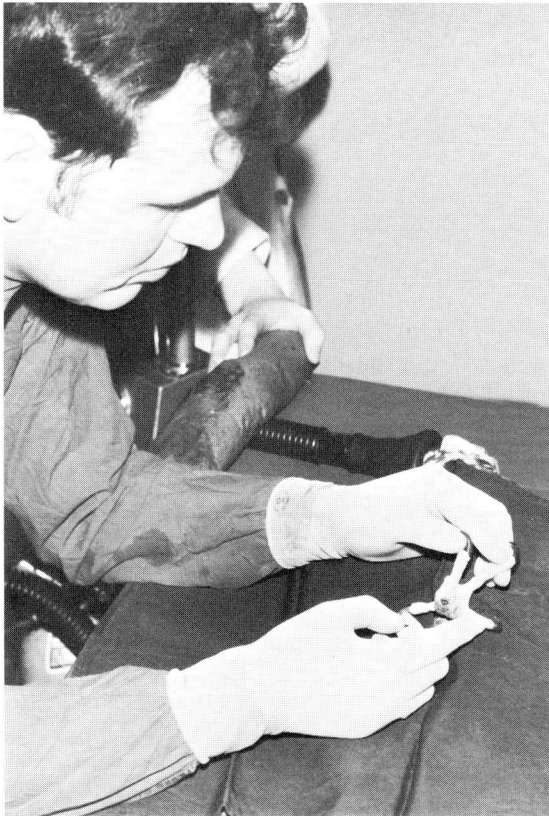

Photo 20a. Bumblefoot surgery on a saker. The anaesthetised bird is covered with a surgical laparotomy cloth and the affected foot, which has been cleaned, is being examined. Not the scab on the sole

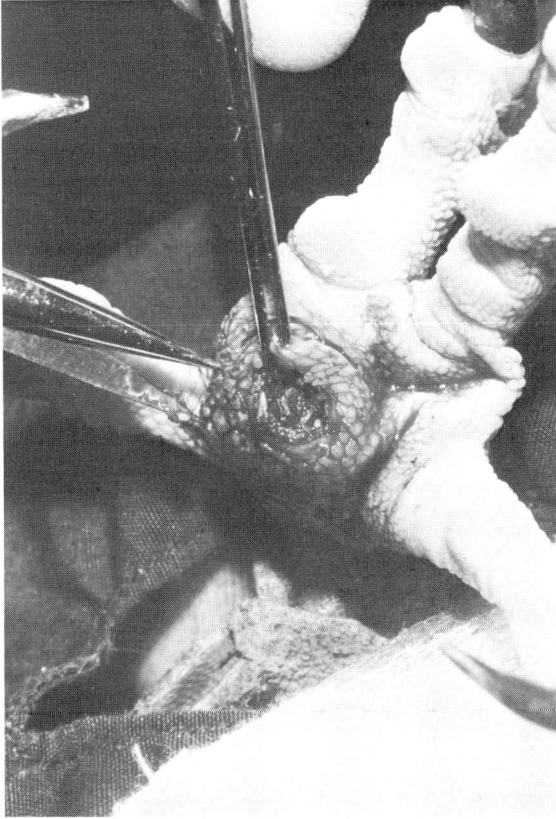

Photo 20b.   Bumblefoot surgery: the scab and a surrounding rim of skin are incised and removed

20b) to remove all infected or necrotic tissue and to prevent re-infection before healing has taken place. Care must be taken to ensure that all necrotic material is removed whilst leaving tendons and nerves intact (Photo 20c). Irrigation with the enzyme trypsin will assist in this respect. I use a 10 ml syringe and a 26 gauge needle and find that the force of the spray helps to dislodge dead tissue as well as moistening the area. If considered desirable an antibiotic can be included in the trypsin solution. The skin wound is closed using silk or nylon mattress sutures, taking care to ensure apposition of healthy epithelium without destroying the normal architecture of the sole too drastically (Photo 20d). A vital part of the operation is the dressing of the wound with a pad of gauze which can be sutured to the skin or held in place with adhesive plaster. This protects the wound and is usually left in place until the tissues are healing, although occasionally I remove the dressing after a few days to inspect the foot. Post-operative care consists of oral or systemic antibiotics, systemic vitamin A and good nursing. The sutures can be

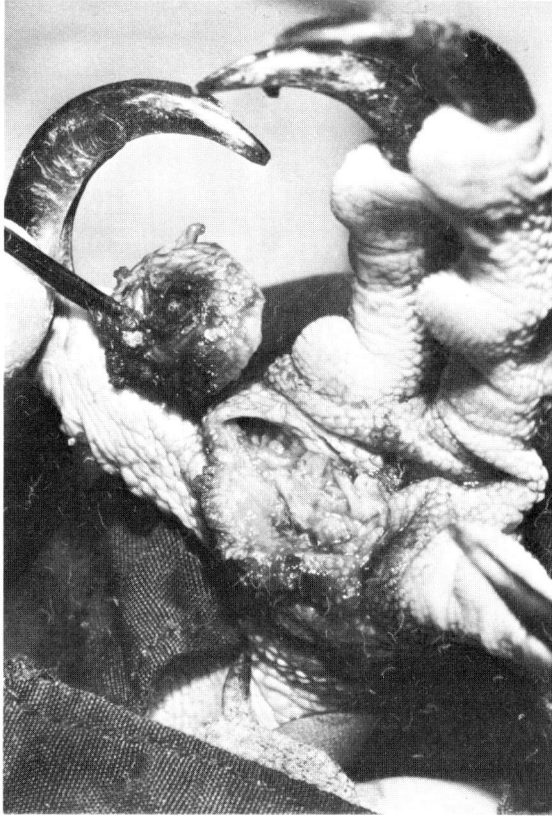

Photo 20c. Bumblefoot surgery: removal of the scab reveals underlying infected tissue which is removed and irrigated

removed at any time after ten days but may be left in place for up to a month. Surgery may need to be repeated later but often (approximately 60% of cases) a successful cure results on the first occasion. If both feet need surgery I usually operate on the second one seven days after the first but occasionally it may be necessary to perform both operations at one time. In such cases the bird may tend to lie down for 3–4 days until healing commences.

I gave an illustrated lecture on the surgical treatment of bumblefoot in Abu Dhabi in 1976 (103); in my paper I particularly emphasised the need for strict asepsis and correct surgical technique if the results are to be successful. Whenever possible, surgery should be carried out by a veterinary surgeon. Far too many falconers, including some in Britain and North America, who should know better, attempt to open infectious bumblefoot lesions in their hawks without anaesthesia and with minimal hygienic techniques; the results are usually poor and in some

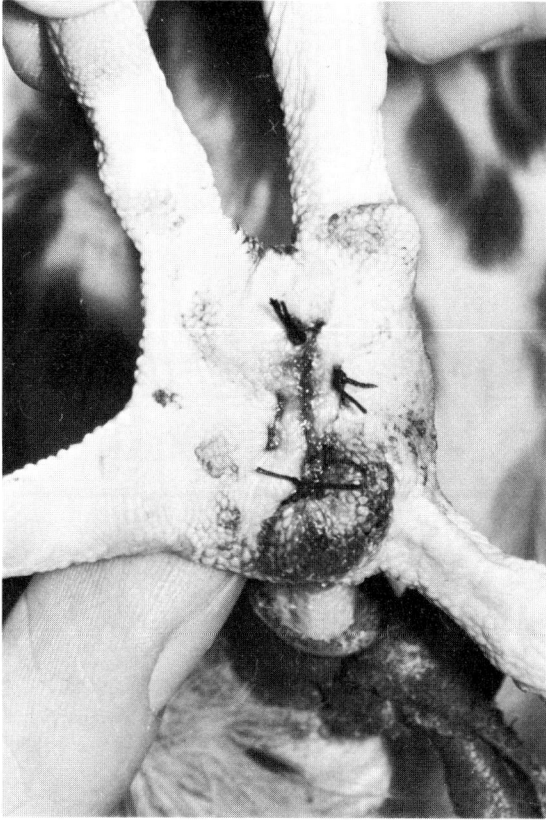

Photo 20d.   Bumblefoot surgery: the skin is sutured before the foot is dressed

cases there may be secondary infection or damage to nerves or tendons.

Prevention of Type 3 bumblefoot consists primarily of prompt attention to milder foot lesions to prevent their becoming chronic.

CHAPTER 8

Nervous disorders

The nervous system of the bird has long attracted the interest of biologists and physiologists and as long ago as 1645 Severino, in his "Zootomia Democritaea" (373), depicted the brains of birds, amongst them a hawk. The history of the subject was reviewed in "The Avian Brain" (331) and this book is recommended to all who are involved in veterinary work with birds of prey. Most of the earlier research was concerned with gross anatomy but in the past 30 years there has been more interest in microscopical structure. More recently brain function has attracted considerable attention, particularly that relating to stereotyped behaviour and the relationship of brain growth and differentiation to the activity of young birds (77, 389). Much of the work has involved the use of experimental birds, particularly the pigeon, and a considerable amount of surgery has been carried out to assess the effect of lesions in different areas of the brain – an example is the work on feeding behaviour by Zeigler and Karten (426).

Despite this history of research on the avian brain, its pathology has been sadly neglected. A number of nervous diseases are recognised in non-domesticated birds but relatively little is known of their aetiology and there has been no attempt to relate them to modern neurology. For example, Arnall and Keymer (15) discussed fits, convulsions, "epilepsy", fainting, vertigo and "hysteria" in cagebirds and emphasised the need for further work on these conditions. Hasholt (201) divided the "diseases of the brain" in cagebirds into three main categories, these being encephalitis, nutritional and toxic encephalomalacia, and functional encephalopathy but he too confirmed that a definitive diagnosis is often not possible.

In the case of birds of prey nervous diseases warrant a separate chapter in view of the fact that "fits" and other disorders have, for a long time, been recognised by falconers, especially in the short-winged hawks or accipiters. For example, in 1619 Bert (32) wrote:

"There is a disease in the head of some, called Vertego, it is a swimming of the braine."

Salvin and Brodrick (361) in 1855 wrote of "fits" which they described as "not necessarily fatal, as the Hawk may live for weeks after experiencing the attack". More recently the majority of authors have described nervous diseases of hawks and they are featured in many falconry books. Woodford (422), writing in 1960, for example, stated that "no one has the slightest idea of the cause of these convulsions or how to treat them".

Clinical features

The clinical signs seen in nervous diseases in birds of prey, vary considerably. In the case of classical fits the bird shows inco-ordination and inability to use its legs (Figure 13). It has a vacant staring appearance and its head is usually on one side, with mouth often slightly open and respiration accelerated and pronounced. Regurgitation of food sometimes occurs. The bird may recover within 2–3 hours and never have another fit, or, more probably, it will have further attacks within the next few hours or days.

A variety of other clinical signs may be seen in raptors and it is not clear whether these represent different syndromes or other manifestations of one disease. Muscle fasciculation is not uncommon and there may be weakness or paralysis of the limbs. In some cases there is opisthotonos and the bird may call out, as if in pain. In one syndrome the bird may be able to stand and walk but holds its head at an angle or upside down.

Other conditions also occur which are possibly of nervous origin. Peripheral nerve lesions, which usually cause more localised clinical signs, are covered separately later in this chapter. Psychological disturbances, some of which may produce marked behavioural changes, are discussed in Chapter 11. Syndromes known as "apoplexy" and "stroke" may result in clinical signs somewhat similar to those in nervous disease but both of these are cardiovascular in origin and are discussed in Chapter 11.

It will be apparent that a variety of clinical features may be encountered by the veterinary surgeon who deals with nervous diseases in birds of prey. As was mentioned earlier, some of the clinical signs seen may be unrelated to the nervous system and this can complicate examination, diagnosis and prognosis.

Neurological examination

Clinical examination of a bird of prey is discussed in Chapter 3. When a nervous disease is suspected the approach is similar but there are some important differences. Full clinical history and records are essential and here the use of a "check card" (questionnaire) is very useful. Important features of history are the age and source of the bird, its previous health, the diet being fed and *detailed* information on the onset, duration and features of the nervous syndrome.

Observation of the bird from a distance is most important since premature handling or disturbance may precipitate a fit or radically influence minor locomotory abnormalities. Much depends upon the severity of the clinical picture. A bird with mild nervous signs, such as muscle tremors, can usually be examined on the falconer's fist or on a table. A bird which is having fits poses problems of restraint and it may be wiser to wait for the fits to subside, or to reduce their severity with diazepam or primidone, before commencing examination. A comatose bird can be handled with relative ease. Subdued lighting should always be used when examining a bird with nervous disease and aids to handling, such as a towel or falconer's hood, must be at hand.

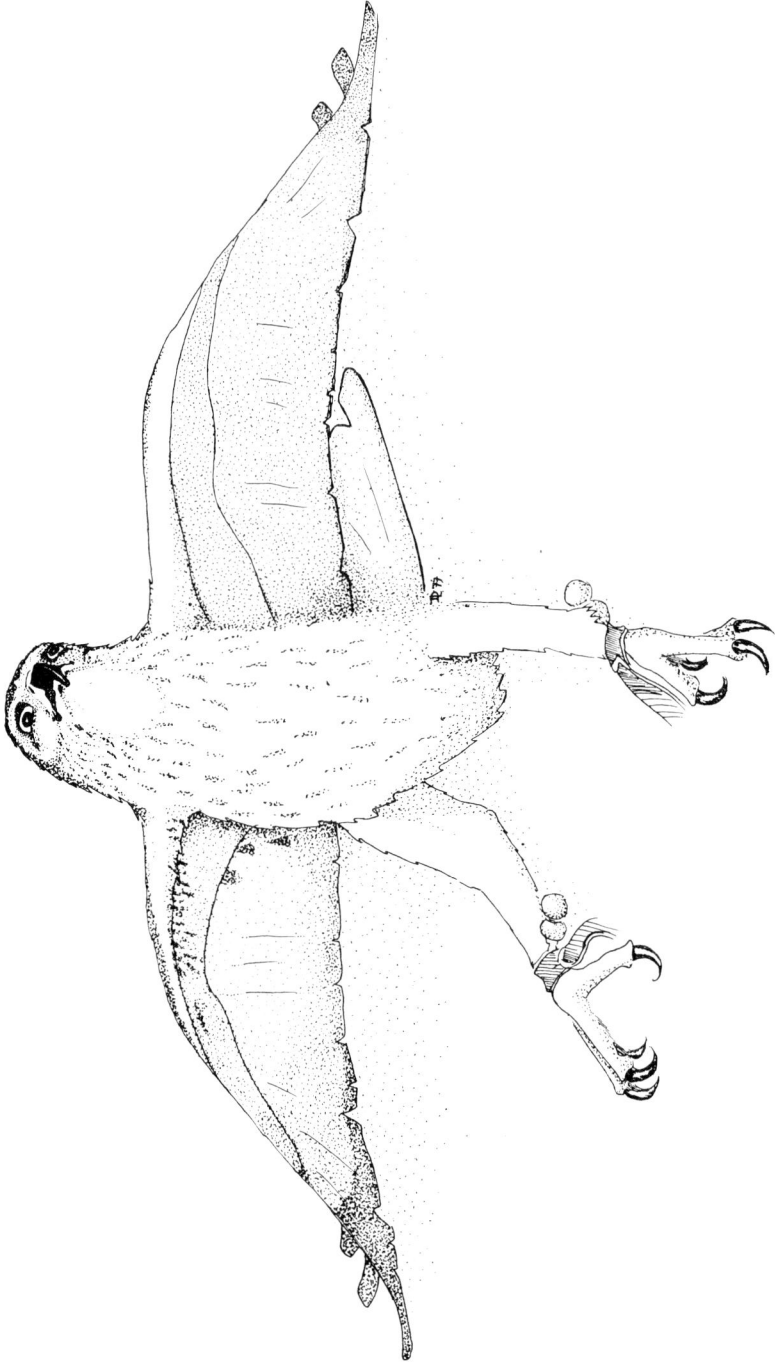

Fig. 13   A hawk eagle having a "fit". The bird is inco-ordinated, with its head on one side, and easily disturbed by external stimuli

At the time of writing there are no sophisticated aids to neurological examination of raptors. Electroencephalography (EEC) and electromyography (EMG) will undoubtedly prove of value in due course. Nerve conduction studies and work on nerve biopsy techniques urgently need investigation. In the meantime one must use standard clinical techniques. In this context it is worth noting that some guide to clinical investigation may be obtained from toxicological studies in poultry where an "ataxia grading" is used to assess the effects of neurotoxicity. Similar criteria could be used in birds of prey and are well worthy of consideration.

General behaviour can be assessed before the patient is restrained and in the case of a falconer's bird a considerable amount of valuable information can usually be obtained from the owner's descriptions. The level of consciousness can also be ascertained from observation. The gait or stance of the bird should be noted and any tendency to hold its head on one side, or to "circle" should be recorded. A word of caution here is that a falconer's bird which is hooded sometimes shows abnormal head movements, particularly if it has some limited vision through the hood. If in doubt the hood should be removed. It is important to see the bird in motion and here again the task is easier with a falconer's bird which will step or fly to the fist. If the bird has come from an aviary it can be released in a suitable room, with reduced illumination, and observed. Important points to note are whether (a) the bird walks or flies into objects, (b) is incoordinated when walking or flying, (c) shows inability to use a limb or limbs properly. The reaction of the bird to sound can be assessed in a falconer's bird by use of a familiar call or whistle and in an aviary bird by sounding a small bell or tapping two metal objects together – the bird should turn its head and show evidence of having heard.

Assessment of postural reactions is again much easier in a trained hawk. There are a number of investigations that can be carried out but tests I regularly use are:

(1) will the bird step on to a perch, or another gloved hand, if pressed backwards so that its legs touch that object?
(2) if the hand carrying the bird is lowered abruptly, does the bird extend its wings and retain its balance?
(3) if a falconer's bird "bates" off the fist, can it return to it satisfactorily?

If the patient is not a trained hawk such tests are not always practicable but it is still often possible to carry out (1) and (2) in a darkened room. Rotating a horizontal bar while the bird is standing on it is another useful technique; normally a bird is able to adjust the position of its feet, and, often with the occasional help of its wings, retain its balance and posture. In many cases of nervous disease it is unable to do so and falls, or flutters, off.

The detailed clinical examination must be systematic. My own approach, with any suspect nervous disease, is to start at the bird's head and progress to the wings, body and legs. When the head is examined it should be checked for evidence of symmetry, for example whether both eyes are equally open. One or both of the nictitating membranes may be conspicuous or perhaps excessively active. The pupillar reflexes should be checked using a pinpoint source of light. The eyes should each be examined ophthalmologically. Nystagmus is rare in birds of prey since the majority cannot move their eyes and instead rotate the head.

The wings, body and legs are gently palpated and sensation assessed with a sterile 21 gauge needle which is used to prick the skin gently. Areas of sensation can be plotted on a rough drawing. Any hyperaesthesia should be noted. If there is evidence of paralysis or impaired use of a limb this must be examined carefully. In particular it is important to assess whether the paralysis is flaccid or spastic. The filming of an affected bird will enable a particular neurological or locomotory sign to be viewed on repeated occasions.

I cannot claim that a detailed examination as outlined above will lead to definitive diagnosis and specific therapy. Very often the treatment finally chosen for the bird is empirical and symptomatic. Nevertheless, there is such a dearth of scientific information on nervous diseases in birds that I feel it essential for each case to be investigated methodically. Only in this way will data be accumulated and some light thrown on the perplexing range of "nervous" conditions seen in raptors.

Terminology and aetiology

As was explained earlier, many layman's terms have been used to describe nervous diseases in birds of prey, and some of these date from the 17th century. The word "encephalitis" was used fairly commonly amongst falconers 20–30 years ago (3), apparently on the erroneous assumption that intraosseous haemorrhages seen in the skull at *post-mortem* examination could be equated with inflammatory lesions in the brain. This is totally incorrect and, with the exception of proven cases of brain infections (for example following otitis media), the term "encephalitis" should not be used.

The word "epilepsy" was used by Salvin and Brodrick (361) 120 years ago and was presumably coined on account of the clinical similarity between fits in hawks and epilepsy in man. However, nowadays the pathogenesis of epilepsy is better understood – the important feature is overactivity of the motor cortex which causes marked locomotory signs – and we do not have sufficient evidence to suggest that this is what occurs in birds of prey. However, in view of the clinical features of fits it is probably justifiable to apply the term "epileptiform" and this description was used by Woodford (422). In this context it is worth noting the useful paper on epilepsy in dogs by Barker (20) who commented that "the veterinary literature shows a strong bias towards listing of the aetiologies and clinical signs with little emphasis on the underlying physiopathogenesis". This is true of all nervous diseases in birds of prey and use of modern neurological terminology and procedures is long overdue.

Since the term "fits" is used commonly by falconers and others to describe any condition where general signs of inco-ordination or nervous derangement are present I shall use the word in that general sense here. I am assuming that "convulsions" and "seizures" are synonymous with fits. Nevertheless, I must emphasise that the overt nervous signs seen in clinical cases are often only one manifestation of an underlying disorder and when improved techniques are available differential diagnoses will, hopefully, be relatively straightforward.

Greenwood (177) divided nervous diseases of raptors into five groups – nutritional, infectious, poisoning, CNS lesions and peripheral nerve lesions. These are convenient headings and will be used here.

Nutritional

I have long suspected hypoglycaemia as being a cause of fits. Birds of prey which are *in extremis* very often have convulsive seizures before death and these are particularly common in birds which are later found at *post-mortem* examination to have died of inanition.

Fits are also seen in birds in low condition which are subjected to exercise, stress or exposure to low temperatures. For example, a falconer's bird will sometimes have a fit after a flight or even following several hours on the fist on a cold windy day when it is expending considerable energy in keeping its balance and maintaining its body temperature. My own results and those of others (189) indicate that the normal blood glucose levels for birds of prey lie between 200 and 400 mg per 100 ml and it is noticeable that birds which have fasted tend to have figures towards the bottom of this range.

It is possible that fits in birds which are not in low condition may also be due to hypoglycaemia if their food intake is being reduced. For example, Woodford (422) mentioned the occurrence of fits at the end of the moult and this may be associated with the reduced or poorer quality food that is usually offered at that time. I have not been successful in obtaining sufficient numbers of pre-mortem blood samples to help confirm the hypothesis that some fits are due to hypoglycaemia but clinical experience (see later) would help support this.

Investigation of blood glucose levels is hampered by the difficulty of getting samples from small birds, especially if they are showing nervous signs, and the possibility that handling and restraint may influence the results. In this context, however, it is worth noting that Nelson and colleagues (315) could detect no influence on blood sugar levels when great horned owls were handled and anaesthetised with phenobarbitone.

Theoretically the initial clinical feature of hypoglycaemia is flaccidity – in contrast to epilepsy, where motor activity is predominant – but in practice this stage is quickly superseded by neuronal activity, possibly on account of hypoxia or metabolite accumulation (327). Specific clinical diagnosis is, therefore, probably not practicable, although premonitory signs of muscle weakness may be suggestive of hypoglycaemia. Probably the bird's history is the most important information.

Glucose can be given to birds by either the oral or parenteral route. If the latter is used, a 10% dextrose solution is injected subcutaneously, intravenously or intraperitoneally. In my experience the administration of glucose is often associated with a clinical improvement although fits may recur some hours later.

In some cases a thiamine deficiency may be involved. The effect of such a deficiency in both birds and mammals has been long recognised; chickens, and later pigeons, were used in experimental work on human beriberi which is characterised by demyelination and other nervous lesions (278). So called "Chastek paralysis" in foxes (*Vulpes vulpes*) and mink (*Mustela vison*) fed on raw fish has also been studied in detail and found to be due to the enzyme thiaminase in the fish. Wallach (405) discussed thiamine deficiency in exotic animals and stated that it "occurs often in ... carnivorous birds (e.g. eagles, penguins, storks, seagulls) because they consume diets high in fish".

In non fish-eating birds of prey the situation is less clear. There is a published account of thiamine deficiency in a peregrine in the United States (408). This bird showed clinical signs of opisthotonos followed by seizures which showed no response to antibiotics, small doses of a vitamin/mineral mixture or sedative drugs; a slow recovery followed the administration of thiamine. The author attributed the thiamine deficiency to the use of day-old cockerel chicks but no other similar cases appear to have been documented. Dr. Vanda Lucke examined the brain of one goshawk which died following fits and described a degree of demyelination of the cerebellum. More recently Mr. L. Cooke and I have seen similar lesions in brains of captive vultures which died after nervous signs. In many cases, however, no such changes have been seen.

Some birds with nervous disease which I have examined clinically or *post mortem* have been fed on chicks but by no means all. In 1977 I investigated fits in hand-reared sparrowhawks fed solely on day-old chicks but was unable to make a definite diagnosis *post mortem*. There was certainly no evidence of demyelination. The only lesions I could detect histopathologically were occasional neurones with intracytoplasmic vacuolation but it is possible that these were artefacts associated with poor fixation. It is of interest to note that young hand-reared kestrels on exactly the same diet showed no nervous signs. The question of thiamine levels in chicks is discussed in Chapter 9.

Nervous signs are well recognised in thiamine deficiency in poultry and certain of the clinical features described in "Diseases of Poultry" (369) are worth repeating: "The chicken characteristically sits on its flexed legs and draws back the head in a 'stargazing' position." Such a posture is similar in some ways to that seen in fits in raptors and might add weight to a diagnosis of thiamine deficiency.

Thiamine can be administered orally or by injection. A B-vitamin complex or multivitamin preparation can be used if the pure compound is not available.

Another probable cause of nervous signs is hypocalcaemia following nutritional osteodystrophy and hyperparathyroidism, as postulated by Wallach and Flieg (407). Unfortunately these authors appeared to recognise no other possible aetiology for such diseases and ascribed both fits and cramp to osteodystrophy. Hamerton (193) reported cases of fits in young buzzards at the London Zoo and described clinical signs "suggestive of tetany"; in view of their age these may have been cases of nutritional osteodystrophy but it is noteworthy that Hamerton reported no significant lesions in the parathyroid. Radiography and clinical chemistry play an important part in the confirmation of a diagnosis of osteodystrophy and hypocalcaemia. The normal serum calcium levels of both falconiform and strigiform birds lie between 7 and 15 mg per 100 ml and, according to Wallach and Flieg, the appearance of "cramps" in the large muscle groups indicates a critically low level of 5 mg per 100 ml.

Administration of calcium in cases of fits should be subcutaneous or intravenous. A 10% calcium boragluconate solution can be used. The newer, more concentrated, calcium preparations which are intended for farm animals appear to be safe but should not be injected into the pectoral muscles in case a reaction should follow. The longterm treatment of hypocalcaemia consists of supplying an adequately balanced diet, but, as is stressed in Chapter 9, the bone changes are often irreversible.

There are other nutritional factors which may possibly cause nervous signs in birds of prey and these include deficiencies of vitamin A and/or E which are known to produce clinical signs of ataxia and inco-ordination in poultry (369). Certain metabolic disturbances, such as hypoxia, uricaemia and electrolyte imbalance, may also be involved and should probably be borne in mind in differential diagnosis.

Infectious

A number of infectious diseases can produce nervous signs. An important example is Newcastle disease and this diagnosis should be confirmed or refuted by serology and attempted virus isolation. Other viruses might also be involved and some examples, including rabies, are discussed in Chapter 5. More likely to be responsible, however, are bacterial infections of the ear, eye or brain. Bacterial otitis media is particularly common; it may occur "spontaneously" or follow trichomoniasis (316).

Protozoal infections do not appear to have been incriminated in nervous diseases of raptors but should be considered in differential diagnosis. Examples are toxoplasmosis and crytococcosis.

Careful clinical examination is necessary to diagnose an infectious cause of nervous disease and must include laboratory techniques such as haematology and microbiology. Therapy of a suspected bacterial infection should comprise intravenous administration of a suitable broad-spectrum antibiotic which is likely to cross the blood-brain barrier and an intramuscular dose of a corticosteroid.

Poisoning

Nervous signs are a feature of poisoning with a number of agents and this subject is discussed in more detail in Chapter 9. In the case of chlorinated hydrocarbon poisoning affected birds are weak and inco-ordinated and may show convulsions. In addition, as will be mentioned later, occasional episodes of nervous disease may be due to sublethal levels in older birds. Greenwood (177) made the important diagnostic point that such poisons produce hypersensitivity and a continuous overall tremor as well as fits.

Many other organic poisons can also produce nervous signs, amongst them organophosphorus compounds, but with all such agents there are problems of relating clinical signs to individual poisons. In addition, there may be species differences in susceptibility and the reaction of a bird to a poison may not be the same as a mammal – on which most toxicological tests are done.

Certain inorganic chemicals can cause similar clinical signs – for example, violent muscular contractions and inco-ordination with strychnine and immobility and loss of righting reflex with thallium sulphate (22). Although lead poisoning appears rare in birds of prey, it may produce nervous signs and should always be considered. Work by Koeman and colleagues (263) showed that a feature of methyl mercury poisoning in captive kestrels was demyelination of the medioventral part of the abdominal spinal cord. Affected birds showed clinical signs of paralysis. Similar clinical and pathological features are seen in poultry poisoned with tri-ortho-cresyl phosphate (TOCP). The extensive studies on this subject have provided data on myelin degeneration in birds (169) which could be of great value in work on nervous diseases in raptors.

Hoerlein (212) referred to carbon monoxide poisoning as a cause of nervous seizures in dogs and the gas could possibly have a similar effect in birds.

Neurological reactions to drugs may be seen from time to time. The compound may be directly toxic to birds or, alternatively, an overdose or impaired metabolism/excretion can result in toxic levels. An important example of the former is procaine penicillin; an injection of the drug into a bird of prey can result in clinical signs ranging from muscle tremors and ataxia to opisthotonos and collapse (see Chapter 10). Overdosage is probably also a hazard. Dr G. J. van Nie has told me that a red-tailed merlin which received 20 mg tetramisole showed ataxia for $1\frac{1}{2}$ days and rather similar clinical signs were seen in a goshawk which was given 1500 mg thiabendazole. Failure to recover fully from parenteral anaesthesia can be manifested by stupor and muscle tremors.

Treatment of poisoning is discussed in Chapter 9. A definitive diagnosis is often difficult and specific therapy is rarely practicable. Symptomatic and supportive treatment should be attempted.

Central nervous lesions

Traumatic damage to brain or spinal cord can result in nervous disease. Some road casualty cases show nervous signs but usually these are characterised by "concussion" – the bird shows reduced response to stimuli, slow pupillar reflexes and depression ranging from unusual tameness to complete unconsciousness. *Post-mortem* examination usually reveals subcutaneous, intraosseous and meningeal congestion and/or haemorrhage. Occasionally the whole head is rotated clinically but, surprisingly, in my experience pathological examination of such cases reveals no specific lesions.

Leadshot in the brain can be diagnosed by radiography. It too can result in rotation of the head.

Treatment of traumatic injuries is discussed in Chapter 4. In the case of nervous lesions supportive treatment should also be given as outlined later.

Tumours of the brain are another possible cause of nervous signs but do not appear to have been reported in raptors; in the budgerigar pituitary tumours produce characteristic clinical signs, including convulsive seizures (363).

General aspects of treatment of central nervous signs

Although I have discussed specific treatment under each of the five headings, it is frequently difficult to distinguish distinct syndromes and general therapy may be necessary.

Initial treatment should be to reduce stimuli by placing the bird in a padded box in the dark or by hooding it. Thereafter therapy may be attempted. My own approach is to administer glucose by mouth with calcium boragluconate and thiamine (or B-vitamin complex) by injection. If poisoning is also considered a possibility I inject atropine (see Chapter 9). Fits may be reduced in severity by the use of phenobarbitone, diazepam or primidone. Corticosteroids may have a part to play in the temporary alleviation of certain clinical signs and can be given by intramuscular injection.

Following initial and supportive treatment attempts at a definitive diagnosis can be made although in some cases therapy will have influenced the results of blood tests and other procedures. A neurological examination should be carried out, as outlined earlier, together with radiography and other investigations.

If a layman has a bird which has a fit he is probably best advised to keep the bird warm, in the dark, if necessary wrapped in a blanket to reduce self inflicted damage. Oral glucose or sucrose should be given, together with vitamins (again by mouth) if available. A number of cases have apparently responded to such therapy and it is well worth following if professional advice is not readily available.

Post-mortem examination

Many birds with nervous disease die and it is important that a *post-mortem* examination and as full laboratory tests as possible are performed. Unfortunately, however, autolytic changes occur quickly in the nervous system and, as Glees (169) in "Experimental Neurology" pointed out, even if material is fixed by immersion immediately after death, the fixative takes some time to penetrate the tissues. It follows that if brain tissue from a bird of prey is sent for examination by post it is usually too autolysed for meaningful interpretation. Under such circumstances it is sometimes wiser to arrange to have samples taken by the owner, or another veterinary surgeon, immediately after death. Perfusion of the bird with formol saline is probably the most reliable method of fixation but, as is mentioned in Chapter 3, this will render it useless for microbiological examination. Often, therefore, fixation by immersion has to be used.

Ideally brain material should be taken for histopathology, microbiology and toxicology. My own technique is outlined in Chapter 3. If the skull is split longitudinally, one half of the brain can be fixed immediately for histopathology and pieces of the other portion kept fresh for bacteriological culture, virus isolation and toxicology. If material for toxicological examination is deep frozen it may be possible to use it again later for microbiology.

I have had only limited success in dissecting and fixing the spinal cord from raptors without damaging it. I prefer to remove a portion of vertebral column, including the cord, from the cervical and lumbar regions. Following fixation and decalcification, transverse sections can be cut. Peripheral nerves should also be taken, preferably the sciatic or brachial, and according to Wallach (405) the vagus is important in the diagnosis of thiamine deficiency.

In addition to the preparation of paraffin sections, nervous tissue should be kept in fixative for fat stains.

Peripheral nerve lesions

Peripheral nerve damage is probably a not uncommon sequal to traumatic injury and is discussed in Chapter 4. The usual picture is impaired use of a wing or leg although care must be taken not to assume that such a clinical picture is always attributable to nerve damage; other conditions can produce similar signs.

Another syndrome which is probably of nervous origin is a bilateral paralysis of the legs which is seen in raptors, especially goshawks, from time to time. The paralysis may be complete or only partial. Usually the digits are tightly clenched and there is considerable tone in the leg muscles. Sensation appears to be present, but impaired. My colleague Michael Williams and I have investigated a number of these cases. Some appear to respond to multiple injections (at 1–2 day intervals) of a B vitamin complex, suggesting that a B vitamin deficiency is involved, as has been described in a golden eagle (384). Some cases treated thus recover fully in 7–10 days. Others, however, show no response and remain paralysed. The digits become abraded, the wing tips damaged and the underparts soiled. There is no response to antibiotics or corticosteroids. Our own approach is to perform euthanasia if there is no response in three weeks. Pathological examination of goshawks which have died or been destroyed has revealed no specific lesions; inflammatory lesions of the legs, including lowgrade lymphocytic infiltration around the sciatic nerves, have been attributed to secondary damage.

There is a report of a syndrome similar to the above in a goshawk by Jack (227). In that case oxytetracycline was administered and the bird made a full clinical recovery. However, as is so often the case, there is no substantial evidence that it was the antibiotic that effected a cure.

Paralysis of the legs may also follow other diseases. For example, it is not uncommon for a bird with severe enteritis to "go off its legs" and lie down; usually it will stand again so long as it receives prompt treatment. "Cramp" may produce similar clinical signs – see Chapter 11. I have also seen lesions of tuberculosis in a kestrel which pressed upon the sciatic nerves and caused complete paralysis of the legs. Needless to say, any intra-abdominal space-occupying lesion may have this effect – even an egg!

Undiagnosed paralyses of wings and/or legs are also seen from time to time in individual birds. In the case of a black kite in Kenya the signs were attributed to traumatic injury but no lesions could be detected radiographically. Wing paralysis of unknown aetiology in a saker with a *Haemoproteus* parasite burden is discussed in Chapter 6.

Damage to nerves may follow surgery and this is mentioned, in the context of bumblefoot, in Chapter 4. Injections into the leg muscles will occasionally produce paralysis of that limb which resolves spontaneously over a period of 5–7 days; one assumes that the sciatic nerve has been damaged in such cases. Trauma to the vagus is more serious and may follow surgery on the crop or thyroid. I have not seen this myself but Voitkevich (402) described clinical signs of "paralysis of the crop" in pigeons and fowls. The patient eats well initially but the crop becomes full of food and is not "put over"; the bird finally dies of inanition. Voitkevich also described impairment of respiratory rhythm following such damage.

Self mutilation is discussed in Chapter 11. This sometimes occurs following surgery or an injury and it is possible that hyperalgesia, due to nerve damage, is a cause.

It will be obvious from the foregoing that very little information is available on nervous diseases in birds of prey. Human neurology has advanced enormously in recent years and standard medical texts cover topics as diverse as embryogenesis, encephalopathies, intoxications, birth defects, malformations and neurosurgery. In veterinary science much remains to be done; Palmer (327) in his "Introduction to Animal Neurology" wrote:

"Animal neurology is still in its infancy; with the course of time the use of sophisticated techniques will improve both diagnosis and treatment".

This is particularly true in avian work and the need for research has been emphasised throughout this chapter. Nervous diseases are a field in which the use of experimental birds is probably justifiable and where, if an affected bird has to be killed, every effort should be made to ensure that full pathology, including clinical chemistry and histopathology, is performed. It is also essential that guidelines are produced on the preparation and subsequent histopathological examination of the central nervous system if improved methods of diagnosis and investigation are to be achieved.

CHAPTER 9

Nutritional diseases, including poisons

The nutrition of birds of prey is an extremely important subject and its relationship to the health of the bird was recognised three hundred years ago (46), when Richard Blome wrote:

> "The wild hawk preserveth herself in all Times and Seasons in a Moderate state by her continual Exercise and Good Feeding".

In a paper on the nutrition of raptors at the 1975 Oxford Conference, I drew attention to the paucity of modern scientific data on the nutritional requirements of these birds. This is still the case, although some advances have been made, especially in our understanding of the deficiency diseases. In this chapter I shall endeavour to outline some such advances and at the same time emphasise the fields in which further work is urgently required.

Birds of prey are, by definition, carnivorous. In the wild they feed upon animals ranging from grasshoppers, snails and earthworms to small gazelle. In captivity they are usually given meat or dead animals, mainly mammals or birds, although (as will be mentioned later) commercial diets have been used in zoological collections. Aviculturists will offer the smaller species a range of insects, such as locusts, while Leese (272) reported, in 1927, that the Arabs fed camel ticks to their falcons. The falconer who has any interest in parasites will, I hope, not follow this example but submit any ticks he finds (even if not from camels) to a specialist for identification!

A few birds of prey will take food other than flesh – for example, the African harrier hawk will eat oil palm nuts (59) – but this is exceptional.

Cannibalism is well recognised amongst the nestlings of free-living birds, particularly the larger species such as eagles, and it can occur in captivity. In very cold climates, such as certain areas of Canada, it may be prudent to separate male and female birds during the winter since, if food becomes frozen, the female may eat the male. A bird that dies in an aviary is very often eaten by one of its peers. Eggs are also devoured from time to time and such behaviour may indicate a nutritional deficiency (341).

Little information is available on the nutrition of captive birds of prey other than limited studies on certain species, mainly in zoos, and scattered reports of diseases supposedly of nutritional origin. This is in contradistinction to free-living birds where studies on food preferences and amount of food taken have often been extensive. More work on captive birds would undoubtedly prove of use to the field biologist as well as the falconer, aviculturist or curator of birds and in this respect it should be noted that in their book "Eagles, Hawks and Falcons of the World" Brown and Amadon (59) referred to work with captive species.

124

The anatomy and physiology of the raptor's gastro-intestinal tract will not be discussed in detail here. Basically it resembles that of the fowl except that the falconiform species generally have small or vestigial caeca and the strigiforms no crop (Figure 5b). Some very valuable work has been done in recent years on the physiology of digestion by Duke and colleagues at the University of Minnesota (133, 134) and the reader is referred to these and more general publications. Developmental abnormalities of the tract appear rare but cystic dilatation of the gizzard has been reported on at least two occasions (95).

Many data are available on the nutrition of poultry but there are significant gaps in our knowledge and correspondence in the "Veterinary Record" in 1974 (404) suggested that even in these species a review of "accepted" levels of nutrients was needed. This, coupled with the important differences between the diet of a fowl and a raptor, makes extrapolation from the field of poultry a risky business.

A diet for captive birds of prey should be:

(1) sufficient in quantity
(2) sufficient in quality
(3) free from deleterious effects
(4) acceptable and digestible
(5) easily and cheaply obtained and stored

Each of these criteria will be discussed in turn.

Quantity

Brown and Amadon (59) gave figures for food consumption for a number of falconiform species in their book and a selection of these is listed below, with the permission of the publishers:

Species	Weight (g)	Daily intake (g)	Approximate % of body weight
Sharp-shinned hawk	100	25	25
Sparrow-hawk	200	53	26·5
Peregrine	683	104	15
Red-tailed hawk	1150	127	10·7
Golden eagle	4047	251	6·25
Steller's sea eagle	7030	240	3·5

Examples of reduction in intake in warm weather are as follows:

Species	From (%)	To (%)
Sharp-shinned hawk	25	23
Peregrine	15	11·5
Red-tailed hawk	10·7	8·6
Golden eagle	6·25	5·26

It will be noted that, the smaller the bird, the greater the % of bodyweight that is consumed daily. Food consumption increases when temperature drops or when a bird is active as opposed to sedentary, or when it is laying eggs. Growth and moulting also require increased food intake. Brown and Amadon's book does not refer to owls but my own observations suggest that they show comparable figures. For example a captive barn owl, weighing 300 grammes, will eat 20–25% of its weight per day.

In captivity a raptor must receive sufficient food to keep it alive and healthy. In the case of falconers' birds the food intake is deliberately controlled so as to make the hawk "keen" and thus more easily trained. As will be mentioned later, under "Inanition", inexperience in this technique can prove disastrous. Overfeeding is more likely in birds maintained in zoological and private collections; it too should be avoided since obesity can also result in disease and death. For example, Fisher (148) postulated that calorific restriction is an important factor in reducing the incidence and severity of atherosclerotic lesions and Wallach (405) discussed the role of excessive calorific intake in producing zoo animals which were obese, lazy, infertile and less resistant to high temperatures. He recommended that "When keeping exotic animals in captivity they should be thought of as animals at rest and fed accordingly". One way of achieving this with raptors is not to feed the birds on one, or possibly two, days a week.

Regular weighing of captive raptors is an important guide to condition but is not usually possible when the birds are maintained for breeding. Under such circumstances it is probably best to feed an excess of food. Indeed, since precopulatory behaviour may include the offering of food to a mate, even when both have full crops, underfeeding may have deleterious effects on breeding. There is also increasing evidence that some species kill surplus food and then hide it – the American kestrel, for example (322). When birds are rearing youngsters underfeeding may result in the offspring being killed and eaten, and again supplying food *ad libitum* is probably desirable. A disadvantage of overfeeding is that uneaten food attracts rats and flies and may harbour disease; a careful check must therefore be kept upon the food supplied.

It may be advisable to maintain a high plane of nutrition throughout the winter for females intended for breeding. It is also important that the diet is optimum prior to, and during, egg-laying – as Frazer (158) stated

"Within the egg . . . the development of the young is confined both spatially and by the food available a few months earlier".

Inanition can probably be defined as "exhaustion from lack of nutrients" and must, regretfully, be mentioned. Starvation probably kills large numbers of free-living birds, for example young kestrels (381) where, as was mentioned earlier, the mortality rate is high in the first year of life. Although a small bird, such as a kestrel, may starve to death in 72–96 hours a large eagle may be able to survive for weeks. Starvation occurs only rarely in raptor collections but in falconry, where a hawk is encouraged to fly by reducing its weight, it can be a cause of death. I have examined many such cases *post mortem*; while the majority of these are due to a reduction in food intake and associated factors, this is not always the case. For example, one peregrine submitted to me died from inanition following damage to the mandible which prevented the bird from feeding; other birds have had a localised infection which has produced the same effect.

Alternatively, a raptor may receive adequate food in terms of weight but its carbohydrate content may be inadequate. As a result the bird fails to thrive and finally dies of "calorific exhaustion" (405). In the case of birds of prey approximately 2,000 total calories per gramme of diet should be provided. An important point here is that the calorific value of whole animal diets may vary. Brisbin (54) reported that wild-caught mice may show significant deviations in "caloric" density from those individuals raised in captivity and referred to work with the rodent *Peromyscus polionotus* which showed that laboratory raised animals had twice as large fat indices as wild-caught specimens (67).

In his book "A Hawk for the Bush" (295) Mavrogordato stated that "lowness of condition" was the chief cause of disaster to trained sparrowhawks and gave an excellent description of clinical features. He drew attention to the change from early signs of being ravenously hungry to a terminal stage of apathy. As he rightly pointed out, the condition should be easily prevented. Hawks which are "low in condition" must be carefully nursed and fed good quality food, without roughage, in small amounts. At the same time they should be kept warm to prevent unnecessary energy expenditure while the administration of oral or parenteral glucose appears to help prevent hypoglycaemia.

Stehle (385) described a rather similar condition ("Verdauungsinsuffiziens") in Germany but in his cases food was retained in the crop and had to be removed manually before treatment (small meals of warm meat in milk) could be commenced. German veterinary surgeons and falconers continue to record this condition but I have not recognised it clinically myself.

Diagnosis of inanition is usually based upon history, clinical signs and the bird's low weight. An estimation of plasma total protein will normally give a low value – less than 2·0 g%. The *post-mortem* findings are largely negative. The bird is thin and may be slightly dehydrated. The pectoral muscles in particular are wasted in appearance; they play an important part in metabolism, and at times of reduced food intake are used as a source of amino-acids. Internally there are usually no fat reserves and either the gastro-intestinal tract is empty or the crop is full of food. The latter is usually due to the owner realising, too late, that the bird is in low condition. The fact that such meals are often not "put over" may explain the rather different syndrome described by the Germans. There may be mild congestion of the lungs and pale internal organs. The gall bladder is usually enlarged. Birds suffering from inanition often ingest vegetation and stones and these are found in both crop and gizzard. However, it should be noted that up to 10% of castings from free-living kestrels may consist of earth in the Winter and early Spring (125). In cases where terminal fits have occurred, or the bird has been tethered on a perch and at death hung from its jesses, agonal intraosseous haemorrhages are seen in the skull. Petechial haemorrhages may be seen occasionally in visceral organs in histological sections but usually there are no significant microscopical lesions.

Green mutes are often a feature of inanition but are also seen under other circumstances. They are usually indicative of a period of low food intake; the green colouration is due to bile. Usually the colour returns to normal once adequate feeding resumes but some birds regularly produce rather greenish faecal material, often intermittently, and this may cause alarm to the owner. No treatment appears necessary but I routinely culture the faeces of such cases bacteriologically and check for parasites.

Although the answer to inanition in practical terms is relatively simple, the whole question of starvation in birds has attracted considerable interest, mainly on account of the unusual features of carbohydrate metabolism in this group of vertebrates. Fisher (148) reviewed the subject in detail and the reader who is interested in the mechanisms involved is advised to read his chapter; it should be noted that Fisher stated that "unfortunately, virtually no information relative to tissue metabolic patterns of non-domestic species is available."

Captive hawks should not suffer from starvation and in the hands of an experienced and conscientious falconer will not do so. It cannot be overemphasised that a trained bird must be weighed regularly; only in this way will a drop in condition be quickly diagnosed. The size of the pectoral muscles is an important clue but, as has been emphasised in other species (325), does not take into account the size of the fat reserves. Another feature that is frequently overlooked is that, while an increase in weight may take several days to achieve, a corresponding drop can occur very rapidly. The Importation of Captive Birds Order 1976 and the Endangered Species (Import and Export) Act 1976 have restricted the importation of birds of prey into Britain and have helped ensure that they only reach the hands of capable people. However one possible disadvantage of captive breeding, particularly of small species such as the kestrel, is that young, inexperienced people may try to use them for falconry – with tragic results.

Quality

A diet may be sufficient to assuage hunger but still be unsatisfactory in terms of content. The important constituents of a diet are water, protein, fat, carbohydrate, minerals, vitamins and roughage and insufficient of excess of any of these may

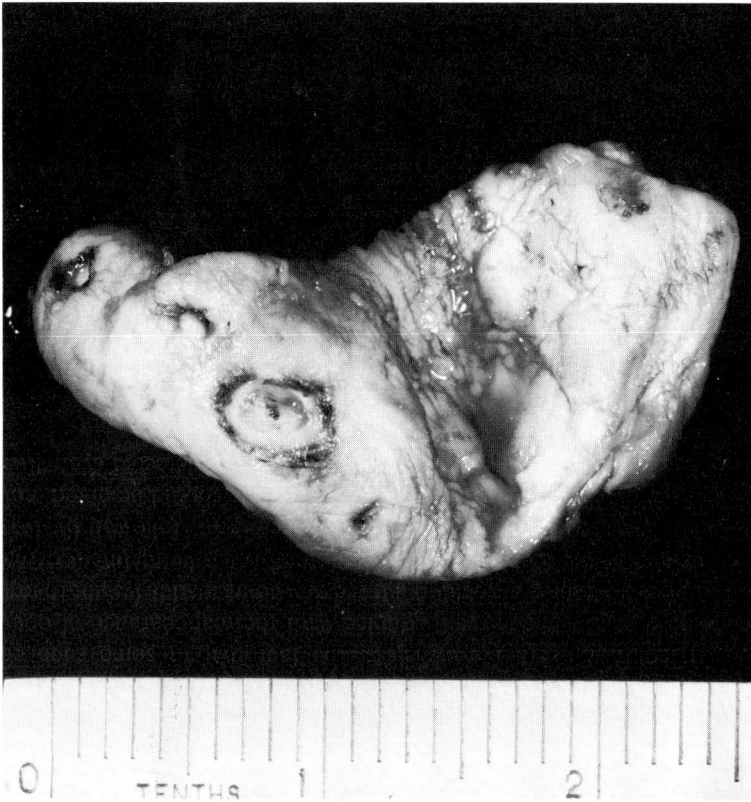

Photo 21.   Ulceration of gizzard of a kestrel. The ulcer is surrounded by a zone of hyperaemia and was associated with a large, retained bolus of indigestible food

result in disease.

Water and roughage are related in that both influence consistency. A diet containing low amounts of roughage for over 14–21 days can result in diarrhoea and birds on such a diet may try to ingest soil or plant material. It is therefore important to ensure adequate feather, fur or artificial roughage such as cotton wool. Impaction of the gizzard occasionally occurs, however, and in one case in my experience it was associated with ulceration (Photo 21). Hamerton (193) reported the death of a falconet due to impaction of a hard ball of mouse fur in the gizzard and consequent obstruction of the intestinal tract. He made the comment that "these insectivorous falcons seem to be unable to thrive on the ordinary meat diet provided for birds of prey." One peregrine I examined died following ulceration of the proventriculus but the cause was not determined; certainly there was no evidence of mechanical damage. Impaction of the crop is even more common; many cases respond to oral liquid paraffin and manual "milking out" of the crop but occasionally surgical removal of crop contents is necessary. Such conditions are less likely to occur if one ensures that the moisture content of the diet is adequate.

Other aspects of the physical nature of the food may influence the health of the bird. Bones can become lodged in the crop or, rarely, penetrate its wall and cause infection. Such bones can be removed surgically or, in some cases, milked out manually. Many raptors are kept on sand and will, inevitably, ingest some with their food. Not only may this reduce palatability but, according to some authors, it can cause enteritis. For example, Hamerton (192) described acute gangrenous gastro-enteritis in a peregrine and reported that "the alimentary tract was packed with fine sand, a condition that is frequently found in acute enteritis among small birds of prey." This has not been my experience; many people maintain raptors on sand without any ill effects and soil is commonly found in the castings of free-living birds (125). Indeed I sometimes find the presence of small amounts of sand in the alimentary tract a useful landmark in radiography! Nevertheless, if complications due to ingesting sand were diagnosed early I would expect liquid paraffin to be of use in treatment.

It is also worthy of note here that occasionally a young bird, especially if hand-reared, appears to swallow air which is then visible and palpable in the crop. The bird may show discomfort, craning its head as if to regurgitate. The condition is recognised by aviculturists in other birds; often it resolves spontaneously but it may be necessary to pass an oesophageal tube through which the air will escape. It is important to distinguish this condition from subcutaneous emphysema, which is discussed in Chapter 4.

When considering consistency it must be remembered that food which has been deep-frozen should be thawed slowly and then, if possible, soaked in water or physiological saline before being used. If this is not done the moisture content may be reduced excessively. Food must not be fed that is still frozen.

Water itself must also be discussed. Falconers rarely give their birds water to drink but in aviaries it should be available and there is increasing evidence that it is taken regularly when birds are egg-laying or rearing young. It is also vital for sick raptors and advisable for those that are moulting. Some sick birds will refuse to feed until they have taken water. Water containers must be kept clean and in temperate climates it must be remembered that they may freeze on particularly cold days.

A subject which should be mentioned is that of "rangle". That captive hawks will swallow small stones was known to the earliest falconers; in 1615 Latham (269) described the way his peregrine would later regurgitate these stones and, if they were placed near the block, swallow them again. Falconers have traditionally believed that rangle stirs up mucus and fat in the stomach and that this has a beneficial effect, as evidenced in Latham's advice:

> "Wash'd meat and stones maketh a hawk to flie,
> but great casting and long fasting maketh her to die"

There is a useful discussion on the history and possible role of rangle in the paper by Fox (154) who concluded that captive birds of prey benefit from having "appropriate stones available to them at all times". He went on to mention captive hawks dying following the use of diets with a high fat content but did not elucidate: stones are occasionally found in the gizzard of birds at *post-mortem* examination or may be detected radiologically.

The protein content of a diet is probably of great importance and in this respect it is probably not unreasonable to extrapolate from the situation in poultry where the protein % used for young chicks is usually 18–20% and this is reduced to 12–14% for growers; layers and breeders require higher levels, usually 14–18%, but adult non-breeding birds will thrive on less than 10%. We do not yet have comparable figures for birds of prey but my own assumption is that a figure of 15–20% is desirable, with young birds receiving higher levels than non-breeding adults. One commercial diet available in the United States contains a minimum of 19% crude protein and this would help support this view. As Bird and Ho (38) pointed out, rodents, chickens and day-old chicks show comparable levels of protein. It is not just protein levels that are of concern, however; the amino acids present are also important and here again scientific data are not available. In poultry the amino acid requirements can differ between strains of fowl and from this one would assume that there are likely to be variations between species of raptor. In the absence of reliable data one should rely on "natural" foods rather than attempt to formulate an artificial diet.

Excess protein must also be avoided. It has been postulated that it may produce visceral and arthritic gout (405).

Even less is known of the importance of dietary fat to raptors. Again, Bird and Ho (38) found little difference in levels in the species they analysed and since raptors appear to thrive on such diets it may be reasonable to assume that a crude fat % (of dry matter) of 20–25% is acceptable. However, I would refer the reader to my comments earlier, under "Quantity", concerning the difference in fat content between free-living and laboratory reared rodents.

A similar situation applies to carbohydrates; figures by Bird and Ho (38) for gross energy, which reflect other constituents as well as carbohydrates, ranged from 5·78–6·02 Kcal per gramme of dry matter and conformed closely with those of Duke and colleagues (133) for mice and young turkeys.

Of the minerals only calcium and phosphorus have been investigated in any detail in birds of prey, largely on account of the prevalence of the disease osteodystrophy. This is usually attributable to a calcium/phosphorus imbalance, and is discussed in detail later in this chapter. Wallach and Flieg (407) recommended a calcium level of 2% of the diet for raptors and Bird and Ho (38) suggested that day old chicks which contain less than this on a dry matter basis should be rolled in bonemeal to increase their calcium content. In Bird and Ho's study rats and mice contained 2·06% and 2·38% calcium respectively. However, the commercial diet mentioned earlier is described as having a minimum of only 0·4% calcium and one wonders if this is adequate for breeding birds. Other minerals may influence calcium metabolism, especially phosphorus and manganese, and as Wallach and Flieg (407) pointed out, exceptionally high levels of these should be avoided.

Bird and Ho (38) also investigated levels of zinc, copper, manganese and iron and, extrapolating from poultry, suggested that rodents and poultry used to feed raptors were adequate in terms of zinc and iron, possibly marginal for copper and very likely deficient in manganese. In view of the known effect of manganese deficiency in infertility of poultry they suggested that supplementation of these diets with the mineral may be necessary. In my view, however, there is as yet no evidence of such an effect in birds of prey and one should be wary of interference with the diet until more information is available.

Vitamins follow the same pattern as minerals – there is only limited information on their importance in birds of prey. Deficiencies have been reported in raptors and these will be discussed later. Bird and Ho (38) were sceptical of the claim that day-old chicks may be deficient in thiamine – in their study comparable figures were obtained for rats and for one strain of chicks. They drew attention, however, to the marked variation in values between strains of day-old chicks and this is an important point to remember whenever the nutritional value of chicks is being discussed. One must also bear in mind that even if the thiamine in the diet is adequate, it may not be available if there is also thiaminase present – for example, in chicks or fish.

Although the indications are that the mineral and vitamin contents of diets fed to raptors are adequate, one must bear in mind that this may not apply when birds are breeding, unwell, or perhaps, when wounds are healing. It must also be remembered that the young growing bird needs a diet of high quality and will fail to thrive on one that appears to be satisfactory for an adult. Another important point is that work in the chicken has shown that abnormal embryonic development, including peaks of mortality, can be due to nutritional deficiencies in the diet of the hen (113). Such deficiencies can include riboflavin (embryonic abnormalities from 9–14 days incubation), biotin (3 and 18–21 days), phosphorus (12–14 days), vitamin B12 (16–18 days), manganese (20–21 days) and vitamin E (2–4 days). Turkey embryos from eggs laid by hens deficient in pantothenic acid do not die in the egg but are unable to pip the shell and show morphological abnormalities. It is reasonable to assume that vitamin deficiencies in raptors could have comparable results – but controlled research is needed.

As was mentioned earlier, nutritional bone disease associated with a relative deficiency of calcium can be a problem in captive birds of prey. There is confusion about the nomenclature used for this condition; many authors speak of "rickets" and "osteomalacia" but these terms are best reserved for vitamin D deficiency. The word osteodystrophy is generally used throughout this book – or nutritional secondary hyperparathyroidism and/or hypocalcaemia when non-skeletal effects are being discussed.

Osteodystrophy is probably not so rare in falconers' birds as Keymer (249) suggested. It is particularly prevalent in young birds which are hand-reared prior to training. It may even occur in captive bred birds on an adequate diet if they are only offered muscle and viscera by their parents instead of bone (98). Small species, such as little owls and falconets, may develop osteodystrophy if fed on a diet of insects, such as crickets, supplemented only with meat; some aviculturists believe, erroneously, that the exoskeleton of such insects contains calcium.

The cause of osteodystrophy is usually an all-meat diet which supplies plenty of protein but offers a calcium/phosphorus ratio of approximately 1 : 15–1 : 40. The optimum ratio is 1·5:1·0 (407) and hence, on the meat diet, a disparity in levels of available calcium and phosphorus results. Serum calcium levels are initially maintained by resorption of calcium from the bones; as a result there is a breakdown of bone structure and spontaneous fractures and locomotory signs may result. Wallach and Flieg (407) discussed the early signs of the disease and described such clinical signs as drowsiness, poor growth, feather pecking and diarrhoea although it is not my experience that these are generally seen in raptors.

Both prevention and treatment are based on increasing the dietary calcium intake; calcium lactate may be used, or bonemeal, or a "natural diet" of adult mice or birds. Vitamin D must not be administered since it may cause further reduction of bone calcium. In severe cases, where bone changes are irreversible, the bird should be killed.

Older birds of prey may on occasion show decalcification of the bones and the clinical signs seen are similar to those in osteodystrophy. This possibly has a different aetiology. For example, Hamerton (193) described "spontaneous fractures due to senile rarefaction of the bones" in a Javan fish owl.

The production of soft-shelled eggs by female birds is another problem which can be associated with an inadequately balanced diet. Work with poultry (11) has shown that the recommended levels of calcium and vitamin D3 (3·6% and 1180 ICU/kg respectively) resulted in high egg production and good eggshell strength. A decrease from 0·55 to 0·26% in dietary phosphorus gave higher egg production and increased eggshell strength but reductions in calcium and vitamin D3 had the opposite effect. It is probable that a similar situation applies in birds of prey and therefore every effort should be made to ensure that breeding birds receive adequate calcium and vitamin D in their diet. Commercial strains of poultry show differences in eggshell strength and it is possible that there are similar variations within raptorial species. Other causes of soft or thin eggshells in birds of prey may include old age, infectious diseases and certain forms of poisoning.

The whole question of calcium metabolism in birds of prey needs more investigation. Cummings and colleagues (121) showed that falconiform birds digest the bones of their prey more thoroughly than strigiforms because of greater gastric acidity and it is therefore possible that an owl is more likely to suffer a calcium deficiency on a low bone diet. There is interest in calcium metabolism in free-living birds of prey and this is a field where captive specimens could play a useful part in research. Mundy and Ledger (306) reported several Cape vulture chicks with broken or deformed limbs, (unfortunately termed "rickets"), apparently on account of insufficient calcium in the diet; they postulated that griffon vultures depend upon carnivorous mammals for a supply of suitable pieces of bone which they feed to their chicks. This is a novel theory since previous authors, such as my friend Dr. David Houston (217) have questioned how vulture chicks, which appear only to eat meat, obtain calcium.

Vitamin deficiencies have been described in birds of prey but only rarely has a full diagnosis been possible. Ward (408) reported a thiamine deficiency in a peregrine which showed nervous signs and this is discussed in more detail in Chapter 8. Wallach (405) stated that thiamine deficiency was common in carnivorous birds fed diets high in fish on account of the high thiaminase content of the latter. He also drew attention to the paper by Friend and Trainer (162) which indicated that thiamine deficient birds frequently die of aspergillosis. Stauber (384) described a syndrome in an immature golden eagle which showed leg paralysis and he postulated that this was a riboflavin deficiency; a rapid clinical response followed the oral administration of a B-vitamin complex. A similar response to B vitamins has been seen in birds showing leg paralysis in Britain, especially goshawks, and I discuss this syndrome in Chapter 8.

I have not myself diagnosed vitamin D3 deficiency (true rickets) in raptors although a number of other authors refer to it, for example Halliwell and colleagues (189). It is important to distinguish rickets from nutritional osteodystrophy since the treatment of the two conditions is very different. Clinically it produces similar lesions but radiographically there is an important distinguishing feature in that the epiphyseal plates are widened and the articular surfaces of long bones enlarged (405). Unfortunately, as with other vitamins, it is possible that there may be a combination of deficiencies and imbalances in which case definitive diagnosis is not always possible. In such instances one often resorts to supplementation with both multivitamins and minerals, sometimes with surprisingly good clinical results.

The possible role of vitamin D in the maintenance of eggshell strength was mentioned earlier. While it is wise to ensure that a diet is not likely to be deficient in this vitamin, it must also be remembered that excess D3 may prove toxic. Some caution must, therefore, be observed. The role of sunlight in the metabolism of vitamin D in raptors is unknown.

I have occasionally noticed small subcutaneous haemorrhages in birds that are in poor condition. These usually overly joints and I tend to attribute them to physical damage but a vitamin K deficiency should perhaps be considered. Unexplained internal haemorrhage in birds at *post-mortem* examination might also be due to a deficiency of this vitamin.

There seems little doubt that vitamin A deficiency plays a part in raptor disease although sound data are again difficult to obtain. I have seen a number of birds with clinical signs of conjunctivitis, swollen eyelids, poor scaling and stomatitis which I consider suggestive of a vitamin A deficiency, possibly combined with other deficiencies. Such birds have usually responded to nursing and dietary supplements. Graham (173) described similar lesions and also attributed "corns" on the feet, anorexia and mouth lesions in hawks on an all meat diet to a vitamin A deficiency. Ocular lesions in hand-reared birds may also be associated with such a deficiency. A young European eagle owl I examined showed partial blindness and was examined clinically by Dr. F. G. Startup: histological examination of the eyes after death helped substantiate his view that an earlier dietary deficiency of vitamin A might have been involved.

Some other diseases show a clinical response to vitamin therapy and it is probable that a deficiency may be involved in the condition, possibly by retarding healing. For example, I treated a goshawk which showed loss of weight, a change of voice and a degree of dyspnoea with intramuscular vitamin A and there appeared to be a rapid and spectacular response. Other respiratory conditions have also appeared to respond to multivitamins by mouth or injection.

The possible role of vitamin A deficiency in foot conditions is discussed in Chapter 7.

Caution must always be taken in the use of vitamins. There is a tendency amongst falconers and aviculturists to assume that, because small quantities of vitamins can be beneficial, large amounts must be even more so. As a result some feed enormous quantities of vitamin supplement to their birds, often seven days a week. I have investigated non-specific diseases in such birds, with vague clinical signs of lethargy or poor condition, and believe that in some cases a nutritional disorder is resulting from *overuse* of vitamins. In a letter to the "Veterinary Record" in 1977 my friend Patrick Humphreys (221) drew attention to the possible hazards of giving a "blunderbuss" concoction of mixed minerals and vitamins to cage birds and my own view is that a similar situation may apply in birds of prey.

A possible exception may be in the newly hatched chick. Broiler chick survival and weight gain appear to be enhanced by the oral administration of multivitamins (211) and it would be interesting to see if a similar situation applies to raptors.

An important point in any consideration of the quality of a diet is that gastric digestion appears to be more efficient in falconiforms than strigiforms. Duke and colleagues (134), using captive raptors of seven species, showed that falconiform birds were able to digest a greater proportion of their diet than owls and as a result a smaller amount of the food consumed reappeared in their pellets.

Deleterious effects

The main deleterious effects of diet are:

(1) infectious and parasitic diseases
(2) poisoning

Diseases due to deficiencies or antagonists in the diet were discussed earlier.

Infectious and parasitic diseases derived from the food

These may be attributable to either infected or contaminated food.

Whilst the feeding of "natural" food, such as dead birds, will probably prevent the development of deficiencies, it can be fraught with danger. A number of infectious diseases may be transmitted thus, amongst them such potentially dangerous conditions as Newcastle disease and tuberculosis, and these and other examples are discussed in Chapter 5.

Certain parasites may be contracted from food, especially if it has become contaminated with faeces but also if the prey item is itself infected, for example with

Syngamus trachea or *Trichomonas gallinae*. These parasites are discussed in detail in Chapter 6. Keymer (249) suggested that *Capillaria* worms might be transmitted from prey to predator, citing as his example ptarmigan (*Lagopus mutus*) and gyrfalcons in Iceland. Certain ectoparasites can also be contracted in this way, especially fleas. At this point I should mention that it is not unusual to find avian lice and fleas in the faeces of raptors fed on wild birds; these parasites are ingested and pass through the intestinal tract and can be a source of considerable surprise to the parasitologist!

Poisoning

Food can also be the source of poisons and the broad subject of poisoning is therefore included in this chapter even though some chemicals may be acquired through routes other than the alimentary tract.

Poisoning is particularly relevant in birds of prey which are at the top of food chains and therefore in a vulnerable position. In free-living raptors the role of poisons is well recognised; for example, in a survey of wild bird deaths Jennings (232) found it to be one of the commonest causes of mortality in the Falconiformes. A similar situation can apply to captive birds. Woodford (422) and Jefferies and Prestt (230) recorded deaths in captive birds due to their being fed on woodpigeons which had ingested seed corn dressed with dieldrin.

The susceptibility of birds of prey to poisoning by chlorinated hydrocarbon insecticides is well recognised following extensive work on free-living birds in Europe, North America and elsewhere and this aspect will not be discussed here. The main hazard to captive birds is from contaminated food or quarry and experimental work with raptors has confirmed this threat (342). Affected birds are usually inco-ordinated and weak and refuse to feed. Fortunately, most falconers and aviculturists are aware of such dangers and acute poisoning is now less common, although, as Wheeldon and colleagues (414) pointed out, it may still occur and diagnosis can prove difficult. Those who keep the smaller species and feed them on insects should be wary of insecticides. I would suggest that the food item should be obtained from a reputable source; there are, for example, registered breeders of crickets in Britain!

In addition, it is possible that a number of birds in captivity may be suffering from sublethal effects. Some falconers in Britain report transient fits or muscle tremors in older birds which resolve spontaneously with supportive treatment. It is possible that these clinical signs are associated with pesticide levels since they often occur following a drop in condition (such as reduction in weight prior to flying) which is not sufficiently critical for hypoglycaemia to be a likely cause. A possible effect of pesticides on breeding is mentioned later.

The only birds I have examined personally in which poisoning was confirmed as the cause of death were owls from the Zoological Society of London, where dieldrin poisoning occurred as a result of using laboratory rodents which had been housed on sawdust impregnated with the insecticide (238). Affected birds either died unexpectedly or were found *in extremis*, often with torticollis or in convulsions. Gross *post-mortem* findings were usually absent although some showed incidental lesions, such as interstitial nephritis, or changes secondary to nervous signs. A falconer who fed his hawks on rodents from the same source also had a number of unexplained deaths and the same negative findings were noted at *post-mortem* examination. In his case it was not possible to analyse the tissues of the dead birds but is is reasonable to assume that dieldrin poisoning was again involved. These incidents have made many falconers and aviculturists aware of the continued danger of pesticides, even from apparently healthy laboratory mice, and it has been postulated that some of the failures to breed birds of prey, and behavioural changes noted in them, might be attributable to non-lethal doses of such chemicals.

Even commercial diets may pose a threat of pesticides. In their 1974 Joint Report F.A.O. and W.H.O. (141) emphasised the need for recommendations relating to residues of pesticides in animal foodstuffs and a paper by Kisling (259) gave figures for chlorinated hydrocarbon levels in a variety of commercial zoo diets. The latter were not high (maximum 0·36 ppm) but they emphasise the point that a "synthetic" product is not necessarily free of those contaminants that one associates with a "natural" diet.

Some of the birds I have examined *post mortem* have had tissues analysed by the Nature Conservancy or Institute of Terrestrial Ecology and a few free-living individuals showed significant residues of chlorinated hydrocarbon insecticides. Unfortunately financial considerations usually preclude the analysis of tissues from captive birds and as a result diagnoses of poisoning may be missed.

A definitive diagnosis of chlorinated hydrocarbon poisoning in birds of prey can usually only be made on the basis of toxicological examination. However, the combination of history and clinical signs may be suggestive of poisoning. Specific *post-mortem* lesions are rarely seen although it should be noted that Bell and Murton (26) reported internal haemorrhage as a common feature of organochlorine poisoning.

The role of polychlorinated biphenyls (PCB's) in birds of prey is still not fully understood although deaths have been reported in a number of non-raptorial species experimentally poisoned with the chemicals. Sileo and colleagues (376) discussed this in some detail and outlined the dilemma that faces the wildlife pathologist in attributing disease or death to this group of chemicals. Insofar as captive birds of prey are concerned the PCB's should probably be classed, together with other chlorinated hydrocarbons, as a potential hazard. A useful general reference to them is the book "PCB Poisoning and Pollution" edited by Higuchi (206).

A possible source of poisoning in captive birds of prey is the use of insecticidal preparations and great care should be taken in their use. An example was reported some years ago (80) when a lanner falcon died of lindane poisoning following the administration of an allegedly "non-toxic" poultry aerosol. In this case the product contained lindane (a form of benzene hexachloride) in addition to its pyrethrum base. It is most important that one checks the constituents of any insecticide intended for use on birds and that the manufacturers' instructions are followed exactly. If in any doubt the compound should not be used and, instead, a safer method of control followed.

It is not only the chlorinated hydrocarbon insecticides that are a hazard to captive birds of prey. A possible danger is alphachloralose used as a stupefying bait for pigeons and other species. In raptors the chemical can produce incoordination and lethargy which will usually wear off, without specific treatment, in 24–36 hours. I have no personal records of alphachloralose being a cause of death but this has been reported in free-living eagles, buzzards and hen harriers (79, 400).

Organophosphorus compounds may also cause disease or deaths. Again a possible source is insecticidal preparations. For example, my friend Dr. Brian Wheeldon told me of the deaths of two lanners within 24 hours of treatment for lice with a dichlorvos/fenitrothion aerosol product ("Nuvan Top": Ciba-Geigy) which is used in veterinary practice to control ectoparasites on dogs and cats. Affected birds can show muscle tremors, limb contractions and/or paralysis and diarrhoea. There is no information on the therapy of such cases in captivity but I have always assumed that atropine sulphate could be used, as is recommended in mammals (386). Shlosberg (374) successfully treated wild raptors which had ingested voles (*Microtus* sp.) containing the insecticide monocrotophos. He used pralidoxime iodide (100 mg/kg bodyweight), given intramuscularly, and drew attention to the apparent varying response in different avian species; this should be borne in mind when treating captive birds.

Contamination with oil is also discussed in Chapter 11. The subject is a complex one and some valuable work on it has been carried out by a number of individuals and institutions, particularly the Department of Zoology, University of Newcastle upon Tyne. Oiling produces both external and internal damage. The former results in heat loss and chilling, or drowning if the bird is in the water. Internally oil can produce enteritis and damage to kidneys, liver and lung. It is vital, therefore, to ensure that a bird which has oil on its plumage does not try to preen and hence ingest it. The bird should be wrapped up to prevent such an occurrence and this will also keep it warm; nursing is most important. In view of the relative rarity of oiling in birds of prey I shall not discuss treatment here but refer the reader to publications by the Research Unit (7, 8) and the chapter by Croxall (120) in the forthcoming book "First Aid and Care of Wild Birds".

Those who feed day-old chicks or rodents to their birds should check as to how they have been killed. I have examined histologically tissues from birds of prey which died in unusual circumstances after being fed chicks killed with excess amounts of carbon tetrachloride; the livers showed severe fatty infiltration. This strongly suggests that carbon tetrachloride may act as a poison to raptors and care should be taken when it is used. Other chemicals used to kill chicks have not, apparently, been associated with toxicity in birds of prey but the use of ether or chloroform may result in the chicks being refused as food, probably on account of their taste. Such agents are also likely to be toxic in large amounts. It is therefore best, whenever possible, to use carbon dioxide to kill chicks and rodents, or to despatch them manually.

Although not true "poisons", antibacterial and antiprotozoal drugs may be present in the food offered to raptors. Excessive quantities could conceivably cause toxicity but, more important, ingestion of low levels of such drugs may result in drug resistance and therefore every effort must be made to avoid their use.

A number of inorganic chemicals are known to pose a hazard to free-living birds of prey, amongst them mercury compounds (145) and thallium (75). Such poisons should be suspected whenever one is dealing with sick birds only recently taken from the wild – casualties, for example. Koeman and colleagues (263) used five captive kestrels to investigate the toxicity of methylmercurydicyandiamide. The chemical was fed to the birds in their diet of laboratory mice. The clinical signs seen in the kestrels consisted of paralysis and *post-mortem* examination revealed heart lesions, demyelination of the spinal cord and mild peritonitis. In the case of thallium, some limited experimental work has been carried out using captive eagles and this suggested that the acute oral LD50 lies between 60 and 120 mg/kg/day. Clinical signs associated with ingestion included inco-ordination, loss of appetite, distress calls and brachypnoea (22).

Lead poisoning does not appear to be an important problem in raptors – probably because ingested lead shot (the usual source of toxicity in other birds) is regurgitated in the pellet. However, Locke and colleagues (277) reported the death of a captive Andean condor due to aspergillosis and lead poisoning; the bird had been fed on shot animals. There were clinical signs of unthriftiness and lead poisoning was originally suspected on finding characteristic acid-fast intranuclear inclusions in kidney tubular cells. More recently Benson and colleagues (27) reported fatal lead poisoning in a captive prairie falcon which had been fed largely on duck heads containing lead shot. The bird showed clinical signs of visual disturbance and, occasionally, ataxia. Gross *post-mortem* findings included an accumulation of sero-sanguineous fluid in the pericardial sac and a green discolouration of the intestinal tract. They suggested that the longterm feeding of material containing lead shot might cause chronic or even acute poisoning. I personally believe this to be uncommon and would think it safe for captive birds of prey to be fed animals that have been shot so long as this is not done excessively. It has long been recognised that lead shot embedded in the tissues is unlikely to be toxic and it is important that surgery is not performed to remove such shot unless it is mechanically interfering with function.

Carbon monoxide can, under certain circumstances, prove hazardous to birds of prey. A bird kept temporarily in a garage can be poisoned if the ventilation is poor and MacPhail (286) described a probable case of carbon monoxide poisoning in a goshawk which was "manned" (accustomed to humans and disturbance) by being carried on a perch in a car. The bird was lethargic and breathless and finally became unconscious and died. The case was not confirmed *post mortem* but was almost certainly due to car fumes.

Toxins from bacteria may cause disease or death in birds of prey. These are discussed in Chapter 5. A toxaemic state may also arise if a bird becomes constipated or suffers an impaction of the intestine or cloaca: the affected bird is depressed and shows abdominal distension and discomfort.

There is a report of toxaemia in two young peregrines which was traced to "toxic" (presumably rancid) halibut liver oil (423). Care should be taken to ensure that any fish oils used are fresh and uncontaminated.

An example of environmental pollution, although not strictly a poison, is that of anthracosis. *Post-mortem* and histopathological examination of birds which have spent much of their lives in a city will reveal black debris in the lungs and air sacs. This is normal and does not appear to be associated with disease.

Although there are specific antidotes for a few poisons, some of which have been mentioned, usually it is necessary to apply general treatment. A useful guide to clinical signs and therapy in mammals is given in the paper by Stevenson and Carter (386) and reference can usefully be made to it. Many of the antidotes recommended in that paper have not been used in birds and are possibly ineffective but can be tried in the absence of more definite information. Nursing is always of importance and a free respiratory passage must be maintained. If there is severe respiratory distress oxygen should be given. Nervous signs can be controlled with phenobarbitone, diazepam or primidone. If the poison has been ingested the crop or stomach should be washed out with saline. A useful emetic is a strong salt solution while liquid paraffin or glycerine can be used as a purgative. A general safe antidote recommended by Andrew Greenwood consists of a combination of activated charcoal, kaolin, light magnesium oxide and tannic acid (101) and although doubt has been expressed in medical circles over such "universal antidotes" (171) it is worth a try. The alimentary tract of birds is very different from that of mammals – particularly in that ingesta passes through very rapidly – and therefore extrapolation from man and domestic species is not necessarily relevant.

There are many other substances which may cause poisoning in birds of prey but on which no information appears to be available. Examples are disinfectants, such as phenols, formaldehyde and many herbicidal and fungicidal compounds. Useful sources of reference in this respect are the chapter by Peckham in "Diseases of Poultry" (332) and the section on poisons in Arnall and Keymer's "Bird Diseases" (15) which should be consulted in the event of poisoning being suspected. Many chemicals have been incriminated in cases of poisoning in domestic and wild birds and the absence of any reports of them in captive birds of prey is no reason to believe that they do not, or will not, occur.

Acceptability and digestibility

If a diet is to achieve maximum results it must be acceptable to the bird and satisfactorily digested by it. The digestibility is related to both the diet itself and the species of bird and will not be discussed here; the reader is referred to standard publications on the subject, especially those dealing specifically with raptors such as the paper by Duke and colleagues (134) referred to earlier.

I assume here that the term "acceptable" includes "palatable". Some items are totally unacceptable to birds; a bizarre example was the piece of sliced orange offered by airline staff to a black sparrowhawk that I transported by air from

Nairobi to London! Even carnivorous diets may, however, prove unacceptable for a variety of reasons. The raptor might not recognise it as food; for example, a newly captured buzzard may ignore a white mouse unless the latter is first opened to expose blood, muscles and viscera. A small bird, such as a merlin, may recognise that a dead hamster is edible but be unable to pierce the rodent's skin with its beak. Some species, which in the wild take only birds, may at first refuse to eat laboratory rodents but this attitude usually changes after a few days, particularly if efforts are made to introduce the new diet gradually. More often it is an individual bird that shows marked distaste for a certain item – I have noticed this particularly when sakers are offered mice – and this must be borne in mind by the veterinary surgeon who hospitalises a sick bird and, perhaps, offers it a different diet. Birds in aviaries will also become accustomed to certain foods and take some time to accept something unusual. A sudden change from chicks to mice, or even (as my friend David Bird has pointed out) the inclusion of black chicks as well as the usual yellow ones, may result in uneaten food being left at the end of the day. If birds are rearing youngsters the result can be hungry nestlings or even cannibalism.

Although live food is used for captive birds of prey in some countries its use is, in general, undesirable and in Britain may lay one open to prosecution under the Protection of Animals Act.

The parts of a dead animal eaten also vary between species and individuals. Much depends on size. A buzzard will swallow a mouse whole while a kestrel tears portion off it and may discard the intestines and stomach. Some raptors pluck a bird before eating it. All these variables have to be considered when investigating a disease problem that may be associated with nutrition.

Under the heading "acceptability" I shall discuss the main diets available for feeding to the larger birds of prey. I shall not refer to the use of maggots, meal worms and other invertebrates, nor the provision of lower vertebrates such as fish, amphibians and reptiles, other than to make the general point that *any* diet must be clean and from a reliable source. Food must be hygienically stored and pests of all types denied access. When using rodents or chicks it is wise to deprive them of food for six hours prior to death; this will result in empty stomachs and the birds are less likely to leave the viscera uneaten.

There are three main groups of diet available for the feeding of captive birds of prey. These are:

(1) Butcher's meat – with or without supplementation.
(2) Commercially prepared diets.
(3) "Natural" diets of either wild or laboratory bred mammals or birds or commercially produced poultry.

Each of these has its devotees; elsewhere in this chapter the pros and cons of each are covered to a certain extent.

Unsupplemented butcher's meat cannot be recommended as a standard diet even though many falconers' birds appear to thrive on it. It can be used for some of the time but must be supplemented. In view of our lack of knowledge of the nutrient requirements of raptors I am sceptical of commercial diets, although I recognise that they have been used successfully (258). Wild birds and mammals are a convenient source of food – they can be shot, trapped or picked off the road – but they constitute an unknown entity and may harbour pathogens or poisons. If they are to be used they should be opened with a knife and any showing pathological lesions, such as white foci in the liver, discarded. I personally prefer a "natural" diet of laboratory bred rodents which can either be obtained from a medical or veterinary institution or bred specifically for the purpose. Mice and rats can be a source of infection to both birds and humans and one must ensure that any used are from a clean source. They should not be purchased from a petshop or private individual but from a recognised laboratory. In Britain it is wise to obtain them from one of the sources approved by the Medical Research Council's Laboratory Animals Centre Accreditation Scheme (393). Commercially produced poultry, especially day-old chicks, were discussed in some detail earlier in this chapter. They are certainly very convenient in terms of storage and allocation of individual rations. Personally, however, I retain some misgivings about them, primarily because there is always the danger (small though it is) of infection with a poultry pathogen. There is also the slight doubt about their nutritive value, especially in view of the variation between strains and, probably, batches. However, many establishments have used day-old chicks successfully, sometimes with a vitamin/mineral supplement, and reported excellent captive breeding results. Doubts over their nutritive value could be reduced if they were reared for a few weeks before being killed but this is both time-consuming and expensive. An alternative approach is to use quail (*Coturnix coturnix*). These too may be a source of infection but this is unlikely if they come from a clean source and have been bred under laboratory conditions. Pigeons are known to be a potential source of many raptor pathogens and, popular though they may be with falconers, I do not recommend them.

Probably the answer to the feeding of captive birds of prey is variety. This should help to eliminate the possibility of dietary deficiencies and may reduce the danger of poisoning from a single source. It will also facilitate a change of diet, if one item becomes unavailable. Much, however, depends upon the size and financial status of one's enterprise, the birds being maintained, and the sources of food available.

CHAPTER 10

Anaesthesia and surgery

Anaesthesia

It must be remembered that competent handling or restraint can sometimes replace the need for anaesthesia. Such techniques are discussed in Chapter 3. However, this is not to suggest that painful procedures should be inflicted upon a raptor without adequate anaesthesia or analgesia. The welfare of the bird should always be paramount.

Enormous advances have been made in the anaesthesia of birds, including raptors, in the past five years and it is now difficult to believe that, even in the early 1960's, general anaesthesia was thought by many falconers to be synonymous with a death sentence for their bird. Gradually, however, the need for efficient and safe anaesthesia grew, and by the late 1960's a number of agents were being used with considerable success (87, 88). New anaesthetic agents appeared for use in mammals and many of these were found to have a place in avian work. At the time of writing (1977) it is true to say that a range of agents, both inhalation and injectable, are available for birds of prey and that improved techniques are dramatically reducing the risks associated with their use. It must be emphasised, however, that very little research has been carried out on the physiological effect of anaesthetic agents in raptors; an exception was the work by Bonath (48, 49) who used buzzards, amongst other birds, in his studies on the effect of inhalation anaesthetics on various parameters.

In his chapter in the book "Small Animal Anaesthesia" Arnall (13) outlined the precautions for avian anaesthesia and the veterinary surgeon who deals with birds should be aware of the particular features of this Class of animals. It must be remembered that birds have a high metabolic rate; as such they usually absorb, metabolise and excrete drugs rapidly. In some respects they are particularly sensitive to anaesthetic agents. Inhalation anaesthesia can be complicated by the presence of air sacs which permit gaseous exchange during both inspiration and expiration (Figure 5c). Assessment of depth of anaesthesia may prove difficult because the abolition of reflexes does not follow a set pattern as in man.

Local analgesia can pose problems in birds since there is evidence of sensitivity to the effects of the procaine group (161). However, in recent years a number of people have suggested that the LD50 of procaine in birds is comparable to that in mammals and the reason for toxicity in the past was overdosing. The safe use of small volumes of 2% lignocaine in larger birds, including raptors, would help substantiate this view but it is obvious that more work is needed. I have not personally encountered toxicity to local analgesics in birds of prey. However, I have seen and treated hawks which have reacted adversely to procaine penicillin. These birds (which were not injected by myself!) developed almost immediate clinical signs of inco-ordination, ataxia and muscle rigidity, including a degree of opisthotonos. In each case a small dose of corticosteroid was administered and there was recovery within 15 minutes. I am therefore wary of the procaine group. I would suggest that great caution is exercised in the use of local analgesics; personally I very rarely use them. A possible exception is for ocular work; Martin and colleagues (293) used 4% benoxinate hydrochloride to anaesthetise the cornea of tawny owls. An ethyl chloride spray can be used to "freeze" an area of skin (for example, on a digit) and I have found this useful for the removal of small lesions or the aspiration of pus. The effect is short-lived, however, and it is probably wise, and less traumatic for the bird, to administer an ultra short-acting general anaesthetic.

There are few sedative or ataractic (tranquilliser) drugs of practical value in birds of prey although diazepam can be useful in some cases. My own experience of phenothiazine derivatives, such as chlorpromazine and acetylpromazine, has been disappointing both orally and by injection; in most cases the birds showed no clinical effect although a combination of acetylpromazine with ketamine appeared to produce smoother recovery than ketamine alone. Low doses of some of the parenteral anaesthetics will produce an hypnotic state and it is to this that I refer when I use the term "sedation" in this book. However, such sedation is sometimes of limited practical value since the bird is usually unsteady on its feet and can be roused. Lumb and Jones (282) referred to Dodge's use of reserpine to quieten newly captured prairie falcons. Following two days oral treatment these birds were in an hypnotic state which lasted 5–6 days; during this time they had to be forcefed. A number of tranquillising agents have found favour in poultry in recent years, for example metoserpate hydrochloride, and these reduce activity and "flightiness" considerably. They could possibly play a part in birds of prey but I have not yet had a chance to investigate them.

There is also no proven analgesic for the relief of pain in raptors. Small quantities of sodium salicylate appear harmless when given orally and may reduce pain or discomfort but there are no reliable data on their action in birds.

I have never used a muscle relaxant in a bird of prey and have been unable to trace any reference to the subject.

General anaesthetics for birds of prey include both inhalation and parenteral agents. Some of the latter, such as metomidate, are probably better termed "hypnotic agents" but are included under the heading of general anaesthetics in this chapter. The effect of such agents depends upon the dose given and the species involved; there is also considerable individual variation in response. The general anaesthetics that I most regularly use are listed opposite.

These and other agents will each be discussed. However, detailed information will not be given since this is available in the published papers to which reference is made.

Inhalation agents may be administered by face mask, intubation or anaesthetic chamber. In the case of the first two, anaesthesia will often already have been in-

Administration	Anaesthetic	Approximate duration of surgical anaesthesia
Inhalation	Methoxyflurane	Varies
	Halothane	Varies
	Ether	Varies
Parenteral		
Intramuscular	Metomidate	15–30 minutes
Intramuscular	Ketamine hydrochloride	15–30 minutes
Intravenous	CT 1341	5–10 minutes

duced, or premedication given, using an injectable agent. Jones (239), in a review of anaesthesia in birds, suggested that inhalation agents should be used alone only when light anaesthesia is required for a few minutes. This is probably sound advice; premedicants, such as ketamine or metomidate, permit balanced anaesthesia to be used with minimum risk. Unfortunately, in the same article, Jones did not warn his readers of some of the contraindications of certain injectable agents in raptors. Ryder-Davies (360) advised against exceeding 2% halothane when anaesthetising birds but this has not been my experience with birds of prey. A small face mask can be applied to the head of a hawk either to induce or maintain anaesthesia; in the case of the former it is preferable if the bird is hooded (for example, on a perch or falconer's "cadge") and the mask not actually allowed to touch the beak or hood. A considerable amount of anaesthetic agent is wasted in this way but if 4% halothane plus O_2/N_2O (50:50) is administered, the bird will gradually become sleepy and unsteady on its feet. It can then be grasped firmly around the wings and anaesthesia continued using 2–3% halothane with the mask tightly against the head. Anaesthesia can be maintained by face mask, but it is cheaper and safer to intubate. Cat endotracheal tubes are suitable for large birds, for example eagles and vultures, but for most species it will be necessary to fashion something suitable from plastic tubing. The tube part of "butterfly" needles can be used for this purpose, or disposable intravenous drip tubing. The glottis is readily visible at the back of the tongue (Figure 14). Local analgesia of the area is not necessary and the tube will slide down with ease to the bifurcation; it should then be withdrawn slightly to ensure that it does not accidentally enter one bronchus only and occlude the other. It is not necessary to use a cuff but careful positioning of the head and neck is important to prevent kinking or obstruction of the tube. Green (175) suggested that inflowing gases should always be warmed and moisturised to help prevent loss of bodyheat. He also recommended a gas flow of approximately three times the respiratory minute volume of the patient – a 300 gramme bird has a minute volume of approximately 250 ml.

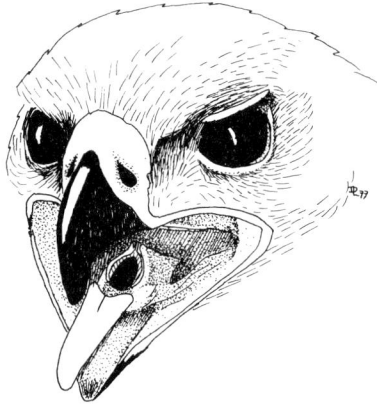

Fig. 14   Head of a tawny eagle showing the open glottis at the back of the tongue and demonstrating
how easily intubation can be carried out

An anaesthetic chamber is useful for induction of inhalation anaesthesia in small birds. Ideally it should be attached to an anaesthetic machine and the agents pumped through. Alternatively a wad of cotton wool can be impregnated with the agent and placed in the chamber but care must be taken (a) to ensure that the bird does not come into physical contact with it, and (b) that there is adequate air to ensure anaesthesia rather than asphyxia. Construction of the chamber is important; many plastic compounds will be damaged by ether. The sides of the chamber should be covered so as not to disturb the bird unnecessarily. The patient should be removed when it is recumbent, with eyes closed and breathing regularly; anaesthesia can be maintained by facemask or tube.

Methoxyflurane is a safe but relatively non-potent agent. It is of great value in wild bird casualties which are often a poor anaesthetic risk. Both induction and recovery tend to be slower than with halothane. Methoxyflurane is valuable for light anaesthesia; for example, for radiography or removal of a plaster, and appears to provide good analgesia.

Ether is a relatively safe anaesthetic which is used by many veterinary surgeons. Its main disadvantage is its inflammability which renders it unsuitable for use when thermocautery is involved.

Halothane is probably the inhalation anaesthetic of choice for surgical procedures. It is, however, potent and must be used with care. It causes a marked reduction in blood pressure in birds, together with a drop in respiration rate and body temperature (48, 49). Bilo and colleagues (36) made a study of halothane anaesthesia in birds and, although their paper is in German, it is worthy of reference. It illustrates techniques of induction and discusses both reflexes and the use of the ECG in monitoring anaesthesia.

Other inhalation agents which can be used include trichlorethylene and cyclopropane. As with all anaesthetics these have their champions. The important point to remember is that experience of an agent counts for a great deal and the veterinary surgeon who feels confident with a certain anaesthetic is often wise to stick to that rather than embark upon another, new, method.

Parenteral agents may be given by the intravenous, intramuscular or intraperitoneal routes. However, the last can be hazardous and I no longer use it in birds of prey other than for euthanasia. For intravenous injection the brachial vein should be used and the technique for locating this was described earlier; it has the disadvantage that the bird must be cast on its back. For intramuscular administration either the thigh or pectoral muscles can be used. Some authors have suggested that injections into the pectorals may impair flight; this has not been my experience but I have seen (on histological examination) severe damage to these muscles following injection of tylosin and oxytetracycline and would therefore suggest that the leg muscles are used in preference.

Barbiturates are of limited value in birds of prey in view of their respiratory depressant effect and their poor analgesia. Sawby and Gessaman (362) used pentobarbitone when implanting electrodes in American kestrels and reported that "a few kestrels died". Nelson and colleagues (315) described pancreatectomy in the great horned owl using sodium phenobarbital and did not report any adverse effects; they noted that owls needed a smaller dose than ducks of comparable weight. I have used thiopentone intravenously and pentobarbitone both intramuscularly and intravenously with relatively good results; such agents can be used, with care, if other anaesthetics are not available.

A combination of pentobarbital sodium, chloral hydrate, magnesium sulphate, propylene glycol and ethanol ("Equithesin" Jensen-Salsbury) has been used successfully in the United States in a wide variety of birds, including raptors (371) and was also recommended by Bonath (49). I have no personal experience of this agent but would draw attention to Seidensticker and Reynold's comment that it probably has a narrow margin of safety (371).

Metomidate was introduced into bird of prey work seven years ago (87) – when it was called "Methoxymol" – and has since proved to be useful in a wide variety of species. The drug appears to be very safe and in Kenya was used at monthly intervals (with occasional exceptions) for 36 months in two African harrier hawks; never were ill-effects observed and regular clinical, haematological and parasitological examinations showed no associated abnormalities. However, Cadle and Martin (65) reported four fatalities in tawny owls. None of these occurred on the first occasion and they suggested that in two cases an antigen-antibody reaction might have occurred. The two deaths were considered a mystery and, unfortunately, neither *post-mortem* examination nor histology was performed. Electrocardiography was carried out during anaesthesia and episodes of asystole and bradycardia were noted. Later in their studies oxygen was given routinely. I cannot account for the fatalities experienced by these authors. My own opinion of metomidate was substantiated by Ryder-Davies (359) who described it as a "very useful drug and a safe one".

Metomidate can be used on its own but on occasion may need supplementation with an inhalation agent. Alternatively a smaller dose can be employed as a premedicant and anaesthesia maintained with halothane. Metomidate is water soluble and solutions of different strengths can be prepared for birds of varying sizes. In low doses it is ideal for minor manipulative techniques and for such procedures as examination of plumage or removal of ectoparasites. It was used successfully by Martin and colleagues (293) in studies on vision in owls and by myself for surgical laparotomy and sexing in a variety of species. A disadvantage of its use is that regurgitation of food or pellets may occur; the bird should be carefully checked for evidence of this and if so, the material promptly removed and the buccal cavity swabbed dry. Another important point is that the optimum dose for Old World vultures appears to be considerably less than for other birds of prey (218).

In the past three years the dissociative anaesthetic ketamine hydrochloride has largely replaced metomidate as the parenteral agent of choice. Its use in birds of prey was first reported by Borzio (50) and several authors have subsequently advocated it in these species. It has similar effects to metomidate and, like it, may need supplementation by inhalation agents. However, incremental doses alone will often prove satisfactory in deepening anaesthesia for surgery.

In Britain ketamine is almost invariably used intramuscularly but in the United States it has been recommended, together with diazepam, by the intravenous route (353). Redig and Duke drew attention to the increased sensitivity of owls to the anaesthetic combination and also emphasised the need to consider the body fat when calculating the dose; the latter point is probably applicable to other parenteral agents. More recently Redig (351) reported that he had found a ketamine-xylazine mixture preferable to ketamine-diazepam, again by the intravenous route. In his paper Borzio (50) pointed out that ketamine is eliminated by the kidney; he recommended fluid therapy in debilitated birds and when the recovery period is prolonged. The possible effects of ketamine on the avian adrenal are mentioned in Chapter 11. In Britain ketamine is available at a concentration of 100 mg/ml or, for human use, 50 mg/ml and 10 mg/ml. Use of these different preparations helps ensure accurate dosage when dealing with birds of varying sizes.

Use of a steroid anaesthetic was first reported in birds of prey in 1973 (106). The drug consists of alphaxalone and alphadalone acetate in polyoxyethylated castor oil and was originally designated "CT 1341"; in the interest of brevity this name is used throughout this book. In the initial work, in Kenya, it proved useful and relatively safe in both chickens and birds of prey. Since then it has established itself, by the intravenous route, as the parenteral agent of choice for ultra-short anaesthesia of raptors. It is best given into the brachial vein; within a few seconds the bird is anaesthetised and duration of anaesthesia is usually 5–10 minutes. Incremental doses of CT 1341 by either the intravenous or intramuscular route will prolong anaesthesia. Alternatively it can be used to induce anaesthesia which is then maintained with an inhalation agent, for example halothane, as described by Holt (215). Very few fatalities have been reported with CT 1341 but Patrick Redig and I encountered adverse reactions to the drug in red-tailed hawks (one of which died) and we later recommended care in its use in this species (110). Abnormal cardiac rhythms were observed in six out of seven birds anaesthetised by my friend Laurence Frank (156). Subsequently Cribb and Haigh (118) carried out electrocardiographic monitoring of birds, including a red-tailed hawk, under CT 1341 anaesthesia and reported a high incidence of sinus arrest and tachycardia. As a result they also urged caution in its use. Despite these reports the drug remains of great value and an important advantage of it is that regurgitation rarely occurs, even if the bird has food in its crop. I rarely use CT 1341 by the intramuscular route but in small raptors this can be of value, particularly if anaesthesia is to be maintained, or deepened, with an inhalation agent.

Other injectable agents have been used in raptors with varying degrees of success. Xylazine has been reported to be useful in a number of species of bird (274) but I have no experience of its use. In 1969 Mr. R. B. Comyn told me that he had used fentanyl and fluanisolone in birds of prey but again I have not tried these agents. Phencyclidine has been used in small numbers of birds by myself and other investigators; my experience was that it produced disturbing and possibly dangerous clinical signs of opisthotonos and severe inco-ordination. There are several other drugs that might be of use in birds of prey and further work is needed on the topic.

The pre- and post-operative care of raptors plays an important role in ensuring successful anaesthesia. Pre-operatively the bird should be observed carefully for 48 hours and, if appropriate, monitored clinically and haematologically. The bird should not be fed in the six hours preceding anaesthesia but starvation for longer than 18 hours in the small birds (e.g. sparrowhawk and merlin) can prove dangerous. My own approach is to feed birds 6–12 hours beforehand but I ensure that this does not include roughage since this can result in regurgitation or increased intra-abdominal pressure. Atropine given by injection 15 minutes before induction will help reduce salivation and is particularly advisable when metomidate is being used.

Induction of anaesthesia in birds is usually not accompanied by marked excitation since even by the intramuscular route induction time is short. During induction with an injectable agent the bird may shake its head, fluff out its feathers and extend limbs. Induction by inhalation may again be accompanied by head shaking and occasionally wing flapping. Once a bird starts to become unsteady on its feet it is often wise to restrain it for further induction.

During anaesthesia the bird must be maintained at a constant temperature, preferably 32°–35°C. An operating light will provide overhead warmth but it may also be advisable to lay the bird on a heating pad or well insulated material. Assessment of depth of anaesthesia depends upon careful observation of the bird and, as was mentioned earlier, the reflexes cannot be used to the same extent as in mammals. Personally I rely on respiratory rate, the response to pressure (squeezing of the foot) and to pain during surgery. In addition, muscle tone (extending a wing or opening the mouth), heart rate and colour of mucous membranes can be used. In some species other indicators may be useful; a rather unusual example to which I have referred elsewhere (96) is the change of face colour in the African harrier hawk from red to yellow as anaesthesia lightened! During surgery observation of the bird may be difficult on account of operating cloths. If possible the head should be exposed. Movement of the base of the tail will correspond with respiration and it is important that this should be visible. Attention must be paid to the respiratory tract to ensure that pellet material, undigested food or mucus is not occluding the glottis. If a bird has obstructed nares it must either have its beak held open or be intubated. The use of an endotracheal tube is always useful, even if no inhalation anaesthetic is being used, since it helps ensure a clear airway and reduces the risk of ingesta being inhaled. In the case of the vultures the positioning of the head is important since asphyxia can occur if the neck becomes twisted (95).

Anaesthetic emergencies occur from time to time. Apnoea is the most common. It is often seen following the use of CT 1341 by the intravenous route but usually respiration recommences within a minute. Occasionally, however, it persists or, alternatively, the bird suddenly stops breathing during surgery and very quickly the tongue appears cyanosed. The first step is to ensure that the mouth and glottis are clear and to place the bird on its breast, when respiration will often resume spontaneously – respiratory embarrassment seems to be more of a problem when a bird is on its back. If breathing does not start oxygen should be given and artificial respiration (squeezing of the rib cage) carried out every 20–30 seconds. If oxygen is not available a piece of tubing can be placed in the trachea (an endotracheal tube can be used) and a 20 ml syringe used to pump air backwards and forwards over the lungs. In cases where an inhalation agent is being used and apnoea occurs it is possible that a reservoir of anaesthetic remains in an air sac – an example of mine was an osprey that took several hours to recover from ether – and in such cases it might be useful to insert a needle into an abdominal air sac and draw off some anaesthetic. This is not, however, a technique that I have yet tried.

Exaggerated breathing movement may indicate airway obstruction: the bird's mouth must be opened to ensure that the glottis is patent. As Green (175) has pointed out, this can be mistaken for a lightening of anaesthesia – with possible fatal results.

Cardiac arrest may also occur. Occasionally it lasts only a few seconds and the the heartbeat recommences but in most instances it persists and, in my experience, shows no response to external massage. I have injected adrenaline into the heart in such cases but with no success. Cardiac arrhythmias are not all all uncommon during anaesthesia: I am uncertain of their significance.

Overdosage of an anaesthetic agent can occur and may result in respiratory depression and failure to respond to stimuli. The former can be treated as outlined earlier for apnoea. Stimulants, such as nikethamide, are used in mammals and may have a place in raptor work but I have no personal experience of them.

Immediately following anaesthesia a raptor should be wrapped firmly in a towel or similar material and kept warm, if possible on a heating pad or in an insulated container. The optimum temperatures are 32–35°C. Administration of oxygen will help accelerate recovery from an inhalation agent. Failure to restrain the bird adequately can result in post-operative trauma since wing flapping and other activity commonly follow the use of injectable agents, especially ketamine. Efficient immobilisation will help prevent this and will also enable the bird to be fed by hand or given fluids. Alternatively a small raptor, such as a merlin, can be placed in a cloth bag which is suspended from a shelf so that the bird inside cannot strike anything. This method may sound crude but is usually very successful. Once the bird is able to stand, it can be returned to its enclosure but is usually best kept warm in a recovery box for at least a further 6–12 hours.

Occasionally it may be necessary to recapture an escaped bird of prey. Although mechanical methods of capture are probably preferable, drugs can be employed: for example, Ebedes (136) used phencyclidine for free-living vultures. I have found oral phenobarbitone or pentobarbitone valuable but somewhat variable in effect. Phenobarbitone is given in tablet form and hidden in the food. Pentobarbitone is best injected intraperitoneally into a mouse or chick and then the dead animal offered to the escaped bird.

Euthanasia should be mentioned. At times it is necessary to kill a bird on humanitarian grounds and it is important that this is done with the minimum of discomfort or pain. Physical methods such as shooting or a blow to the head are often the most humane and rapid but are frequently repugnant to laymen. If a chemical method is to be used then an overdose of an anaesthetic agent is permissible. Pentobarbitone or ketamine can be injected by any route but CT 1341, thiopentone and methohexitone should be used intravenously. Of the inhalation agents halothane, ether or chloroform are probably best and these can be pumped into an anaesthetic chamber or similar container. Under no circumstances should a bird be disposed of until it has undergone *rigor mortis*, and, in any case, the carcass should, whenever possible, be submitted for *post-mortem* examination.

Surgery

Surgical techniques in birds of prey do not differ greatly from those used in other birds and some examples of the latter were described in "Bird Diseases" by Arnall and Keymer (15). Most of the more important procedures in raptors are discussed elsewhere in this book – for example, fixation of fractures (Chapter 4) and surgical treatment of bumblefoot (Chapter 7). Others will be described briefly in this section and mention will be made of general considerations when performing surgery on raptors.

Although asepsis is important in surgery, there is little doubt that post-operative infections are relatively rare in birds compared with mammals. For this reason one can afford to be less fastidious over the preparation and protection of the surgical site. This is important since over-enthusiastic plucking of feathers or use of disinfectants can result in considerable loss of bodyheat and the possibility of shock.

The positioning of a bird for surgery has been mentioned previously and my friend Colin Green, in his book (175) discussed this subject in some detail. He stressed that birds should not be kept on their backs for long periods since hypotension can develop due to reduced venous return. Nor should limbs be overextended too forcibly. All movements during surgery should be made slowly and gently.

In the smaller birds of prey blood loss can be a problem. Every effort must therefore be made to control haemorrhage using artery forceps or, if the method of anaesthesia permits, thermocautery. If considerable blood loss is expected the bird should be given glucose-saline subcutaneously prior to surgery.

Some procedures can hardly be described as "surgical" but should be mentioned. Most present no problems to the experienced falconer or aviculturist but occasionally a veterinary surgeon will be asked for advice, especially over difficult cases. The regular clipping ("coping") of talons and beak is an example. In my opinion coping is best carried out using sharp (veterinary) nail clippers or even a pair of garden secateurs. A strong light will help localise the blood vessels – which should not be cut! In the case of the beak, manicuring can be carried out with a scalpel blade or sharp knife and a nail file or piece of sandpaper. If there is extensive damage to the beak, it is often helpful to anaesthetise the bird lightly during the procedure. Falconers' birds that are kept on stone blocks will tend to keep their own talons and beak short.

Falconers have a long tradition of experience in the care, and to a certain extent repair, of their birds' feathers and some of the techniques used are discussed in Chapter 11.

Increasingly large numbers of falconers' birds are now telemetered and the use of a short-acting anaesthetic will make the attachment of the transmitter to a leg or tail much easier.

Deflighting of captive raptors may be requested, especially involving large species such as vultures and eagles in safari parks. The simplest method is to clip the primaries (or even alternate primaries in some species) on one wing; the outer primary should be left intact on aesthetic grounds and since it helps protect the other feathers. This technique will usually prove successful, and is of course painless, but flight will be possible again once the bird has moulted. Amputation of a wing at the carpus is an irreversible alternative and should be performed under general anaesthesia. Other techniques are used in waterfowl, amongst them a patagiectomy whereby a portion of the patagial membrane, on the leading edge of the wing, is removed surgically so that the bird is unable to extend the treated wing (358). This and other procedures may be of value in raptors but I have no experience of them.

In recent years there has been great concern over the theft of captive birds of prey and the falconer, in particular, may seek advice over methods of marking his hawks. It is possible that identification of an individual bird will become an important subject if statutory control over the keeping of raptors is introduced. Tattooing is carried out as in mammals, using the skin of the feet or wing. Other methods of recognising birds include close-up photographs of the soles of the feet – these are usually different in each individual, especially if it has had foot lesions – and radiography, which may reveal the presence of lead shot, healed fractures or skeletal abnormalities (104).

With the increase in interest in captive breeding the veterinary surgeon may be asked for assistance with artificial insemination. I do not propose to discuss this in detail since information is available from many publications. Collection of semen may be cooperative – in which case veterinary attention is unlikely to be needed – or by massage. The latter involves a certain amount of physical stress and smaller volumes of semen are collected than by voluntary ejaculation. A useful paper for reference is that by Bird and colleagues (40). For insemination, inversion of the oviduct is useful and increases the chance of fertilisation. A detailed description, with a line drawing, is given in the paper by Boyd and colleagues (53) and reference should be made to it.

Minor surgery may be required for the removal of unsightly or pathological lesions, such as papillomata, or for histological diagnosis. Cautery is very useful in such work and cryosurgery is likely to prove valuable in future. I must repeat how important it is that a raptor is anaesthetised for a surgical procedure, even if the latter is only brief. As long ago as 1655 Markham (288) writing about the surgical suturing ("seeling") of hawks' eyelids stated:

"But this manner of seeling of Hawkes, is both troublesome, painfull and dangerous to the Hawke".

One still hears disturbing reports of raptors being operated upon without anaesthesia and this is, in my opinion, quite unacceptable in the second half of the 20th century.

It may be necessary to operate upon the crop in order to remove impacted material or to clean and suture traumatic injuries. The procedure is similar to that in the fowl. A stab incision is recommended and the crop and skin must be sutured separately.

Occasionally veterinary surgeons receive requests for a raptor to be "de-voiced" because it makes too much noise. The usual cause is a bird taken too early from the nest – a so-called "screamer". I refuse to perform this operation on ethical grounds but I know that it has been carried out, with varying success, in Britain and the United States. The technique first described for the fowl by Durant (135) would appear to be applicable.

A laparotomy may be necessary for the purpose of diagnosis or treatment. It can be carried out safely so long as the operator is aware of the anatomy of the bird, and avoids delicate internal organs and air sacs. I have used a midline incision, with the bird on its back; careful dissection is necessary to avoid damaging the underlying gastro-intestinal organs, especially if there is much fat present. Alternatively the lateral approach can be used, as described for sexing of birds of prey (96). The latter technique is likely to be superseded by other, less traumatic, methods (see Chapter 11) but at the present time still plays an important part in sexing of certain species. It can also be used to investigate gonad activity. The bird is placed on its right side; the left wing is raised and the left leg drawn back. The incision is made, after appropriate plucking of feathers and aseptic precautions, just in front of the left femur and anterior to the sartorius muscle. For sexing, the incision is made between the 7th and 8th ribs but this can be varied for other purposes. I do not usually suture the air sacs but I use 000 or 0000 catgut for muscles and subcutaneous tissues and silk or nylon mattress sutures for skin wounds.

A muscle biopsy is of value in studies on pesticides and a technique used successfully in East African species was described by my colleague Laurence Frank and myself (157). The biopsy is taken as a wedge lateral to the keel and in a bird of 500–1000 grammes bodyweight can measure 2 cm long × 4 mm wide × 3–4 mm deep. The wound is treated topically with antibiotic and the skin sutured with catgut. The technique described takes under five minutes and is easily performed under CT 1341 anaesthesia. Infection of the wound is rare and haemorrhage is not a problem so long as the incision is made in the position described and not more caudal or lateral.

The subject of experimental surgery should be mentioned. It is not new. For example, the preparation of a gastric fistula was reported 50 years ago (354) and pancreatectomies in birds of prey as long ago as the 1890's (referred to by Nelson and colleagues (315)). These and other techniques may be required in experimental work in future and it is important to be aware of them.

Nelson *et al* (315) performed pancreatectomies on great horned owls under phenobarbitone anaesthetic and stated that "little difficulty was experienced in removing the gland which is quite discrete and located in the loop of the duodenum".

The Russian biologist Voitkevich carried out thyroidectomies in a wide range of birds, amongst them short-eared owls and kestrels, as part of his investigations into feather development. Surgical techniques used were described in the book "The Feathers and Plumage of Birds" (402) and will only be summarised here. Feathers were plucked from the ventral aspect of the neck and a midline incision made. The crop (when present) was displaced and the interclavicular air sac either incised or pushed aside. The thyroid was removed by blunt dissection, care being taken to minimise haemorrhage and to avoid touching the vagus nerve. Voitkevich made the point that owls, in common with certain other species, have a very tough thyroid capsule. Ligation of blood vessels was not considered essential, speed of operation being more important. Sutures were placed only in the skin. Voitkevich referred to surgical procedures used by other authors and stressed the importance of ensuring that all thyroid tissue has been removed; if any remains, it may regenerate.

It is increasingly probable that surgical techniques for the implantation of telemetry equipment and indwelling cannulae will be requested by experimentalists. Sawby and Gessaman (362) described the implantation of electrodes for electrocardiography in American kestrels; their approach was midline, just posterior to the sternum, and the electrodes inserted inside the body cavity, dorsal to the sternum. The lead wires were then threaded under the skin to exit points on the flank and back. The use of this and other techniques is likely to yield valuable data on physiology and will contribute to improved diagnostic techniques.

A number of other experimental procedures have been used in poultry and it is likely that some of them may find their way into raptor work. Such techniques as castration, ovariectomy and abligation of the caeca were described in some detail in the fifth edition of "Diseases of Poultry" (366) and reference can usefully be made to this. I have listed caponising as an "experimental" procedure but it has been postulated by my friend Dr. Robert Kenward that such an operation might in due course be advisable in captive red-tailed hawks in Britain to ensure that they could not establish themselves and breed on release or escape. This would certainly raise ethical problems!

CHAPTER 11

Miscellaneous and emerging diseases

Under this heading is included a number of diseases which are not discussed fully in other chapters, together with others which are "emerging" in the sense that it is only in recent years that they have come into prominence. The latter comprise some conditions which have probably escaped notice in the past plus others which have increased in prevalence or importance – often on account of new systems of management, especially captive breeding. Birds of prey maintained in captivity may live to a considerable age and some examples of this were given in the "International Zoo Yearbook" in 1970 (324). Amongst birds listed in that paper were a bateleur eagle that lived to be 44 years and 4 months, two buzzards (still alive) in their sixteenth year and a Javan fishing owl (also still alive) of 36 years. Birds kept for falconry probably live less long although in recent years I have treated a number of peregrines and lanners of 12 years or older. It is interesting to contrast this with the comments in "Falconry in the British Isles" in 1855 (361) where the authors stated that they had "met with several trained peregrines which reached the ages of five, seven, eight and ten years." However, Brown (57) pointed out that the life of a falconer's bird is probably healthier than that of its counterpart in a zoological collection and this may be relevant when considering disease. Some of the conditions discussed in this chapter are likely to be associated with this increased longevity.

Old age itself can produce clinical signs of lethargy, stiffness of movement (particularly if the weather is cold or wet) and a tendency to "doze" with the eyes closed. Recovery time may be extended if the bird is anaesthetised. If an old bird deteriorates too drastically in physical condition it is best to kill it humanely. A raptor which has died of natural causes at an advanced age usually shows no specific lesions. The plumage may be frayed and lustreless and the feet often show calluses. Internally there are often extensive fat deposits within the body cavity itself and on the heart. On histological examination there may be evidence of interstitial nephritis and infiltration of the liver by excess numbers of chronic inflammatory cells.

Ageing an old bird is not easy and some clinical or pathological guidelines would prove useful. Care should always be taken in the anaesthesia of aged birds and a combination of agents is recommended. Nevertheless, it can usually be carried out safely; I have frequently operated upon birds of 12–13 years of age for bumblefoot.

Feather conditions

Feather abnormalities are a common cause of concern to the falconer whose bird's performance may depend on the state of its plumage. Such conditions are of

156

less importance in aviary birds but traumatic injuries, such as damaged wing and tail feathers, are usually much more common in the latter. In addition, breeding birds may damage one another's plumage during courtship. For example, for two years in succession, I have examined a male Harris's hawk which, while not showing any obvious physical injury, ends the breeding season with a neck plucked bare of feathers. Clinical and laboratory examination have failed to demonstrate any aetiology and it is the opinion of the owner and myself that the bird's mate has been responsible. An interesting sequel to this case is that, following isolation of the male, it was found to be developing bare areas on its flanks and the indication was that it was beginning to remove its own feathers! It is possible therefore that, in addition to being pecked by their companions, raptors may pluck themselves (as do psittacine birds) on account of "boredom" or lack of stimulation.

Falconers are extremely knowledgeable on the care of a bird's plumage. Bent feathers are straightened by immersion in warm water. Broken feathers are mended by "imping" on a new piece of feather and this technique has been described by many authors throughout the years; the veterinary surgeon may like to refer to Blaine (44), Cooper (82) or Woodford (422). The word "imp" is one of many falconry terms used by Shakespeare, for example in Richard II:

> "If, then, we shall shake off our slavish yoke
> Imp out our drooping country's broken wing ....."

The technique could be used to advantage by those who wish to return a casualty or captive bred bird to the wild and who are reluctant to wait until the next moult before being able to give the bird exercise. Imping of feathers can be facilitated by appropriate anaesthesia or sedation.

Injury to a wing can result in the production of feathers of poor quality which may be misshapen; this is a common sequel to bursitis of the carpus ("blain") which is discussed in Chapter 5. Skin granulomas can have the same effect. There is no remedy other than to wait until the next moult during which time the tissues will, hopefully, have healed. Sometimes one feather is damaged – for example by striking a projecting object in the mews – and as a result it protrudes at an angle. It can be attached to the adjacent feathers with a stitch but the latter must be removed in time for the moult.

Occasionally the plumage of a raptor may be damaged by oil. I have treated an osprey contaminated with oil from the sea and would advise the use of a warm solution of washing-up liquid, repeated if necessary, and followed by rinsing and drying. It is imperative that such birds are kept warm and not permitted to ingest the oil – for example, by the use of a collar to prevent preening. Wilson (417) reported the oiling of a trained hawk by fulmar oil and Clarke (74) suggested that oiling by fulmars (*Fulmarus glacialis*) might even be a significant cause of mortality in free-living peregrines; such oiling should be treated as outlined above.

Mallophaga (biting lice) may cause mechanical damage to feathers giving a typically moth-eaten appearance; the eggs or "nits" may also be seen on the feather barbs. The condition is easily diagnosed and treated. Care must be taken not to incriminate these or other parasites when *dropped* feathers are found to be infested. The culprits in such cases are almost invariably non-pathogenic and may even include clothes moths (*Tinea* spp.)

Less straightforward are non-specific conditions of the feather which result in poor feather growth and, often, breakage. A low plane of nutrition or some other stress factor in early life may produce areas of weakness termed "hunger traces", "fret marks" or "fault bars". These defects in the feather are common in young birds reared in captivity and have also been reported in free-living birds of prey of a number of species. Possibly similar in origin is a condition I call "pinching off", where the young vascularised feathers fall out prematurely and on examination are found to have a marked constriction at the base of the shaft. There is no treatment for these syndromes other than to wait for new feathers to grow; removal of affected tail feathers will initiate rapid replacement but primaries will usually not develop until the next moult.

A number of other conditions may also be encountered, the aetiology of which remains obscure. Some involve the whole feather, others only the shaft or barbs (Photo 22). I investigated a "bald thigh syndrome" at one establishment where several birds lost feathers from the medial surface of the legs (Photo 23). No parasites were seen in scrapings or skin sections and there was no improvement following a dietary change from day-old chicks. The condition eventually resolved spontaneously and no diagnosis was ever made. Similar cases of feather loss occur from time to time in individual birds or collections and I have had a report of

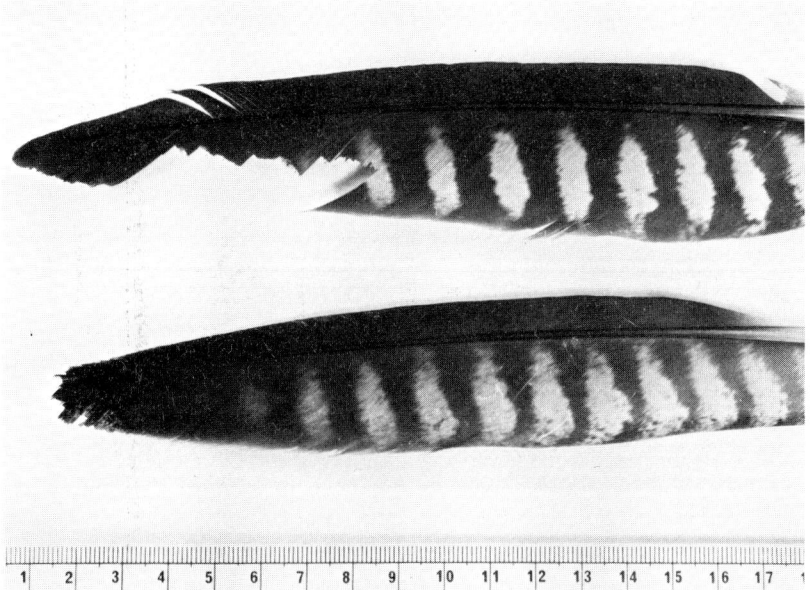

Photo 22.   Feather abnormality, of unknown aetiology, in a peregrine. Note ragged lesions of barbs

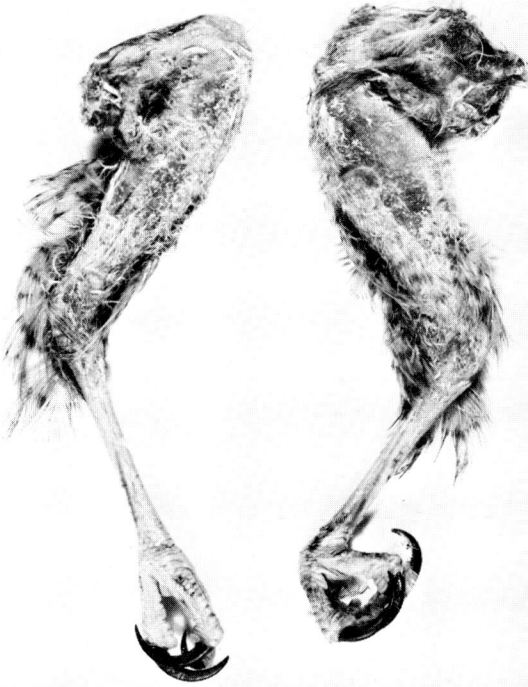

Photo 23. Baldness of medial surfaces of legs of a sparrowhawk, of unknown aetiology

it in a sparrowhawk from Dr. G. J. van Nie of Holland. Nutritional supplements may be tried as treatment but often are to no avail. Some early cases of feather abnormality appeared to respond to dietary additions of hydrolysed feather meal – a protein supplement used in poultry (123) – but I have been less impressed with subsequent results. A recent paper (346) described the successful use of medroxyprogesterone acetate by injection to treat areas of feather loss in psittacine birds and the drug should perhaps be tried in raptors. A number of products are available on the market which, it is claimed, will improve the skin and plumage of birds and these usually contain vitamins, minerals (especially zinc) and polyunsaturated fatty acids. I have no experience of their use. An important point to remember in the investigation and treatment of any feather condition is that one is examining lesions which reflect an abnormal situation many weeks or months previously, when the feather was growing. The feather itself is a dead structure.

The uropygial (preen) gland should always be examined in cases of poor feathering. A healthy gland is usually firm to the touch and not painful. If it is functioning properly the small feathers around the external orifice appear slightly oily.

Although some species such as African vultures shed feathers continuously, the normal moult in birds of prey is annual and lasts between five and seven months. In the Northern Hemisphere it commences in the late Spring or Summer and the feathers are generally dropped in sequence. As can be imagined, the moult can pose problems for the practising falconer if it is delayed or prolonged since birds should not be flown until their plumage is complete. Feather development is closely linked to thyroid activity and moult can be induced by the use of oral thyroxine. Voitkevich (402) discussed the use of thyroxine and referred to experimental work with pigeons which showed that a large single dose had less deleterious effects than several small doses, which tended to cause weight loss. Nevertheless, my own experience with raptors has been restricted to the daily use of small quantities at the dosage given in Appendix IX. I have not encountered any obvious side effects associated with thyroxine but, until controlled trials have been carried out, I would urge caution in its use. The treatment should certainly be stopped if there is any evidence of marked weight loss, palpitation of the heart or hyperaesthesia (15). Other drugs have been recommended by a number of authors, amongst them Beebe (23), who advocated the use of progesterone; I have no personal experience of these medications.

As has been explained, an irregular or slow moult can pose problems to a falconer but it is suggested that the use of drugs to "hasten the moult" be undertaken only in special cases. Use might instead be made of changing the lighting pattern as suggested by Lawson and Kittle (270); controlled studies are needed on this subject. Progression of a moult may be retarded when the bird is treated – especially, I believe, with corticosteroids – and it may be necessary to bear this in mind with falconers' birds in the Summer and Autumn. Woodford (422) reported that hawks moulted faster if kept warm and this appears to be correct. I have encountered a premature moult (early Spring) in birds which have been kept indoors, in the warm, during the Winter.

It will be apparent from the foregoing remarks that the whole question of feather development is a complex one. There have been no detailed investigations reported into feather conditions in hawks and this is a topic that warrants further research. The monograph entitled "The Feathers and Plumage of Birds" by Voitkevich (402) gave an excellent introduction to the subject of feather growth and development and referred to work, including experimental studies, in raptors. The reader may also like to refer to an article I published in 1972 (90) which discussed in more detail some of the feather abnormalities described above.

Musculo-skeletal conditions

Many of the conditions affecting the musculature and skeleton have been described elsewhere in this book.

Both acute and chronic inflammatory lesions of the muscles may follow irritant injections and bacterial infections. Traumatic injuries to the muscles can cause myofibrillar degeneration and chronic inflammatory cell infiltration.

Clinical signs which appear to relate to the musculo-skeletal system are not uncommon in birds of prey. For example there is a syndrome resembling rheumatism which is seen particularly in older birds. This condition appears to bear no relationship to hypocalcaemia or other nutritional diseases. One or both legs are stiff and may be unwilling to bear weight. There is no palpable swelling and usually no lesions on radiography. The condition may resolve spontaneously, often to recur later. Some birds thus affected also show intermittent signs of collapse, resembling a "stroke", suggesting that this could be a disease of old age and possibly associated with the cardiovascular system.

Cramp itself is a disease of young birds and has been recognised for a long time. Cox and Lascelles (116) in "Coursing and Falconry"(1892), stated that:

> "Hawks that are taken too young from the nest or that have been much exposed to cold when taken are sometimes seized with *cramp* in the legs; this will completely paralyse the limbs and render the bird useless".

Unfortunately the term "cramp" probably refers to a number of different disorders, all of which are manifested by stiffness or paralysis of limbs. Hypocalcaemia is probably the most common cause and is discussed in Chapter 8. Salvin and Brodrick (361) in 1855 described cramp as "the most fatal of all the diseases to which Hawks are subject" and referred to it as "Tetanus" in parentheses. Blaine (44) stated that:

> "Cramp frequently attacks young peregrines taken from the nest at too early a stage. The attack may be so violent as to break the leg bones".

These and other examples would add weight to a diagnosis of hypocalcaemia.

The term cramp is still commonly used by falconers and in many cases the cause is probably not hypocalcaemia. Woodford (422) grouped cramp and paralysis together and, amongst other things, postulated that fowl paralysis (Marek's disease) or a neuritis might be involved in their aetiology. He suggested that the disease might be prevented by keeping young birds warm and dry and feeding a diet of birds and mammals. Hurrell (223) used the word cramp when he reported a juvenile sparrowhawk "with tightly clenched feet and flexed legs, unable to stand or feed, and supporting herself on outstretched wings". The bird recovered following the administration of calcium, vitamin D, prednisolone and chlordiazepoxide but, as with so many cases, one does not know which, if any, of these drugs played a part in treatment.

My own view is that the term "cramp" should be avoided whenever possible. It probably covers many syndromes and it is far preferable to describe the bird's clinical signs and to try to relate them to a particular organ system or systems.

Tendon damage is mentioned in Chapter 7 as a possible sequel to bumblefoot. Halliwell (186) discussed this in some detail and illustrated his paper with drawings of the foot. He emphasised how relatively easily the flexor tendons of the digits can be stretched or torn.

Studies on musculo-skeletal disorders in birds of prey would be facilitated if improved diagnostic aids were available. Electromyography (EMG) has been used to investigate muscular dystrophy in chickens (214) and is a technique which could prove valuable in raptors.

Ocular conditions

The eyes of birds of prey play an extremely important part in the detection and capture of their quarry. In captivity the situation is rather different but, nevertheless, impaired vision will have a significant effect on the health and welfare of the bird. The ophthalmoscope should be used in clinical examination but it should be noted that constriction of the pupil often renders examination of the fundus difficult. Of more general value are tests on response to stimulation and pupillar reflexes when a pinpoint source of light is used in a darkened room. Ocular disorders are usually quickly noticed in falconers' birds – where vision is so important – but may be missed for some time in others.

There has recently been considerable interest in the vision of raptors, and experimental studies, especially in owls (291, 292), may help improve diagnostic techniques as well as yielding valuable scientific data. For example, Martin and colleagues (293) used benoxinate hydrochloride for analgesia of the cornea and 1% cyclopentolate hydrochloride to dilate the pupil, neither of which appears to have been employed in routine clinical work.

The eyes are prone to injury and such conditions as corneal ulceration and intra-ocular haemorrhage are common. A young snowy owl at the Hawk Trust was found to have intra-ocular haemorrhages but there was no obvious cause. The lesions resolved spontaneously over a period of 4–5 weeks. The practice of "seeling" the eyes of falcons by sewing their eyelids together is no longer carried out as an aid to training in Britain but occurs in the Middle East and imported birds may be found to have small scars on their lids as a result.

Blindness occurs from time to time, often following a traumatic injury. Total blindness is usually relatively easy to diagnose on the basis of clinical signs and the total absence of a pupillar reflex. Partial loss of sight is less easily detected although slow or only partial pupillar reflexes and excessively dilated pupils are usually a feature. Examination of the internal chambers of the eye will sometimes reveal a blood clot and/or opacity.

Cataracts were reported in birds of prey by Arnall and Keymer (15) and were said to occur primarily in old age. In a survey of non-domenticated birds from the Zoological Society of London Keymer (253) recorded more cataracts in the Falconiformes than in any other Order of birds but, interestingly, none was seen in the Strigiformes. I have never diagnosed cataracts myself but they will possibly be reported more frequently now that birds of prey are living longer in captivity. Ocular opacity, which occurs often after traumatic injury, should not be mistaken for cataract; it usually involves disruption of the whole eye and the lens is not affected *per se*.

There is very little information on diseases of the other special senses of birds of prey. Otitis is discussed earlier in the book. There has been considerable research on the ears of owls, largely on account of their asymmetry (321) and this is likely to provide useful groundwork for future studies on aural pathology.

Cardiovascular conditions

In the first edition I reported several cardiovascular conditions in birds of prey, amongst them an unusual case of circulatory failure in a red-headed merlin, endocarditis and hydropericardium. Oedema was seen in a number of cases including pulmonary oedema associated with hydropericardium and oedema of the head and feet (Photo 24) following mechanical obstruction. Some similar cardiovascular lesions were recorded by Keymer (249).

Since the first edition of this book appeared Dr. Ariela Pomerance and I have examined the hearts of many birds of prey, both macrosopically and

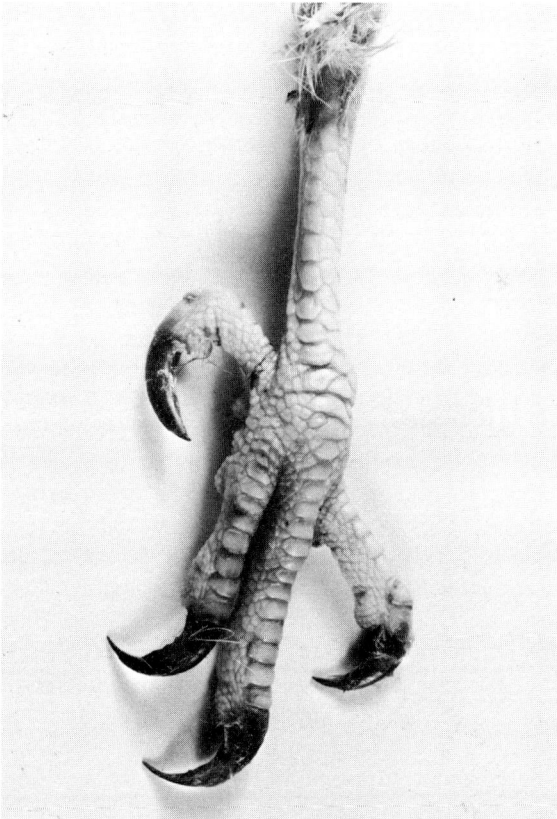

Photo 24.   Foot of a kestrel showing oedema of metatarso-phalangeal joint associated with a necrotic mass of tissue (due to injury) at the head of the femur

histopathologically. A number of interesting lesions have been seen and a review of these will be published elsewhere. Our findings have included myofibrillar degeneration, focal myocarditis, atheromatosis, a thrombus in an epicardial vein and pericarditis. In few of these has the lesion been considered contributory to death and we have not been able to associate them with clinical signs of disease. The exceptions were severe atheromatosis, which killed an eagle and a hawk eagle and an acute purulent pericarditis which, together with pneumonia, was considered the cause of death in a kestrel. Our findings suggest that while clinical signs of cardiovascular disease are either rare, or difficult to detect, in birds of prey, their occurrence in *post-mortem* material is not uncommon. Further work is needed to ascertain the significance of heart lesions in a clinical context.

Clinical investigation of cardiovascular conditions would be much facilitated by use of electrocardiography. Several authors have reported ECG work in raptors in both experimental and diagnostic work, for example Martin and colleagues (293) and Wingfield and DeYoung (418) respectively. The latter authors also described the use of a Doppler flow probe to detect arterial blood flow and this is a technique which may prove useful in the future.

The finding of arteriosclerosis and atheromatosis in raptors is not unexpected, these conditions having been first recorded over fifty years ago (152). Finlayson (147) examined birds from the Zoological Society of London collection and found that there was a higher percentage of atherosclerosis in the Falconiformes than in any other Order. A number of raptors with arterial lesions, in some cases associated with myocardial degeneration, are included in the book "Comparative Atherosclerosis" (357), including a free-living kite. Clinical diagnosis of such conditions is probably impossible although the indications are that an overweight, underexercised bird is most likely to be at risk. Typical atherosclerotic lesions are found at *post-mortem* examination and, if the cause of death, are usually associated with pulmonary and visceral congestion.

Heart lesions may be due to other causes. Infections can result in pericarditis, epicarditis, myocarditis or endocarditis; although bacteria usually are involved, *Aspergillus fumigatus* will also produce such lesions. Sometimes focal myocarditis is seen on histopathological examination of birds that have died of other causes. In visceral gout the pericardium, and sometimes the epicardium, become coated with urates. Heart pathology can also be a feature of some poisons; for example Koeman and colleages (263) described changes in the muscle fibres of kestrels experimentally poisoned with a methyl mercury compound.

A disease known as "apoplexy" is of interest. It has long been recognised in cagebirds and Arnall and Keymer (15) described its possible aetiology. Mr. E. Boughton told me of a case in a captive peregrine; the *post-mortem* picture was characterised by marked internal congestion and haemorrhage. I have encountered similar cases on a few occasions and in none of mine, despite careful dissection, have I been able to ascertain the source of the haemorrhage. In a classical case the bird suddenly struggles, coughs up blood and dies within a minute. No treatment is likely to be of any avail and there are no obvious predisposing factors. In their book "Falconry in the British Isles" Salvin and

Brodrick (361) recognised apoplexy and made the interesting observation that it was "fatal to nine-tenths of the merlins and sparrow-hawks trained every season." Unfortunately they gave no description and it is possible that they were describing nervous "fits" – but I personally doubt this since in the same book they also referred to "epilepsy". It should perhaps be mentioned that such a mortality does not occur amongst falconers' birds nowadays; Kenward (245) reported that 12 out of 14 merlins in his survey were either lost or released.

A condition resembling "stroke" is recognised in raptors, particularly old birds, and is probably cardiovascular in origin. The affected bird suddenly collapses or falls off its perch and shows weakness and inco-ordination. It usually recovers within a few hours (sometimes within minutes) but may remain partly paralysed or unsteady on its feet. Occasional birds are comatose and die within 12 hours. Unfortunately I have not had an opportunity to examine such a case *post mortem*. A similar disease in cagebirds is associated with *post-mortem* findings of a dilated, thin-walled heart and a pale myocardium and valves (56) but I have never observed such lesions in birds of prey.

Ischaemia of the feet or legs can occur following trauma or frostbite and is discussed in Chapter 4. In a paper on frostbite in captive birds Wallach and Flieg (406) reported that some severely affected individuals developed valvular vegetative endocarditis.

There are scattered reports of cardiovascular "accidents" in birds of prey; for example, an owl died at the London Zoo in 1939 from "rupture of the left auricle and haemopericardium" (193) while Dr. G. J. van Nie has told me of an aneurysm of the aorta in a red-headed merlin. I have not encountered such lesions myself.

Urinary conditions

Diseases of the urinary tract are not uncommon but are often only diagnosed *post mortem*. There had been little work on diagnostic tests in birds although plasma uric acid levels can be assayed; this technique has been used in poultry (323) and in budgerigars (364) but not, as far as I can tell, in birds of prey. It is of interest in this context to note that as long ago as 1923 Fox (153) found nephritis to be more common in the Falconiformes than in any other Order of birds and there are many examples of renal disease in raptors in the Pathologists' Reports at the Zoological Society of London.

Impaction of the cloaca is seen, especially in birds which have been recumbent for some time, but the condition may also occur spontaneously. Clinical signs include soiling of the vent region and the passing of blood in the mutes. Some cases may show paralysis of the legs. The largest cloacal calculus I have seen was 6 cm in diameter and when analysed by Dr. D. E. Kidder of the University of Bristol was found to consist of uric acid and ammonium urate; it caused the death of a goshawk and histological examination revealed cloacitis and severe nephrosis. Mr. E. Boughton has told me of a similar case of cloacal impaction and nephrosis he diagnosed in a sparrowhawk and cloacal impaction and visceral gout in a kestrel. All cloacal calculi should be submitted for analysis; usually they consist of ammonium urate, which is a normal waste product in birds, but may contain traces of other minerals, such as apatite.

A diagnosis of a cloacal calculus may be confirmed by radiography or by digital exploration of the cloaca. For the latter, the finger, preferably in a finger stall, must be well lubricated with liquid paraffin. Following such examination small calculi may be voided spontaneously; larger ones will need to be removed.

In the first edition five birds were diagnosed as having died following a kidney condition and there were significant kidney lesions in four others. Of the former five, four were captive birds and these had combinations of nephritis, nephrosis, visceral gout and a blood clot over the kidney.

Visceral gout has been reported in hawks before. Its cause is obscure but it probably can be secondary to renal damage and the latter may, according to Ward and Slaughter (411) be brought about by an unbalanced diet. Wallach (405) attributed both visceral and articular gout to an excess of dietary protein and the role of this (and, incidentally, of starvation) in raising blood uric acid levels in chickens was demonstrated by Okumura and Tasaki (323). Halliwell and colleagues (189) listed other possible causes including vitamin A deficiency and neoplasia and distinguished between primary uricaemia, where excess uric acid is produced, and secondary uricaemia due to impaired blood clearance by the kidneys. Deprivation of water has been incriminated as a cause of visceral gout in reptiles (114) and it is possible that a similar situation might apply in birds.

There appear to be no specific clinical signs in raptors with kidney disease or even visceral gout, although birds which drink excessively or have watery droppings are possibly suspect. Such clinical signs were seen in a few birds in my series some of which later, at *post-mortem* examination, were found to have kidney lesions. However, in the majority of my cases there have been only general signs of inappetance and lethargy or the birds have died suddenly.

I have not personally seen cases of articular gout despite careful examination of material from swollen joints. Stehle (385) reported the finding of urates in some such conditions and Boughton's kestrel had "gross arthritic gout" in addition to the visceral gout and cloacal impaction mentioned earlier.

Histopathological lesions are not uncommon in the kidneys of raptors but it is difficult to be sure of their significance. A degree of interstitial nephritis is seen relatively frequently in birds which have died of other causes but may also be a primary condition. For example, a laughing falcon from the Zoological Society of London died of kidney disease associated with *E. coli*. On histological examination there was a severe interstitial nephritis in which eosinophils predominated. Other pathological lesions seen commonly in kidneys, although not necessarily a cause of death, include calcification, glomerular lesions, cystic dilatation of renal tubules and tubular degeneration.

Immunological disorders

Despite the prominent role played by the fowl in our understanding of the immune response – particularly lymphocyte function – very little information exists on immunological disease in non-domesticated birds. Arnall (14) listed "allergy and anaphylaxis" amongst respiratory diseases of pigeons and he and Keymer (15) discussed the possible part played by allergy, anaphylaxis and hypersensitivity in diseases of cagebirds. In both publications, however, the absence of any reliable data on the subject is emphasised.

The role of humoral and cellular defence mechanisms in birds of prey may be very significant. For example, it has been suggested that the apparent failure of rabies virus to establish itself in birds may be due to the rapidity with which immunity develops, including antibodies bound to the central nervous system (172). The work by Jorgenson and colleagues (240) in which antibody titres to rabies virus in a great horned owl rose following corticosteroid administration would help support this.

I have been unable to trace any records of truly immunological disease in birds of prey. However, if one includes reactions to foreign antigens under this heading there are some conditions worthy of note. For example, unexplained swellings of the head, which usually resolve spontaneously within 48 hours, are probably due to bites of mosquitoes. Bee sting can kill birds of prey and is discussed in Chapter 6. Adverse reactions to drugs such as procaine, are covered in Chapters 3 and 10.

I have not diagnosed anaphylactic shock in birds of prey but it could prove a problem if the use of hyperimmune serum ever became prevalent. I have suggested elsewhere (99) that, like vaccines, such sera may have a part to play in the control of certain infectious diseases.

Neoplasia

Marek's disease is discussed in Chapter 5, under viral infections.

Other neoplasms ("tumours" or "cancers") have been reported only rarely in birds of prey although several authors, amongst them Fox (153), Jennings (231), Blackmore (41) and Keymer (249), have described small numbers of cases.

My own findings have been restricted to the diagnosis of a metastasising adenocarcinoma in a 12 year old captive buzzard (105), a mixed cell tumour in a free-living fledgling Seychelles kestrel and an oviduct adenocarcinoma in a Mauritius kestrel. In addition I have removed proliferative lesions from the feet and eyelids which on histological examination have proved to be benign papillomata. Eyelid lesions in one such case occurred following severe traumatic damage to the bird's head in an aviary (Photo 25); hypertrophy of the cere was another feature of the case (see Chapter 4). Some stomatitis lesions show epithelial proliferation but I do not believe that these are neoplastic; possibly they are associated with trauma or chronic inflammation.

Neoplasms are amongst the conditions that are likely to be recognised more frequently as birds are kept longer in captivity. At the present time there is no specific treatment that can be recommended for such lesions. The surgical removal of subcutaneous tumours is a well recognised procedure in psittacine birds and might be applicable to raptor work.

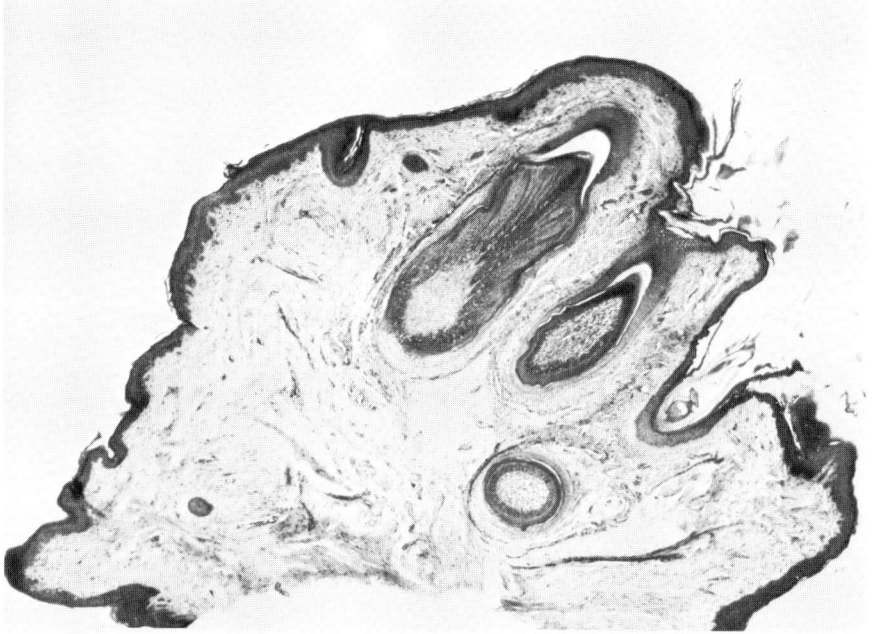

Photo 25.   Low power photomicrograph of a papilloma removed surgically from the eyelid of a lanner. In this case the lesion was probably the result of trauma

Shock and stress

In the first edition only four birds were diagnosed as having died of "shock" but a number of others showed a degree of circulatory collapse associated with different conditions. Since then I have dealt with many more wild bird casualties and it has become apparent how often shock can supervene, especially after injury or fluid loss. The term shock should really only be applied in cases where there are changes associated with circulatory failure and the prevention and treatment of this condition is discussed in Chapter 3.

"Stress" is equally difficult to define, though von Faber (403) discussed its aetiology in poultry and drew attention to the changes seen in the pituitary and adrenal glands, lymphoid tissues and blood. He listed a number of stressors which may produce the "general adaptation syndrome" in poultry and these include fatigue, excess cold or heat, starvation, crowding or restraint. He also discussed the use of vitamins, antibiotics, hormones and tranquillisers in countering stress. There has been a considerable amount of subsequent work in the fowl, for example by Freeman (159) and it appears that the first (alarm) stage is characterised by the release of such chemicals as glucagon, adrenaline and nor-adrenaline into the circulation. The adrenal cortex is stimulated via the hypothalamus and pituitary.

The significance of these findings to work with birds of prey is unknown and far more research is needed. For example, can stress play a part in preventing apparently healthy birds from breeding in captivity? What role does it have in predisposition to such diseases as aspergillosis? Can the response of a bird of prey to stressors be modified by the use of drugs, such as antibiotics, as has been suggested in the chicken? What effect does lack of stressors have? As Freeman and Manning (160) pointed out, the subject is still little understood in the fowl, and it is likely to be a long time before we have much data on non-domesticated birds. In the interim I think it is reasonable to assume that, while regular exposure to stressors is probably both normal and desirable, excess or prolonged stress in captive birds is likely to prove deleterious. Practical recommendations for reducing stress include the avoidance of excess heat and cold, adequate nutrition and prompt attention to disease. Unnecessary disturbance should be avoided and the construction of aviaries and other enclosures should take into consideration the species and temperament of the bird. For example, stress can be minimised by using higher aviaries and reducing unnecessary stimulation. In this respect one may have to strike a balance between disturbing the birds and a build-up of potential pathogens since regular cleaning of an aviary, while advisable in terms of disease prevention, may cause considerable disturbance to the inmates.

Green (175) has pointed out that acute cardiovascular failure may occur in birds if they do not have time to adapt to the first (alarm) stage of the general adaptation syndrome. He emphasised the need to reduce trauma associated with anaesthesia, including careful positioning of the patient and "neural shock" which may result from stretched nervous plexuses. These factors are discussed in more detail in Chapter 10.

Some birds appear to be suffering from "stress" on account of a previous prolonged period of poor management, intercurrent disease or chronic injury. Such birds often have lustreless, brittle plumage, pale rather dry legs and fail to put on weight. Laboratory investigation may show a depressed PCV and/or haemoglobin level and both endo- and ectoparasites are often present. Such birds show no obvious immediate response to treatment but will often gradually improve in condition following better management, a varied diet and vitamins. Some cases, however, continue to deteriorate and either die or have to be killed on humanitarian grounds. At *post-mortem* examination they appear in poor condition, anaemic, with varying degrees of hydropericardium. Histopathological examination sometimes reveals chronic inflammatory cell infiltration of the kidneys and liver but not, in my experience, any other lesions that might help support a diagnosis of stress.

The adrenal glands may occasionally appear enlarged *post mortem* and histological examinations have shown such abnormalities as haemorrhage and cellular hypertrophy as well as infectious lesions, especially tuberculosis. Further work continues on this subject. There has been an increase in interest in the avian adrenal gland in recent years and one paper of particular relevance is that of Chiasson and colleagues (71) who reported atrophy of the adrenal in poultry following the use of the anaesthetic agent ketamine hydrochloride. It is not known whether a similar situation applies in other birds but if it does, this may be of relevance to reproductive performance. Possibly it should be a warning against the anaesthesia of birds for such techniques as artificial insemination.

Ulceration of the alimentary tract, which may be associated with stress, is seen only rarely in birds of prey; some examples are discussed in Chapter 9.

A condition which will be mentioned here but which is equally relevant to "Musculo-skeletal conditions" is that of exertional rhabdomyolysis, also called capture myopathy, overstraining disease and a variety of other terms. Although well recognised in a number of mammals, in birds it has only been diagnosed in flamingoes (Phoenicopteridae), where the clinical signs are leg paralysis following capture (424). The pathology of the condition is complex but is characterised by muscle necrosis and myoglobinuria.

Other endocrinal conditions

There are relatively few endocrinological disturbances recognised in birds of prey other than infectious disease, such as pancreatitis, and hyperparathyroidism associated with osteodystrophy. There has been interest in the avian pancreas since the 1890's and, as is mentioned in Chapter 10, the early work even included pancreatectomies in birds of prey. In contrast to other birds, this operation resulted in hyperglycaemia with blood sugar levels as high as 1200 mg/100 ml.

As was mentioned earlier, feather development is closely related to thyroid function and routine *post-mortem* examination of thyroid glands, especially from birds that clinically show poor or abnormal plumage, might prove rewarding. The only lesions I have detected in the thyroid have been cysts which were possibly developmental in origin. Hamerton (192) reported acute thyroiditis in an Eleanora's falcon but I have been unable to trace any other references. Possibly, as with other "rare" conditions, some endocrinological diseases go unrecognised.

The effect of photoperiod on raptors is related to the endocrine system and is likely to prove of increasing interest in future. Birds kept at latitudes different from those in the wild, or under conditions of artificial lighting, may need extra illumination to encourage reproductive activity. In due course it may be possible to induce extra breeding seasons by the use of appropriate lighting patterns; this might also influence the moult, as discussed earlier.

Psychological disturbances

In recent years there has been great interest in ethology, the study of animal behaviour, and such research has extended to birds of prey. Particular interest has been shown in the behaviour patterns relating to courtship and breeding; valuable work has been done using captive falconiform and strigiform birds, together with studies on free-living species. A useful and very practical paper on the subject was that by Nelson (317); this included discussion of behavioural changes during egg-laying and the thorny problem of "imprinting". The latter has attracted particular attention and was first described in birds by Lorenz (280). Imprinted birds are usually ones that have been hand-reared in isolation, away from the company of the same species; as a result they become imprinted on humans. Man is accepted first as a parent, then as a social companion and finally as a sexual partner. Some birds of prey remain imprinted for life but in other cases hand-reared birds have finally mated successfully with their own species. The whole subject is a complex one which is not strictly within the realms of "disease" but is mentioned here since it is an aberration of normal behaviour. Imprinted birds can be used for artificial insemination, as described by Berry (31) and Boyd and colleagues (53) and it is probable that the veterinary surgeon will see more of them in future.

There is need for more detailed research on the behaviour of captive birds of prey, especially those bred in captivity. After several generations it will be interesting to see what effect "domestication" has had on behaviour. Similar work has already been performed on quail, chickens and ducks (185).

Differences in behaviour patterns have long been recognised by falconers, for example between birds taken as "eyasses" (nestlings), "haggards" (adults) and "passagers" (subadults). An example is the description given of Beatrice in Shakespeare's "Much ado about nothing":

> "She is too disdainful.
> I know her spirits are as coy and wild
> as haggards of the rock".

Changes in behaviour can be a useful early clue to the presence of disease. The failure of a falconer's bird to perform well is often the first indication of ill-health. Likewise, unexpected docility in a bird which is usually rather wild and unmanageable should be regarded with suspicion.

Variations in individual temperament are worthy of comment. While probably often due to genetic factors, poor management may be contributory. Some captive birds are extremely nervous and this may be reflected in "shivering", poor feathering, damaged cere and rather loose mutes. Such birds are often difficult patients and, unlike those of a more placid nature – which will possibly even permit intramuscular injections to be administered while on the fist – will usually need to be cast for the most minor procedures. Temperament may well play an important part in predisposition to disease and must be borne in mind whenever case histories are considered. Highly strung birds should be restrained as infrequently as possible since repeated contact with man can reinforce "neurotic" conditions. There is also the danger of injury during capture and a tendency to lose condition rapidly on account of excess physical activity.

One aspect of behaviour which appears to have attracted little interest in raptors is that of sleep. Work on the domestic fowl has shown that sleep in this species is closely related to the light/dark cycle and less clearly defined than in mammals (220) but there has been no detailed investigation of the role of sleep in the normal metabolism of the bird. Such studies could be of great interest in birds of prey, especially those used for falconry, whose performance might be influenced by disturbed rest. Hawks differ considerably in their tendency to sleep, some appearing to need to do so far more than others.

A number of behavioural disturbances have been noted in captive birds of prey, of which self mutilation is perhaps the most significant. The disease "aggresteyne" was first described in 1486 in "The Boke of St. Albans" (30) and undoubtedly referred to such mutilations:

> "when ye se youre hawke hunte his fete with his Beke and pullyth her tayll, then she hath the aggresteyne".

This condition is still occasionally seen. Some raptors peck their own or other birds' feathers for no apparent reason, as mentioned earlier in this chapter. Birds also peck at sutures or at exposed wounds and in some instances may damage themselves so badly that euthanasia is necessary. In milder cases the use of an "Elizabethan collar" round the neck may prove an effective deterrent. Proprietary products, usually in the form of aerosols, are used to discourage feather pecking in poultry but I have no experience of their use in raptors. Birds that mutilate themselves are, however, in the minority and most will not interfere with natural or surgical wounds.

Interaction between raptors of the same or different species can also be an important problem. Some species are relatively peaceable while others will kill one another readily. There is tremendous variation between species and individuals and the degree of aggression may relate to different times of the year. Some species can usually be mixed but care must always be taken. Females may kill males, or less commonly, vice versa. If one of a pair has an old injury this may result in its being less able to fend for itself. Marked incompatibility by an individual may be a characteristic of imprinting as shown in junglefowl by Kruijt (266) who described abnormal behaviour (in terms of aggression and escape) in birds raised in isolation. My friend Carl Jones has seen very similar disturbances in captive bred raptors and those hand-reared in "psychologically non-stimulating" environments. Kruijt also described "hysterical fits" in his junglefowl and it is not impossible that some cases of nervous disease in raptors may be psychological in origin.

Prevention of fighting and aggression is based on managemental factors. Whenever birds are kept together in an aviary there should be ample opportunity for them to avoid each other, especially by the provision of vegetation and other forms of cover. If one raptor is particularly aggressive it should not have another bird placed in its enclosure. An injured male bird should not normally be put with an intact female, which is larger. If mixing does have to be carried out the dominant bird should first be removed and only introduced again 7–10 days after the newcomer. If there is any doubt about the response of a bird to others it should be introduced to them cautiously and kept under careful scrutiny. Other techniques that can be used include the initial tethering of a dominant bird in order to restrict its activity but this must be undertaken with great care.

The possible role of circadian rhythms should be mentioned. Daily cycles in body metabolism have already been recorded for raptors and can be related to their day or night time activity (167). Changes in circadian rhythm following, for example, disease or transportation may therefore result in behavioural abnormalities.

A relevant feature of breeding behaviour is that birds may appear clinically unwell; this particularly applies following copulation and prior to egg-laying when, as has been emphasised before (104), a female bird will look ruffled and depressed, often with eyes glazed or half-closed (Figure 15). The bird's abdomen may well appear swollen and the mutes tend to be larger than normal. This combination of features is now commonly termed "egg-laying lethargy".

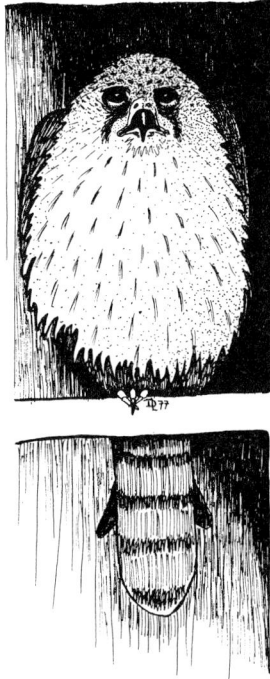

Fig. 15   Female kestrel prior to egg laying. The bird is hunched, with feathers ruffled and eyes half-closed

Reproductive disorders

At one time there would have been little or no place for discussion of reproductive disorders in a book on captive birds of prey but the great advances in recent years have resulted in concern over reproductive abnormalities, particularly the relatively high percentage of birds that still fail to breed in captivity.

I have diagnosed a number of abnormalities of the reproductive tract since the first edition of this book appeared. Egg material is not uncommonly passed *per cloacam* (Photo 26) and may be associated with an infection of the reproductive tract. Cases of oviductitis and egg peritonitis have also been diagnosed *post mortem*, usually associated with *E. coli*, but in one interesting case, a rare Mauritius kestrel, a *Streptococcus* sp. was involved. I have not yet diagnosed

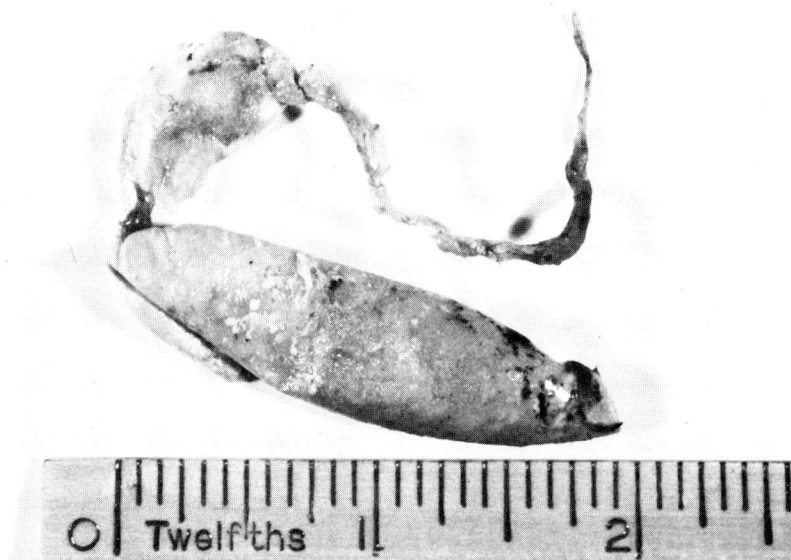

Photo 26.   Egg material from a kestrel, passed *per cloacam* and possibly associated with a chronic infection of the reproductive tract

cases of egg impaction in raptors but they occur – for example an eagle owl died at the London Zoo from this cause (192) – and this must always be a differential diagnosis in birds that show abdominal discomfort or straining. Treatment should be as in smaller birds – warmth, liquid paraffin and, if necessary, surgery.

Failure to breed in captivity may be due to a number of factors, amongst them failure to sex the birds properly, incompatible pairs and birds that are too immature for breeding. Generally speaking, the larger the bird the slower its maturation.

Whenever birds of prey are examined *post mortem* the size and activity of the gonads should be noted and histological sections prepared. Little is known of reproductive physiology in birds of prey, despite advances in the past few years, and further research is needed. Occasionally an unusual lesion is noted in gonadal tissue when examined histologically; for example, the protozoan parasite *Leucocytozoon* (334).

Sexing

Although not a "disease", the problem of sexing some raptors is one that is likely before long to confront all those who deal with the health of these birds. In some species there is distinct sexual dimorphism in the plumage and no problem is likely to occur. In others, however, the only tangible difference may be one of size and here overlap can occur so that one is uncertain as to whether the bird in question is a large male or a small female!

A chemical test for sexing was described by Dieter (129) but this technique needs sophisticated laboratory equipment. Chromosomal tests are also possible but are as yet at only an early stage of development (298). A faecal steroid technique was described by Czekala and Lasley in 1977 (122) and this seems promising although they used only one species of raptor. At the time of writing the Zoological Society of London has started a "bird sexing service" using faecal steroid analysis and details are available from them. A problem is that samples must be examined during the breeding season, when the gonads are active, and in the case of raptors this may pose difficulty in collection as well as being too late for any action that season.

A surgical laparotomy is possibly the most reliable method (96) and this was discussed earlier; however, it involves subjecting the bird to anaesthesia and surgery and should not, in my opinion, be used until other options have been tried. Its value in captive birds of prey was emphasised by myself and Andrew Greenwood (178) following criticism from professional ornithologists over its possible use in free-living birds (150).

More use could possibly also be made of cloacal examination in order to distinguish the different anatomy. Alternatively Hamerstrom and Skinner (191) described "cloacal sexing" of birds by inducing them to prolapse their cloaca. Ejaculation of semen will follow in the male and, with experience, this can be distinguished from urates. In the female prolapsing reveals the rosette-like opening to the oviduct. Unfortunately this technique also has to be carried out in the breeding season.

Genetic and developmental disorders

There is an old Gaelic saying that "All birds cannot be noble falcons, neither can all men be great men". This serves as a useful reminder that there is inevitable biological variation between individuals of the same species. Those who breed or train birds of prey should not assume that differences in size, plumage, temperament or ability are necessarily due to some organic disease. Nor should veterinary surgeons be tempted to try anabolic steroids or other "growth promoting" drugs unless there is a clear clinical indication for such therapy.

Little is known of the genetics of birds of prey though it is to be hoped that the current intensive work on captive breeding will result in greater understanding of the subject. In view of the shortage of breeding stock there has as yet been little opportunity for conscious selection of certain traits in birds of prey, but this will inevitably occur. It is important that the subject is approached scientifically if undesirable characteristics are not to be perpetuated although it should be noted that considerable controversy exists as to whether one should select traits that are advantageous in the wild (such as fear of man) or in captivity (such as tameness). The important consideration is, of course, whether offspring are to be released or retained, although even this is a gross over-simplification since other factors also have to be taken into account.

The hybridisation of species has also been criticised although in my view there are scientific arguments for the production of such hybrids in captivity in order to learn more of such subjects as behavioural genetics and taxonomy of the various species.

Inbreeding is already being practised to some extent, largely on account of the few birds available. There is not, as yet, any evidence that it is proving deleterious but it must be remembered that, generally, inbreeding tends to result in animals of lower viability and fertility. Nevertheless, inbreeding has been used extensively, and usually successfully, in both agriculture and laboratory animal work and it would be wrong to assume that it is always detrimental. Inbred birds of prey could prove of enormous value in studies on physiology and pathology and it is not impossible that strains might be developed that are either resistant or particularly susceptible to certain diseases. I must stress here that I am referring to birds intended for maintenance in captivity and preferably under laboratory conditions. In my opinion repeated inbreeding and other generally undesirable manipulations should not be contemplated by those breeding raptors in small numbers for falconry or release to the wild.

There is much confusion over the terminology used when discussing genetic and developmental abnormalities. The word "genetic" implies some disturbance of the genes and this may be due to a mutation or detrimental genes acquired from the parents at conception. A "congenital" abnormality is one present at birth and it may or may not be genetic in origin. An "inherited" disease is a genetic condition that is transmitted to a bird from one or both of its parents or, through them, from a previous ancestor; it may be passed to a subsequent generation. A "developmental abnormality" is one that occurs during the process of growth and development and this includes the period within the egg. It will be apparent that there can be considerable overlap between the terms used above. For example, an owl which has no tail when it hatches from the egg has a congenital abnormality which is developmental in character. The condition may or may not be due to a genetic abnormality and if it is, the condition might or might not have been inherited.

In view of the almost complete absence of data on these abnormalities in birds of prey I shall discuss the subject only very briefly and in general terms. The reader is referred to standard text-books on genetics, particularly those relating to livestock, for more detailed information. Much work has been carried out on poultry, pigeons and (to a lesser extent) certain cagebirds and some of this is likely to prove relevant to raptors (61).

Although plumage changes, such as albinism, melanism and erythrism are recognised in birds of prey (59), other abnormalities are either rare or undiagnosed. Lesions are not infrequently seen on histopathological examination which are probably developmental in origin, an example being fluid filled cysts in the thyroid gland. Some clinical conditions also appear to be developmental but whether they are genetic in origin is open to question. For example, I have a black kite with a congenital abnormality of the wings; both are bowed at the tip and the bird flies with difficulty. The kite shows no radiological evidence of skeletal abnormality. In the Raptor Research Pathology Committee Report for 1972–73 two cases of "congenital deformity" were listed but no details were given.

Other congenital abnormalities are reported verbally by aviculturists but, alas, are not documented nor is material submitted for professional examination. For example, in 1977 I was told that a pair of lanners had produced five youngsters, three of which were lacking a cloaca.

With the advent of artificial insemination it has become increasingly important that abnormalities and traits noted in captive bred birds are recorded. In most cases they will be attributable to environmental or disease factors but any chance of a "stud" bird disseminating undesirable genetic material should be prevented as soon as possible.

Embryonic death and problems affecting the nestling

Increased interest and experience in the captive breeding of birds of prey has opened up a whole new spectrum of problems which may confront the veterinary surgeon. Some of these are discussed elsewhere in the book and the subject as a whole was reviewed in a paper presented at the Second World Conference on Breeding Endangered Species in Captivity (104). Captive breeding of raptors has been described as an art, rather than a science, and the indications are that some people have good results while others do not.

Despite extensive work on the embryology of the domestic fowl and the causes of embryonic death in chicks, there is little information on the subject in birds of prey. As a result, much of the material in this section is extrapolated from work with poultry and a little from experiences in aviculture. It is vital that those who breed birds of prey in captivity keep comprehensive records and submit unhatched eggs and dead chicks for *post-mortem* examination; only in this way will substantial progress be made. I intend shortly to carry out a study on the normal embryology of a bird of prey, probably the kestrel, and this will hopefully provide some baseline data.

I shall not discuss such subjects as the various techniques for breeding raptors in captivity and of incubating the eggs. Suffice it to say that artificial incubation, while a valuable tool in management, can also lead to problems and frustrations. Only those who are willing to take the subject seriously and scientifically should involve themselves in this and other artificial techniques. Unfortunately, despite many publications, there are not, at the time of writing, authoritative data and guidelines on the optimum requirements for captive breeding. For example, considerable differences of opinion are expressed over such factors as types of incubator, temperature and relative humidity for artificial incubation and how often the eggs are turned. In other species research has been carried out using telemetered eggs to monitor such parameters under "natural" conditions (131); similar studies with raptors are limited (367) but likely to prove of great potential value.

The pathological examination of eggs is discussed in Chapter 3. Failure to hatch is probably the most common problem at present, and is usually due to the egg being infertile. Many factors can lead to infertility of the eggs as discussed in a useful paper on the problems of captive breeding of birds of prey by Mendelssohn and Marder (297). Amongst the factors involved are behavioural problems in the adults, such as imprinting or nervousness, which may result in a degree of courtship but not culminate in mating. The birds may be too young or too old. Alternatively the aviary may be unsuitable or there is so much disturbance that mating never takes place. Conversely, the *absence* of humans may be responsible for the failure of partially imprinted birds to copulate.

These and other problems have been discussed by a number of authors. It is also possible that an individual bird is of low fertility or even sterile; this is often difficult to ascertain in view of the other factors which may have complicated the picture. However, it is not unreasonable to assume that a bird that has had a reproductive disorder, or is nutritionally deficient, may show reduced fertility.

Obesity is probably an important cause of poor fertility since many captive raptors are grossly overfed. It is also possible that excessive use of a male bird for breeding may lead to reduced fertility but I have been unable to trace any information on this in raptors. There has been some limited work on the onset and duration of fertility in female birds of prey; for example Berry (31) and Bird and Buckland (37) reported 4 and 8·1 days for goshawks and American kestrels respectively. Stimulation of sexual behaviour in the male prairie falcon has been attempted by intramuscular injection of testosterone propionate (2·5–5·0 mg) (53) but in their discussion the authors questioned its value.

Various other factors can be involved in low fertility in poultry and are possible causes in birds of prey. Examples are poisons, unsatisfactory lighting patterns, lethal or sublethal genes, extremes of temperatures, use of certain drugs and poor artificial insemination techniques.

Examination of semen samples is discussed briefly in Chapter 3. Birds of low fertility may show sperm abnormalities, such as swollen heads or kinked tails, or the motility may be poor. The latter can be a feature of old samples and therefore a second specimen should be obtained and examined as soon as possible after collection.

Eggs are sometimes soft and abnormal in shape. It is important that such features are recorded since they may indicate disease or immaturity in the hen or be signs of an inadequate diet. Various factors may result in thin eggshells and some of these were discussed (as differential diagnoses for pesticide poisoning) by Ratcliffe (350); more detailed data are available from poultry textbooks. The possible role of heat stress is mentioned in Chapter 4.

Fertile eggs may fail to hatch for a variety of reasons. They can be damaged by the hen bird or by rough handling. They may become infected with bacteria or fungi. There may be embryonic mortality on account of dietary deficiencies in the female bird (see Chapter 9). Most important of all, the eggs may become chilled on account of neglect by the hen bird or, more commonly, because the incubator is at fault. An incorrect temperature and/or relative humidity can easily result in embryonic death. Genetic features probably also play a part but as was emphasised earlier, information is lacking.

Infection of eggs may occur on account of poor hygiene in breeding quarters. Heintzelman (203) discussed the possible role of bacteria-contaminated nestboxes in embryonic death of free-living and captive American kestrels and Porter and Wiemeyer (341) suggested that a number of organisms, amongst them *Proteus* spp., might cause such mortality. Far too little work has been done on this subject, another reason for ensuring that unhatched eggs are examined pathologically.

Prevention of the above problems is not easy, but some simple guidelines may help. Eggs should always be handled with extreme care so as not to damage the embryo or other contents. Hygiene is vital since pathogenic organisms may enter an egg through the pores in the shell. The use of protective clothing, especially gloves, is recommended and incubators should be fumigated at the end of a season. Incubator technique is particularly important and the novice is strongly advised to seek advice before embarking on artificial incubation of eggs. The hen bird which is sitting on eggs must be exposed to as little disturbance as possible.

Some eggs begin to hatch but the chick is unable to emerge and will, unless assisted, die in the shell (Photo 27). In such cases the relative humidity (which is often at fault) should be increased and careful efforts can be made to help remove the chick. Small portions of the shell should be chipped away until the chick is free but special care must be taken not to cause haemorrhage; if this occurs the procedure is being carried out too early. Incubation requirements depend upon the ecology of the bird, and the reader who requires further information on this subject is referred to the paper by Drent (131). For example, some species such as the gyrfalcon, which nests where the ambient humidity is low, can tolerate a lower humidity than others. An oedematous chick or an unabsorbed yolk sac may be an indicator of too *high* a humidity although the latter is often also a manifestation of other managemental problems.

The newly hatched chick is susceptible to a number of diseases, many of which have been mentioned elsewhere in the book. In the case of some infectious diseases the chick may be protected for a certain length of time by maternal antibodies acquired from its yolk sac; this might be an argument in future for the use of appropriate vaccines in breeding stock.

It is particularly important to remember the young bird's susceptibility to hypothermia; it *must* be kept warm. It can be maintained at incubator temperature for the first 48 hours; thereafter it should be kept at a constant temperature of 32–35°C for the first week. As a general rule the larger the bird the lower the temperature needed but if in doubt it is best to adjust the temperature according to the reaction of the birds. Chicks that are too hot pant and those that are too cold appear hunched and shiver. Accommodation which provides a temperature gradient is probably best; the chick can then move to its preferred temperature.

The chick is also prone to traumatic injuries and greenstick fractures and subcutaneous emphysema commonly occur. Young chicks must be handled with the greatest care, especially when being weighed or examined.

Nutritional disorders can occur, ranging from an impacted crop or transient diarrhoea to oesteodystrophy. Confinement on a slippery surface may result in splayed legs which, without treatment, can lead to irreversible damage. The bird should be put on a rougher surface and a figure-of-eight bandage tied temporarily

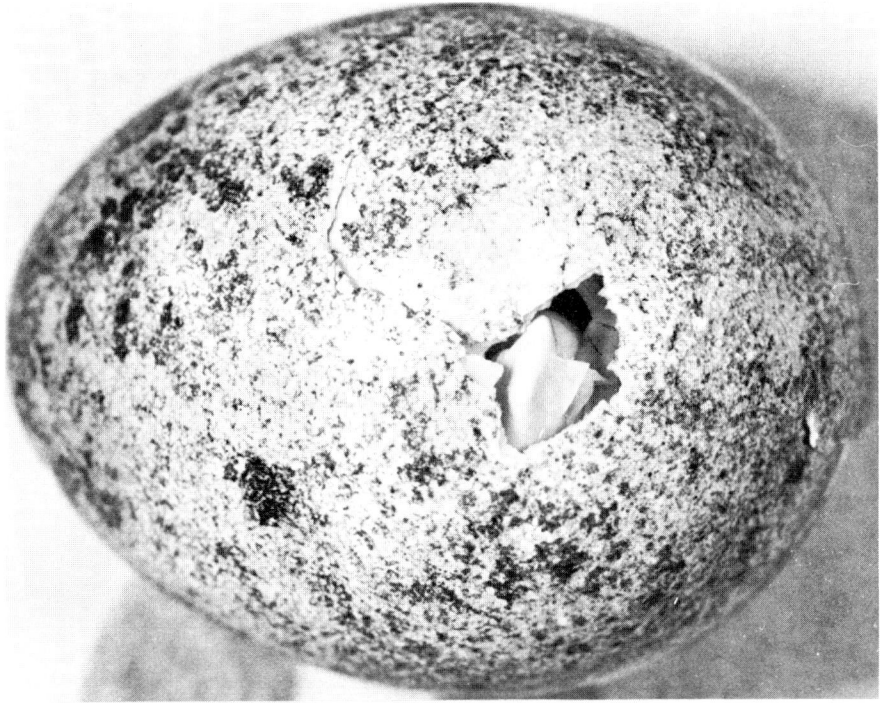

Photo 27.   Peregrine egg containing dead youngster which was about to hatch. The young bird's beak and "egg tooth" can be seen. The causes of death in such cases are still little understood.

round the legs in order to adduct them.

The hand-reared young bird must be treated as an individual and given as much personal attention as possible if disease problems are to be prevented or diagnosed and treated promptly. The subject of captive breeding is rapidly expanding and many of the problems associated with its practice are related to health and veterinary care. Much remains to be learned and a vital part of this is that detailed records are kept by all those involved in captive breeding. An example of a record card is given in Appendix II, but it should be noted that this is very basic; many features can be expanded if necessary.

Unfortunately, certainly in Britain, there is a tendency for aviculturists to "go it alone"; often they have, or claim to have, considerable success in breeding various species of raptor but all too often the emphasis seems to be on quantity, rather than quality, and the results are not published. Note should be taken of the point made by Prestwich, in the preface to his book "Records of Birds of Prey Bred in Captivity" (344) when he said:

> "The compiler ... would impress on breeders the importance of recording *all* their results in one of the recognized avicultural or ornithological journals".

CHAPTER 12

Discussion and conclusions

In the earlier chapters of this book I have endeavoured to show that veterinary attention for captive birds of prey does not differ greatly from other avian species. It should be apparent that a considerable amount of useful information can be extrapolated from cagebirds and, to a certain extent, from poultry. Most of the common conditions of birds of prey also occur in other birds and while the practical significance of some (e.g. bumblefoot and feather abnormalities) may be different, the veterinary approach remains the same. A wide variety of drugs may be used for such work, ranging from some of the falconer's old remedies to modern antibiotics, corticosteroids and anthelmintics. In a few cases special care is needed in the selection of drugs on account of toxicity but these contra-indications usually also apply to psittacine and other cagebirds. Anaesthesia and surgery of birds of prey pose no unique problems and a wide range of techniques can now be carried out routinely and successfully.

However, a word of warning must be sounded here. In common with other authors I have tended to write of "birds of prey" as if they are one genus or family. In fact, as was explained earlier, they comprise two Orders which, although similar in that they are predatory, have very different internal anatomy and physiology and which probably show considerable variation in reaction to drugs and infectious agents. A quail and a fowl are more closely related than a barn owl and a merlin and yet it is recognised that some diseases are unique to them as a species. It is not unreasonable to asume that, in the course of time, some specific diseases of the barn owl, merlin and other raptorial birds will also be recognised. Already there are indications that some conditions are particularly prevalent in certain birds of prey and one is therefore wise not to lump the species together unnecessarily.

Whilst treatment of the sick raptor is of value the emphasis must, always, be on preventive medicine. This hinges largely on management factors since by alteration or improvement of management many health problems can be avoided. Examples are the provision of well-designed perches to reduce trauma to the feet and the avoidance of poorly-ventilated accommodation where *Aspergillus fumigatus* spores may flourish. Hygiene is important in reducing the numbers of pathogens in the environment and there seems little doubt that vaccination is going to prove of increasing significance. Captive breeding is likely to bring with it many problems and the relatively intensive management used for such purposes will necessitate improved hygiene and health programmes.

Although the management of the trained and caged raptor differ considerably, the common feature is that in both cases the bird is confined under unnatural conditions. As such the health problems encountered are very similar and prevention is based on the same criteria. Some conditions are peculiar to trained hawks (for example, abrasion of the legs by jesses) and others, possibly, to caged, or unexercised individuals (for example, atheromatosis) but in general it is true to say that both falconer and aviculturist are confronted with a similar spectrum of diseases in their charges. More liaison between them and others working with birds of prey is urgently needed.

Birds of prey are attracting increasing attention from both scientist and layman. As was stressed in Chapter 1, the disastrous decline of some species in the wild has drawn attention to their highly significant ecological role. They are at the top of the food chain and as such are particularly prone to poisoning and diseases acquired from their prey. Few people now doubt the value of scientific studies on the status, ecology and causes of mortality of free-living birds of prey and veterinary involvement in such projects is increasingly being sought. Much remains to be learned of the diseases and infections of free-living raptors and such information is also likely to prove relevant to captive birds. More work should be performed on the carriage of bacteria and other organisms by free-living birds; this would involve the swabbing of the cloaca, skin, mouth and nasal cavity. Likewise there is need for more research on the haematology and clinical chemistry of wild birds. I would suggest that ornithologists and others who trap and handle raptors regularly should be encouraged to take appropriate samples.

Captive birds of prey are no longer kept solely for sport, pleasure or education; many are used for scientific investigations in an attempt to learn more about the hazards mentioned earlier or in attempts to retard their decline in numbers in the wild. In addition, birds of prey have been utilised for research in other fields and there seems little doubt that they will be used increasingly for studies on diseases. The maintenance of hawks in captivity for research purposes requires high standards of management and many problems are encountered upon which expert advice is regularly required.

Even if a veterinary surgeon is unfamiliar with raptors he is usually able to refer the case to a more experienced colleague or a veterinary college and should be encouraged to do so. He should also be asked to submit raptors that die for a full *post-mortem* examination with which a veterinary college, research laboratory or (in Britain) a Veterinary Investigation Centre will be able to assist.

My own study of birds of prey over the past ten years has never been full time and has usually had to be fitted into a busy work programme. However, during this period I have endeavoured to improve our knowledge of clinical and pathological aspects of bird of prey diseases. In so doing I have maintained close co-operation with others, especially veterinary surgeons, zoologists and ornithologists and also with falconers and laymen.

In the first edition I listed the cases examined and the diagnoses which I had made over the previous six years. As a result of that survey it was possible to throw light on the possible aetiology of some diseases, to put forward suggestions about others and to study various techniques of treatment. The continued co-operation of falconers and aviculturists has permitted the investigation of various drugs, such as cloxacillin and lincomycin in the treatment of bumblefoot, methyridine and levamisole for capillariasis and metomidate, CT 1341 and ketamine for anaesthesia. Similar progress has been seen elsewhere and a number of important advances have been made. There are, however, many unanswered questions and problems which could be solved if sufficient work and time were devoted to them. The advances to date have been largely due to the personal interest of a small number of enthusiasts who, often against considerable odds, have involved themselves in hawk medicine.

Other benefits have accrued from my own and other people's work on bird of prey disease. In particular, the maintenance of health in raptors kept for captive breeding has been improved considerably and conservation projects, such as that with the Mauritius kestrel, have benefited from the increased store of knowledge on disease prevention and therapy. As a result of *post-mortem* examinations it was possible to submit data (5) to the British Home Office as evidence to support the introduction of legislation restricting the importation of birds of prey. Relevant information has also been made available to other bodies, including organisations concerned with conservation and animal welfare.

As I mentioned in Chapter 1, the past decade has seen the appearance of many publications on bird of prey disease. These have included not only papers in scientific journals but also less technical articles in publications intended for falconers and other laymen. The appearance of such material has enabled those concerned with captive birds of prey to approach the subject of raptor diseases scientifically and methodically. It is not only in this country that such advances have been made. Important publications have appeared in Europe and in North America and many of these are included in the References at the end of the book. It is imperative that liaison with those working in other countries is sought. In view of this I have always tried to maintain close contact with overseas bodies, in particular the Raptor Research Foundation in the United States, of whose Pathology Committee I am fortunate enough to be a member. Such interchange of information is vital if knowledge is to be disseminated and progress made.

A particularly encouraging feature of the past five years has been the upsurge of interest, more especially among veterinary surgeons but also wildlife biologists and conservationists, in the treatment of sick and injured wild raptors. It is increasingly being realised that such work can play a role in conservation and education as well as being justifiable on humanitarian grounds. Recognition of this fact has resulted in public and private support for schemes and practical assistance to those involved in them.

In North America in particular, the study of raptor biology has become a respected branch of animal science; papers of high quality regularly appear in "Raptor Research" and other journals. Increasingly these deal with problems related to health, amongst them nutrition, physiology and pathology.

As a result the whole field of bird of prey medicine is expanding and it is reasonable to assume that the next ten years will see dramatic developments in such fields as clinical chemistry, anaesthesia, surgery and pathology. Those involved in raptor medicine are likely to become more specialised in their various disciplines and it is probable that future editions of this book will include contributions by experts in different fields. It is not impossible that developments in captive breeding may result in the production of strains of birds that are, amongst other things, resistant to certain disease. Improved techniques of artificial insemination may result in the recognition of venereally transmitted diseases or, conversely, the procedure may find acceptance as a means of *preventing* disease spread, by direct contact, between birds. Increased numbers of birds in captivity will enable more detailed studies of disease to be carried out and, hopefully, controlled trials on drugs of various types. These and other possibilities offer an exciting challenge.

There also seems little doubt that experimental work using captive raptors or other birds as laboratory "models", will assume increasing importance. Such an approach is essential if many of the problems relating to raptor disease are to be elucidated. The use of germ-free birds may become possible in the study of infectious disease and the "normal" anatomy and physiology. In Britain at least, experimental work on raptors will receive a mixed reception, since there is considerable public concern over the use of animals in research. Those who involve themselves in such studies must ensure that the work cannot satisfactorily be performed by using any non-living system and that attention is paid at all times to the welfare of the birds.

Birds of prey have been associated with man for centuries and considerable knowledge has been acquired on their care and management. Much remains to be learned, however, of the diseases, infections and causes of death of these species. With the increasing interest in the maintenance of raptors in captivity the need for veterinary attention and advice has become vital and it is encouraging to note that more members of the profession are prepared to treat such cases. If the veterinary surgeon is to play a full role then he must have access to data on these species. It is hoped that this book will go some way towards meeting those demands.

List of species

These species are those birds of prey to which reference is made elsewhere in the book. Other scientific names are given in the text.

English name	Scientific name
FALCONIFORMES	
Turkey vulture	Cathartes aura
King vulture	Sarcorhamphus papa
Andean condor	Vultur gryphus
Osprey	Pandion haliaetus
Black-shouldered kite	Elanus caeruleus
Black kite	Milvus migrans
African fish eagle	Haliaeetus vocifer
White-tailed sea eagle	Haliaeetus albicilla
Steller's sea eagle	Haliaeetus pelagicus
African white-backed vulture	Gyps africanus
Cape vulture	Gyps coprotheres
Lappet-faced vulture	Torgos tracheliotus
Bateleur	Terathopius ecaudatus
African harrier hawk	Polyboroides typus
Crane hawk	Geranospiza caerulescens
Hen harrier	Circus cyaneus
Dark chanting goshawk	Melierax metabates
Pale chanting goshawk	Melierax canorus
Gabar goshawk	Melierax gabar
Northern goshawk (Goshawk)	Accipiter gentilis
Black sparrow-hawk	Accipiter melanoleucus
European sparrow-hawk	Accipiter nisus
Sharp-shinned hawk	Accipiter striatus
African goshawk	Accipiter tachiro
Shikra	Accipiter badius
Cooper's hawk	Accipiter cooperii
Grasshopper buzzard eagle	Butastur rufipennis
Harris's hawk	Parabuteo unicinctus
Red-tailed hawk	Buteo jamaicensis
Common buzzard	Buteo buteo
Augur buzzard	Buteo rufofuscus
Tawny (and steppe) eagle	Aquila rapax
African hawk eagle	Hieraaetus fasciatus

English name	*Scientific name*
FALCONIFORMES	
Wahlberg's eagle	*Aquila wahlbergi*
Golden eagle	*Aquila chrysaetos*
Martial eagle	*Polemaetus bellicosus*
Secretary bird	*Sagittarius serpentarius*
Laughing falcon	*Herpetotheres cachinnans*
Falconet	*Microhierax* sp.
Red-legged falconet	*Microhierax caerulescens*
American kestrel	*Falco sparverius*
Common kestrel	*Falco tinnunculus*
Mauritius kestrel	*Falco punctatus*
Seychelles kestrel	*Falco araea*
Red-headed falcon (or merlin)	*Falco chicquera*
Merlin	*Falco columbarius*
Eleonora's falcon	*Falco eleonorae*
Lanner falcon	*Falco biarmicus*
Prairie falcon	*Falco mexicanus*
Lagger (or lugger) falcon	*Falco jugger*
Saker falcon	*Falco cherrug*
Gyrfalcon	*Falco rusticolus*
Peregrine	*Falco peregrinus*

STRIGIFORMES	
Barn owl	*Tyto alba*
Great horned owl	*Bubo virginianus*
European eagle owl	*Bubo bubo*
Spotted eagle owl	*Bubo africanus*
Verreaux's eagle owl	*Bubo lacteus*
Javan fish owl	*Ketupa ketupa*
Spectacled owl	*Pulsatrix perspicillata*
Snowy owl	*Nyctea scandiaca*
Red-chested owlet	*Glaucidium tephronotum*
Little owl	*Athene noctua*
Barred owl	*Strix varia*
Tawny owl	*Strix aluco*
African wood owl	*Strix woodfordi*
Short-eared owl	*Asio flammeus*
Marsh owl	*Asio capensis*
Saw-whet owl	*Aegolius acadicus*

Subspecies are not usually differentiated in this book. Thus, for example, the European peregrine (*Falco peregrinus peregrinus* Tunst.) and the black shahin (*Falco peregrinus peregrinator* Sund.) are both listed as "Peregrine – *Falco peregrinus*". The only exceptions are the tawny and steppe eagles, which are referred to separately by their English names but both of which are listed as "*Aquila rapax*".

Bird of prey record card

Species: Reference Nos.
(English and scientific names)   Subspecies:
                                             (if known)

Sex: Age: Date of hatching:
                                             (if known)

Where obtained: Origin:
(if known)

Date obtained:

Health when obtained:
   Clinical examination:

   Laboratory tests:

   Treatment (if any):

Weight on arrival: Wing measurement:
                                   (carpus to tip of longest primary)

Other data:

Management on arrival:

188

Subsequent history (general):

DATE	COMMENTS

Breeding Records:

(a) *Courtship and reaction to owner*

DATE	COMMENTS

(b) *Egg laying*

DATE	COMMENTS

(c) *Hatching and rearing of young*

DATE	COMMENTS

(d) *Other comments (e.g. diet, use of A1, artificial incubation etc.)*

Ultimate fate of bird:

Clinical examination

Clinical No. ....   Pathology No. ....
Species...   Sex .... Age ....
Owner ....   Address ....
Veterinary Surgeon ....   Address ....
First examined..............................   Location ....
Indications for examination ....
Radiography performed .... Weight ....

HISTORY AND RELEVANT DATA

RESULTS OF CLINICAL EXAMINATION

FURTHER TESTS, RADIOGRAPHY

LABORATORY RESULTS

SUBSEQUENT INVESTIGATIONS

COMMENTS

Post-mortem examination

Clinical No.	Pathology No. ....
Species..	Date of examination......................
Sex.................. Age	Pathologist ....
Owner	Address ....
Veterinary Surgeon	Address ....
Specimen...................Died/killed.........................Destroyed by ....
Post-mortem state	Nutritional state ....
Radiography performed	Weight ....

HISTORY AND RELEVANT DATA

EXTERNAL FINDINGS

INTERNAL FINDINGS (GENERAL)

DIGESTIVE CANAL

LIVER AND OTHER GLANDS

URINO-GENITAL

RESPIRATORY

CARDIOVASCULAR

MUSCULO-SKELETAL

NERVOUS

FOR FURTHER INVESTIGATION

LABORATORY RESULTS:

(a) Microbiology

(b) Histopathology

(c) Toxicology

(d) Other

PROBABLE CAUSE OF DEATH

COMMENTS

Egg examination

Ref. No..

Species.. Date laid .... Storage ....

Owner .... Address ....

Veterinary surgeon .... Address ....

Date received .... Date examined ....

HISTORY AND RELEVANT DATA (including method of incubation, age and origin of parents, details of clutch)

RESULTS OF EXAMINATION

Weight.. Length .... Width ....

Weight of empty dried shell...

External appearance

Internal appearance

Comments on embryo

Microbiology

Histopathology

Toxicology

Other tests

COMMENTS

Key to major clinical diagnoses

Locality	Clinical sign or lesion	Possible diagnoses
Head	Swelling	Trauma, pox, sinusitis, insect bite, stomatitis, abscess.
	Rhythmical distension of soft tissue in front of eyes	Upper respiratory infection or physical obstruction.
	Ocular lesions	Trauma, conjunctivitis, ophthalmitis, vitamin A deficiency, pox, cataract.
	Eyes closing	A sign of many diseases including (sometimes) tuberculosis and low condition.
	Sneezing	Rhinitis, sinusitis, irritation by dust or chemicals.
	Nasal discharge	Rhinitis, sinusitis.
	Nasal haemorrhage	Trauma or hypertensive (?) rupture of blood vessels.
	Mouth lesions	Trichomoniasis, capillariasis, pox, stomatitis (see text).
	Fluid from mouth	Capillariasis or other mouth lesions, some types of poisoning.
	Blood from mouth	As for nasal haemorrhage (above).
	Damp feathers on side of head	Otitis, trauma.

Locality	Clinical sign or lesion	Possible diagnoses
Head (cont.)	Head on one side	Otitis, trauma, encephalitis or other nervous disease.
	Head hanging low	Blindness (see later).
	Blindness (complete or partial)	Trauma, poisoning (especially chlorinated hydrocarbons), vitamin A deficiency.
	Voice change	Respiratory disease, syngamiasis, starvation, several other conditions.
Wings	Wing hanging or paralysed	Fracture, dislocation, tendonitis/arthritis, traumatic damage to joint, nerve, tendon or ligament, osteodystrophy, irritant injection in pectoral muscles.
	Blood on feathers	Compound fracture, skin wound, damaged young feathers.
	Swellings	Fracture, abscess, granuloma, tuberculosis, bursitis.
	Missing or drooping feathers	Moulting, feather abnormalities (see later), gangrene.
Legs	Swelling or displacement	Osteodystrophy, rickets, fracture, dislocation, bursitis, abscess, granuloma, tuberculosis, oedema.
	Haemorrhage	Trauma, poor fitting jesses.
	Paralysed	Trauma, internal lesions, egg-laying, vitamin deficiency, Marek's disease?
	Absence of feathers	Ectoparasites, feather abnormality, possibly an underlying hormonal or metabolic disorder.

Locality	*Clinical sign or lesion*	*Possible diagnoses*
Feet	Swelling	Bumblefoot, articular gout, arthritis, trauma, jesses or ring too tight.
	Pale in colour	Low dietary carotene.
	Localised lesions	Pox, Type 1 bumblefoot, trauma, vitamin A deficiency, papillomatosis.
	Paralysed	As for nervous signs, may occur in conjunction with enteritis.
	Knuckling over	Nervous damage.
Body	Swelling	Fracture, abscess, tuberculosis, granuloma, haematoma, obesity, neoplasia, subcutaneous emphysema, irritant injection.
	Abdominal distension and discomfort	Egg peritonitis, impacted cloaca, damage during insemination, other abdominal lesions.
	Soiling of cloaca	Enteritis, cloacitis, prolonged recumbency.
	Sternal lesion	Trauma, prolonged recumbency.
Feathers	Missing	Moult, trauma, nutritional deficiency, metabolic disturbance, non-specific factors.
	Broken	Trauma, metabolic disturbance, nutritional deficiency.
	Frayed	Ectoparasites, metabolic disturbance, nutritional deficiency.

Locality	Clinical sign or lesion	Possible diagnoses
General signs	Chronic weight loss	Tuberculosis, aspergillosis, various types of parasit
	Dyspnoea	Foreign body in upper alimentary or respiratory tract, syngamiasis, rhinitis, pneumonia, air sacculitis, aspergillosis.
	Hyperpnoea	Overheating, septicaemia, pneumonia, air sacculiti anaemia.
	Excessive drinking	Tuberculosis, kidney disease, other infections, Dehydration, egg-laying.
	Anorexia	Overweight, several infectious diseases, food unpalatable.
	Dysphagia	Pellet not cast, foreign body, any condition affecting buccal cavity or causing dyspnoea.
	Flicking of food	Stomatitis and certain other conditions, food unpalatable.
	Regurgitation	Oesophageal capillariasis or other crop lesion, gastritis, air sacculitis. May also occur under stressful conditions.
	Wet, foetid casting	As for regurgitation.
	Failure to cast, or delay in casting	A sign of many diseases. Also associated with overfeeding and dry food.
	Diarrhoea	Bacterial or parasitic infection of intestine, cloacitis, low roughage diet, air sacculitis, unsuitable food, non-specific factors (e.g. chilling).
	Poorly formed mutes	Enteritis, cloacitis, egg-laying.
	Green mutes	Low food intake.
	Yellow faeces	Previous administration of certain drugs (e.g. 2-amino-5-nitrothiazole).

Locality	Clinical sign or lesion	Possible diagnoses
General signs (cont.)	Dysentery (fresh blood)	Trauma, cloacal calculus, cloacitis, constipation (straining).
	Dysentery (partly digested blood)	Coccidosis, capillariasis, other causes of haemorrhage in upper tract.
	Unabsorbed yolk sac (chicks)	Chilling or other environmental stressor.
	Nervous signs	Poisoning (especially insecticidal), vitamin B1 deficiency, hypocalcaemia, hypoglycaemia, bacterial otitis or encephalitis, trauma.
	Trembling	Nervous temperament, various nervous diseases.

Key to major post-mortem diagnoses (Macroscopical)

Locality	Lesion	Possible diagnoses
External	As in previous Appendix	As in previous Appendix.
Internal Body cavity	Inflammation Caseous lesions	Peritonitis, septicaemia. Aspergillosis, tuberculosis, nocardiosis.
	Haemorrhage	Trauma, electrocution, poisoning, apoplexy.
	Pale colour, watery blood	Anaemia.
	Bright pink colour Hyperaemia of organs Internal swellings	Carbon monoxide poisoning. Septicaemia, poisoning. Haematoma, abscess, neoplasia, tuberculosis, aspergillosis, egg in oviduct or body cavity.
	White deposits on serosae and elsewhere	Visceral gout, intraperitoneal barbiturate.
Respiratory tract	Inflammation	Rhinitis, bronchitis, air sacculitis, pneumonia.
	Clouding or thickening of air sacs	*Post-mortem* degeneration, air sacculitis.
	Nematodes	*Cyathastoma, Syngamus* or *Serratospiculum* infestation.
	Lesions in lung or air sacs	Pneumonia, air sacculitis, aspergillosis, inhalation pneumonia, abscess (extension from fractured rib), trauma.

Locality	Lesion	Possible diagnoses
Respiratory tract (cont.)	Black or dark material in lungs or air sacs	Anthracosis, inhalation of certain drugs.
Alimentary tract	Inflammation	Enteritis of bacterial or other aetiology.
	Nematodes Cestodes Trematodes }	Helminthiasis (various species).
	Haemorrhages	Coccidiosis, capillariasis, poisoning, electrocution.
	Green material	Low food intake, lead poisoning.
	Stones and fibrous material in gizzard	Impacted gizzard, presence of rangle, inanition.
	Constipation	Impacted cloaca, high roughage diet, mechanical lesion of intestinal tract e.g. intussusception.
Cardiovascular system	Flabby heart Oedema Hydropericardium }	Anaemia or other circulatory disturbance.
	Lesions of pericardium	Pericarditis, septicaemia, visceral gout.
	Lesions of myocardium	Myocarditis.
	Lesions of endocardium	Atheromatosis, endocarditis.
	Lesions of blood vessels	Vasculitis, atheromatosis, arteriosclerosis.
Liver	Foci	Tuberculosis, aspergillosis, viral hepatitis, other infections.
	Other parenchymal lesions	Septicaemia, viral hepatitis, trauma, neoplasia. fatty change.

Locality	Lesion	Possible diagnoses
Liver (cont.)	Capsular lesions	Septicaemia, air sacculitis, aspergillosis, visceral gout.
Kidney	Swollen	Nephritis, nephrosis.
Cloaca	Distended	Cloacal calculus.
	Wall thickened or inflamed	Cloacitis.
	Fresh blood	Cloacal calculus, cloacitis, constipation (straining) or traumatic injury (e.g. associated with artificial insemination).
Adrenal glands	Enlarged	Adrenal hypertrophy, infection.
Nervous system	Lesions on nerves	Tuberculosis, Marek's disease?
	Congestion of brain and meninges	Nervous disease, infection, trauma, bird in abnormal position before or at death.
Locomotory system	Muscle atrophy	Lack of use of muscle, starvation.
	Pale muscles	Anaemia.
	Soft, pliable bones	Young bird, osteodystrophy.
	Multiple fractures	Osteodystrophy, trauma.
	Swelling of bones or joints	Arthritis, osteitis, healing fracture.

Locality	Lesion	Possible diagnoses
Locomotory system (cont.)	Intraosseous haemorrhages of skull.	Agonal, trauma.
	Pale bone marrow	Anaemia.
	Bright pink bone marrow	Carbon monoxide poisoning.

Parasites identified from birds of prey 1966–77

The authorities for these parasites are not listed and for more detailed information the reader is referred to Chapter 6 and the appropriate References. The order in which the Hosts are listed reflects the relative frequency of identification of the parasite.

Group	Species of parasite	Hosts
PROTOZOA	Trypanosoma sp.	Peregrine
	Leucocytozoon sp.	Peregrine
	Leucocytozoon toddi	Augur buzzard Goshawk Sparrowhawk Peregrine
	Leucocytozoon ziemanni	Barn owl Tawny owl Red-chested owlet
	Haemoproteus sp.	Peregrine Saker Goshawk Grasshopper buzzard
	Haemoproteus cellii	Verreaux's eagle owl
	Haemoproteus figueiredoi	Tawny eagle
	Haemoproteus syrnii	Red-chested owlet Tawny owl
	Haemoproteus tinnunculus	Saker

Group	Species of parasite	Hosts
PROTOZOA (cont.)	*Plasmodium fallax*	Tawny eagle
	Plasmodium subpraecox	Red-chested owlet
	Plasmodium ?subpraecox	Snowy owl
	Haemogregarine	Snowy owl Black kite
	Trichomonas gallinae	Kestrel
	Coccidia (not identified)	Many species
NEMATODA	*Porrocaecum* sp.	Many species
	Porrocaecum angusticole	Goshawk Buzzard Lappet-faced vulture
	Porrocaecum spirale	Buzzard
	Porrocaecum depressum	Sparrowhawk Buzzard
	Cyrnea sp.	African goshawk
	Syngamus sp.	Several falconiform species
	Cyathastoma ?americanum	Goshawk
	Serratospiculum sp.	Peregrine Lanner Prairie Lagger
	Serratospiculum guttatum	Lanner

Group	Species of parasite	Hosts
NEMATODA (cont.)	*Serratospiculoides alii*	Saker
	Desmidocercella sp.	Red-chested owlet
	Synhimantus ?laticeps	Tawny owl
	Ascaridia sp.	Goshawk Sparrowhawk Buzzard Merlin Kestrel Red-headed merlin Lagger
	Capillaria sp.	Goshawk Merlin Peregrine Kestrel Lanner Red-headed merlin Sparrowhawk Red-chested owlet Lagger Gabar goshawk Shikra
	Capillaria contorta	Red-headed merlin Kestrel Peregrine Tawny owl
	Habronema tulostoma	Tawny owl Lappet-faced vulture
	Monopetalonema sp.	Crane hawk
	Microfilariae	Red-chested owlet

Group	Species of parasite	Hosts
NEMATODA (cont.)	Not identified	Goshawk Lagger Merlin Peregrine African goshawk Tawny owl Shikra
CESTODA	*Cladotaenia* sp.	Lagger
	Cladotaenia globifera	African hawk eagle Goshawk
	Physaloptera ?alata	African hawk eagle
	Hymenolepidae	Lagger
	Dilepididae	African hawk eagle
	Not identified	Many species
TREMATODA	*Neodiplostomum spathula*	Goshawk
	Not identified	Merlin Buzzard Sparrowhawk African goshawk Peregrine Lagger American kestrel Kestrel African white-backed vulture
ACANTHOCEPHALA	Unidentified	Lizard buzzard Black kite

Group	Species of parasite	Hosts
MALLOPHAGA	*Colpocephalum napiforme*	African fish eagle
	Colpocephalum turbinatum	Lanner
	Colpocephalum zerafae	Peregrine
	Laemobothrion sp.	Steppe eagle
	Laemobothrion maximum	Black kite African hawk eagle
	Laemobothrion tinnunculi	Merlin Lagger
	Laemobothrion vulturis	African white-backed vulture
	Strigiphilus sp.	Barn owl
	Craspedorhynchus sp.	African hawk eagle
	Craspedorhynchus platystomus	Buzzard
	Craspedorhynchus spatulatus	Black kite
	Degeeriella fulva	Buzzard African hawk eagle
	Degeeriella rufa	Lanner
	Degeeriella regalis castanea	African fish eagle
	Degeeriella discocephalus aquilarum	Steppe eagle

Group	Species of parasite	Hosts
MALLOPHAGA (cont.)	*Nosopon lucidum*	Kestrel
	Falcolipeurus suturalis	Steppe eagle
	Falcolipeurus lineatus	African white-backed vulture
	Not identified	Tawny owl African fish eagle
DIPTERA	*Ornithomyia avicularia*	Kestrel
	Stenepteryx hirundinis	Peregrine
	Pseudolynchia canariensis	Pale chanting goshawk
	Not identified (hippoboscids)	Tawny owl African white-backed vulture Mauritius kestrel
	Lucilia sericata	Kestrel Peregrine
	Calliphora sp.	Peregrine
SIPHONAPTERA	*Echidnophaga gallinacea*	Black-shouldered kite
ACARINA	*Ornithonyssus sylviarum*	Barn owl Goshawk
	Argas sp. (larvae)	Lanner

Drugs and other agents used in treatment

The drugs listed are those that have either been used by myself or for which reliable data, such as published papers, are available. Dosages are on a daily basis unless otherwise stated. For further information on the use of any agent listed the reader is referred to the text.

Condition	Drug	Route	Dose	Comments
Bacterial infections	Tetracycline Oxytetracycline Chlortetracycline	Oral Oral Oral	250 mg/kg	Capsules or powder in food or water. Chlortetra-cycline powder often eaten readily.
	Tylosin	Oral	250 mg/kg	—
	Spiramycin	Oral	250 mg/kg	—
	Lincomycin	Oral	Up to 50 mg/kg	Occasionally results in regurgitation.
	Ampicillin	Oral	250 mg/kg	—
	Cloxacillin	Oral	250 mg/kg	—
	Flucloxacillin	Oral	250 mg/kg	Not yet used by injection in raptors.
	Streptomycin	Oral	15 mg/kg	Often given with kaolin or sulphonamide.
	Neomycin	Oral	15 mg/kg	—
	Sulphonamides	Oral	500 mg/kg	—

Condition	Drug	Route	Dose	Comments
Bacterial infections (cont.)	Tetracyclines (as above)	i-m or i-v	15 mg/kg	May be painful by i-m injection.
	Tylosin	i-m	15 mg/kg	—
	Crystalline penicillin	i-m or i-v	Up to 100,000 units/kg	Do not use procaine penicillin.
	Spiramycin	i-m	20 mg/kg	—
	Ampicillin	i-m	100–250 mg/kg	—
	Cloxacillin	i-m	100–250 mg/kg	—
	Various other antibiotics (e.g. sodium fusidate)	Topical	As required	—
Fungal infections	Amphotericin B	Intra-tracheal	1 mg/kg	May be side effects. Usually given together with a broad-spectrum antibiotic.
	Other antifungal agents	Topical or by inhalation	Varies	See text.
Helminth parasites	Piperazine	Oral	100 mg/kg	—
	Thiabendazole	Oral	500 mg/kg	—
	Diethylcarbamazine	Oral	50 mg/kg	—
	Bunamidine hydrochloride	Oral	25 mg/kg	—
	5-chloro-N-salicylamid	Oral	150 mg/kg	—

Condition	Drug	Route	Dose	Comments
Helminth parasites (cont.)	Rafoxanide	Oral	10 mg/kg	—
	Methyridine	Oral or i-m	0·15 ml/kg	—
	Levamisole	Oral or s-c	15 mg/kg	—
	Tetramisole	Oral	100 mg/kg	—
Anti-protozoals	Sulphadimidine	Oral	500 mg/kg	Coccidiosis. Use for 3 days and then repeat after a break of 2 days.
	Acinitrazole	Oral	40 mg/kg	Trichomoniasis.
	Dimetridazole	Oral	100 mg/kg	Trichomoniasis.
	Metronidazole	Oral	100 mg/kg	Trichomoniasis.
	2-amino-5-nitrothiazole	Oral	20–40 mg/kg	Trichomoniasis.
Ectoparasites	Derris dust	External	As required	Care should be taken in the use of all insecticides for birds of prey.
	Pyrethrum powder	External	As required	
	Piperonyl butoxide	External	As required	
	Malathion (5% powder)	External	As required	
	Coumaphos, propoxur and sulphanilamide ("Negasunt": Bayer)	External	As required	
	Trichlorphon	External	0·15% solution	
Dehydration or shock	Glucose-saline or similar fluid replacement	Oral or by s-c or i-p	Plasma volume (4% BW) s-c or half this i-p	s-c is the route of choice. In emergency cases the i-v route can be used.

Condition	Drug	Route	Dose	Comments
Dehydration or shock (cont.)	Protein hydrolysate ("Protogest": welcome)	Oral	Up to 10 ml/kg	—
	Corticosteroids	i-m	See later	—
Inanition	Vitamin preparations	Oral or by i-m	See later	—
	Protein hydrolysate	Oral	As above	—
	"Complan" (Glaxo)	Oral	Up to 10 ml/kg	An oesophageal tube is recommended.
	Dextrose (glucose) solution	Oral	Up to 10 ml/kg	—
	„ „	s-c	Up to 5 ml/kg of 10% solution	—
Wounds	Gentian violet/ crystal violet	Topical	As required	—
	Tincture of iodine	Topical	As required	—
	Quaternary ammonium disinfectant	Topical	As required	Solution in warm water.
	Sulphonamide powder	Topical	As required	—
	Crystalline penicillin	Topical	As required	For irrigating deeper wounds.
	"Negasunt" (Bayer)	Topical	As required	Wounds where maggots present.
	Oxytetracycline/ gentian violet spray	Topical	As required	—

Condition	Drug	Route	Dose	Comments
Local analgesics	Ethyl chloride	Spray	—	Effect superficial.
	Lignocaine (2% solution, preferably diluted 1/10 in saline)	Injection	0·5 ml/kg	Use, with caution, in large birds only.
General anaesthetics	Pentobarbitone sodium	i-m or i-v	30 mg/kg	Not usually recommended.
	CT 1341	i-v	10 mg/kg	—
	Metomidate	i-m	10 mg/kg	Smaller doses are recommended for vultures.
	Phencyclidine	i-m	1 mg/kg	Not recommended; side effects can be marked.
	Xylazine	i-m	7 mg/kg	Reported to be effective and analgesic.
	Ketamine	i-m	50 mg/kg	—
	Ketamine	i-v	Up to 30 mg/kg	Smaller doses are recommended for owls.
	Ether	Inhalation	As required	—
	Halothane	Inhalation	As required	—
	Methoxyflurane	Inhalation	As required	—
	Trichlorethylene	Inhalation	As required	—
"Sedatives"	Pentobarbitone	Oral	Up to 20 mg/kg	Effect is variable.
	Phenobarbitone	Oral	Up to 30 mg/kg	
	Diazepam	i-m	10 mg/kg	
	Diazepam	i-v	Up to 2 mg/kg	Can be used in conjunction with ketamine in anaesthesia.
	Xylazine	i-m	Up to 2 mg/kg	

Condition	Drug	Route	Dose	Comments
"Sedatives" (cont.)	Metomidate	i-m	5 mg/kg	—
	Primidone	Oral	125 mg/kg	—
	Ketamine	i-m	25 mg/kg	—
	Reserpine	Oral	2–4 mg/kg	Produces prolonged sedation.
Hormones and similar agents	Prednisolone	Oral	Up to 0·5 mg/kg	Slowly increased and decreased.
	Methylprednisolone acetate	i-m	5 mg/kg	Given weekly.
	Betamethasone	Oral or i-m	Up to 0·05 mg/kg	Slowly increased and decreased.
	Thyroxine	Oral	Up to 1 mg/kg	To induce moult: slowly increased and decreased.
	Adrenaline (1/10,000 solution)	i-m or i-c	0·5 ml	Emergency use only.
	Atropine	i-m	0·05 mg/kg	—
Emetics	Salt solution	Oral	Up to 20 ml/kg	Provide water *ad lib.* after use.
	Mustard seeds	Oral	Up to 1 g/kg	An old-fashioned remedy.
Purgatives	Liquid paraffin	Oral	Up to 5 ml/kg	Also *per cloacam* for impaction.
	Glycerine	Oral	Up to 5 ml/kg	
	Sucrose in water	Oral	Up to 10 ml/kg	A mild purgative.

Condition	Drug	Route	Dose	Comments
Anti-diarrhoeals	Kaolin (or kaolin/bismuth) suspension	Oral	Up to 15 ml/kg	Avoid mixtures which contain morphine.
	Kaolin and neomycin ("Kaobiotic": Upjohn)	Oral	2–5 ml/kg	—
	Also see Bacterial Infections			
Vaccines	Newcastle disease vaccine (inactivated)	s-c	As for poultry	Repeat regularly.
	Pigeon pox	Scarification	As for pigeons	—
	Staphylococcus toxoid	i-m	Up to 1·0 ml	Of doubtful value.
Vitamins	"Abidec" (Parke Davis & Co.)	Oral	0·5 ml/kg or one capsule	—
	Multi-Vitamin (C-Vet)	i-m	Up to 0·5 ml/kg	—
	Vitamin A injection (C-Vet)	i-m	Up to 0·5 ml/kg	—
	Thiamine hydrochloride	i-m	1·0 mg/kg	—
	"SA-37" (Intervet)	Oral	Up to one teaspoonful	Do not give continuously.
	"Vionate" (Squibb)	Oral	Up to one teaspoonful	Do not give continuously.

Condition	Drug	Route	Dose	Comments
Minerals	Sterilised bonemeal	Oral	Small quantities on food	Do not give continuously.
	Calcium boragluconate (10% solution)	i-v or s-c	Up to 5 ml/kg	—
Miscel-laneous	Trypsin solution	Topical	—	Irrigation of bumble-foot lesions.
	Silver nitrate	Topical	—	Proliferative lesions of mouth or feet.
	10% sodium chloride solution	Topical	Up to 10 ml/kg	Granulating lesions and old wounds.
	Feather meal	Oral	Up to one teaspoonful	A general supplement: possibly valuable for feather conditions.
Disinfectants	Formalin (1–2%)	—	As required	Very effective but irritant. Rinse afterwards.
	Washing soda (2–5%)	—	As required	Cheap and effective. Rinse afterwards.
	Cetrimide (1%)	—	As required	Very effective against bacteria. No need to rinse.
	Phenol compounds (1–5%)	—	As required	Effective against bacteria but irritant and toxic. Rinse afterwards.
	Methyl or ethyl alcohol (70%)	—	As required	For instruments.

The following drugs are not, in general, recommended for use in birds of prey:

Drug	Reason
Chloramphenicol	Danger of infective resistance (4)
Streptomycin (injection)	Toxicity (15, 56)
Neomycin (injection)	Toxicity (Cooper, unpublished data)
Procaine penicillin	Toxicity (15)
Local analgesics (procaine group)	Toxicity (161, 339)
Chlorinated hydrocarbon insecticides	Toxicity (51, 80)

Many chemical agents may also prove toxic and several of these are discussed in Chapter 9.

Suggested drug and equipment list

This list is not comprehensive but includes the main drugs and equipment that are likely to prove valuable for the treatment of birds of prey. It is particularly intended as a guide for those working on raptor projects in isolated areas where regular veterinary attention is not always available.

Those items marked with an asterisk can, at the time of writing, be obtained in Britain without a prescription.

All drugs should be stored at +4°C, *except* CT 1341 anaesthetic.

Brilliant green/crystal violet*
Oxytetracycline powder
Spiramycin injection
Tylosin injection
Ampicillin capsules 50 mg and 250 mg
Cloxacillin/ampicillin injection
Lincomycin injection
Ophthalmic (antibiotic) ointment
Levamisole
Piperazine tablets*
Thiabendazole tablets or suspension*
Bunamidine hydrochloride tablets*
Sulphaquinoxaline or sulphadimidine solution
Dimetridazole tablets
Trichlorphon insecticide*
Pyrethrum powder insecticide*
Atropine injection
Adrenaline solution
Corticosteroid injection and tablets
Liquid paraffin*
Neomycin/kaolin suspension
Calcium boragluconate injection*
Multivitamin injection*
Glucose saline solution*
Glucose powder*
Sterilised bone meal*
Phenobarbitone tablets
Steroid (CT 1341) anaesthetic
Metomidate anaesthetic
Ketamine anaesthetic

Methoxyflurane anaesthetic
Halothane anaesthetic
Avian tuberculin
Newcastle disease vaccine
Pigeon-pox vaccine
Formalin solution 10%*
Quaternary ammonium or ampholytic disinfectant*
Vacuum flask and ice*
Distilled water*
Phosphate buffered saline*
Methyl alcohol 70%*
Scalpel blades*
Needles and syringes*
Surgical appliances and diagnostic aids*
Plaster of Paris*
Oesophageal tube*
Gloves*
Hood or small piece of cloth or canvas*

Relevant law

This is a brief summary of the legislation most relevant to the veterinary aspects of captive birds of prey. In applying the law to individual circumstances reference should be made to the legislation itself and to the relevant literature; professional advice should be sought where necessary. The law stated is that applying to England and Wales at the time of writing and may be subject to subsequent amendment.

Veterinary Surgeons Act 1966

Veterinary surgery is the diagnosis and treatment of illness and injury in animals.

Veterinary surgery may only be practised by registered veterinarians. Except that:

(a) an unqualified person may give an animal first aid treatment to save life or relieve pain,
(b) the owner of an animal or a member of his household or their employee may treat his (the owner's) own bird,
(c) a doctor, dentist or physiotherapist may carry out treatment at the request of a registered veterinarian.

Medicines Act 1968

This Act controls the production and supply of medicinal products.

Poisons Act 1972

This Act controls the storage and supply of poisons, whether medicinal or not.

These two Acts are gradually being brought into force, replacing the Therapeutic Substances Act 1956 and the Pharmacy and Poisons Act 1933.

Misuse of Drugs Act 1971

This Act regulates the supply and possession of controlled (formerly called dangerous) drugs, particularly those of addiction.

Protection of Birds Acts 1954–67

These Acts make it illegal (subject to certain exemptions) to kill, injure or take any wild bird. Nests, eggs and young birds are also protected. It is illegal to have in one's possession a bird recently taken or killed unless this was done legally. It is legal to take or kill a bird, often under licence, for certain sporting, educational and pest control purposes. It is legal to take a sick or injured wild bird for the sole purpose of tending it and releasing it when it has recovered or to kill a bird which is beyond hope of recovery. However, the harm must not have been caused by the person taking the bird for attention.

There are restrictions on the sale and importation of birds (see later) and a licence is required to take certain birds in the course of falconry.

The rarer birds, including all indigenous British birds of prey except the kestrel and the buzzard are listed in the First Schedule and thereby attract higher fines on conviction for an offence involving them.

Protection of Animals Acts 1911–64

It is an offence to cause unnecessary suffering to domesticated or captive animals, including birds. This can include positive maltreatment and the failure to attend to a bird's needs, failure to obtain necessary treatment and the performance of a surgical operation without due care and humanity.

Abandonment of Animals Act 1960

An animal, including a bird, must not, without reasonable cause, be abandoned in circumstances likely to cause it unnecessary suffering. To do so will amount to an offence of cruelty under the Protection of Animals Acts. When releasing a wild bird, therefore, consideration must be given to its ability to survive.

Cruelty to Animals Act 1876

It is an offence to perform painful experiments upon vertebrate animals, including birds, except under the authority of a Home Office licence.

Diseases of Animals Act 1950

Zoonoses Order 1975
The Ministry of Agriculture, Fisheries and Food has power to investigate an outbreak of salmonellosis in any species of bird although the reporting of an outbreak is compulsory only in food-producing species.

Transit of Animals (General Order) 1973
Birds, inter alia, must be protected from injury and unnecessary suffering and provided with their general welfare needs, such as food and water, during transportation.

Endangered Species (Import and Export) Act 1976

Many species of bird of prey are listed in Schedule 1 of the Act and their importation and exportation require a Department of the Environment licence as well as documents from the overseas country involved.

Importation of Captive Birds Order 1976

All captive birds and hatching eggs must be imported into Great Britain under a Ministry of Agriculture licence and will be subject to 35 days' quarantine under veterinary supervision. There is an exemption from the licencing requirements for the import of up to two caged pet birds accompanying a person entering Great Britain (not merely on a holiday trip); imports under licence of up to 12 birds must undergo isolation and veterinary supervision although they are exempt from the stricter requirements of quarantine.

The Theft Act 1968

A free-living (wild) bird is no-one's property and cannot therefore be stolen. Once it is taken into captivity it has an owner and unlawfully to deprive him of the bird is theft.

There are many aspects of the law which are in some degree relevant to birds of prey which cannot be included here, in particular, the game laws which must be observed by those practising the sport of falconry and the civil law, which governs the rights between individuals, particularly regarding compensation for loss, injury and damage. More detailed information can be obtained from the literature listed in the bibliography.

Bibliography

Anon. (1971). *Wild Birds and the Law*. The Royal Society for the Protection of Birds, Sandy, Beds.

Anon. (1975). *Legislation Affecting the Veterinary Profession in Great Britain*. The Royal College of Veterinary Surgeons, London.

Anon. (undated). *Cruelty to Animals and the Law*. The Royal Society for the Prevention of Cruelty to Animals, Horsham, Sussex.

Boyd, H. (1972). Legal requirements. *Laboratory Animal Handbook* **5**, 91–100.

Cooper, Margaret E. (1977). Birds of prey and the law. Occasional paper published by the Hawk Trust, Hungerford, Berks.

Cooper, Margaret E. (in press). Wild bird hospitals and the law. In Cooper, J. E. and Eley, J. T. Editors. *First Aid and Care of Wild Birds*. David and Charles, Newton Abbot.

Field-Fisher, T. G. (1964). *Animals and the Law*. Universities Federation for Animal Welfare, London.

Halsbury, Lord (1973). Editor. *Laws of England*. Volume 2, 4th Edition, Butterworths, London.

North, P. M. (1972). *The Modern Law of Animals*. Butterworths, London.

Porter, A. R. W. (1975). Pet animals and the law. In Anderson, R. S. Editor. *Pet Animals and Society*. Ballière Tindall, London.

Thomas, J. L. (1975). *Diseases of Animals Law*. Police Review Publishing Co. Ltd., London.

Anaesthetic and surgery consent form

Owner's name and address..

....

Species of bird ....

Name or reference .... Age .... Sex ....

After explanation by my veterinary surgeon of the procedure, I authorise the administration of a general anaesthetic to the above bird and the performance of such surgical and/or other procedures as may prove necessary.

Signature of owner or authorised agent.......................................
Date.......................................

Despatch of pathological specimens

Articles Sent for Medical Examination or Analysis

Deleterious liquids or substances, though otherwise prohibited from transmission by post, may be sent for medical examination or analysis to a recognised medical laboratory or institute, or to a qualified medical practitioner or a registered dental practitioner or veterinary surgeon by first class letter post, but on no account by parcel post, under the following conditions:—

1. Any such liquid or substance must be enclosed in a receptacle, hermetically sealed or otherwise securely closed, and this receptacle must itself be placed in a strong wooden or metal case (or other case which has been approved by the Post Office) in such a way that it cannot shift about, and with a sufficient quantity of some absorbent material (such as sawdust or cottonwool) so packed about the receptacle as absolutely to prevent any possible leakage from the package in the event of damage to the receptacle. The package so made up must be conspicuously marked FRAGILE WITH CARE and bear the words PATHOLOGICAL SPECIMEN.
2. Any packet of the kind found in the parcel post, or found in the letter post not packed and marked as directed, will be at once stopped and destroyed with all its wrappings and enclosures. Further, any person who sends by a post deleterious liquid or substance for medical examination or analysis otherwise than as provided by these regulations is liable to prosecution.
3. Receptacles supplied by a laboratory or institute must be submitted to Postal Headquarters (PMk 1), St. Martin's-le-Grand, London, EC1A 1HQ, in order to ascertain whether they are regarded as complying with the regulations.

(Extracted, with permission, from
Post Office Regulations).

APPENDIX XIV

Notes on the collection and submission of material for laboratory investigation

General

The following notes are intended only as a guide. Those who regularly submit material from birds of prey for pathology and/or parasitology will usually be advised appropriately by their veterinary surgeon or laboratory.

Strict hygienic precautions should *always* be followed when pathological material is being handled. It is a wise precaution to wear gloves. Pathological material must be packed in suitable containers. Carcasses should be wrapped in two plastic bags surrounded by several layers of newspaper. Tissues should be enclosed in a clean, preferably sterile, container which is then wrapped in several layers of newspaper. Under no circumstances should an old medicine bottle be used since it may contain a drug which can affect laboratory results. Parasites should be placed in bottles.

Labelling is of great importance. A full clinical history should accompany a carcass but it must be wrapped separately and *not* enclosed in the same plastic bag as the specimen. Bottles should be clearly labelled and the tops sealed. The most important data required are:

Species
Reference (if any)
Date of death or of sampling, and
Name and address of owner.

All material sent by post should be well-packed and despatched by first class mail, marked 'URGENT. PATHOLOGICAL SPECIMEN'. Those who regularly send or receive such material are strongly advised to consult the Post Office Regulations (see Appendix XIII).

Dead birds for post-mortem examination

These should reach the Pathologist as soon as possible, preferably within a few hours of death. In the event of any delay, the specimen should be chilled at a refrigerator temperature of approximately +4°C.

Deep freezing will preserve a specimen, and certain bacteria and other organisms within it, but will damage the tissues and render histological examination extremely difficult. In certain cases, however, it may be necessary to freeze a

227

specimen before it can be examined or despatched. In such cases, it should be *rapidly* frozen, by placing it in a deep freeze which does not contain large amounts of other material.

Fixation of a specimen in formalin will preserve its tissues, thus making histology possible, but the formalin will kill bacteria and other organisms. Bacteriology and certain other tests will therefore prove unsatisfactory. Again, however, it may be necessary to use this technique under certain circumstances. It is particularly useful where a non-infectious disease e.g. a wound or a tumour, is present.

To fix a specimen in formalin use a 10% solution. This is made by purchasing concentrated formaldehyde from a chemist; although the bottle is marked 40% it should be considered as 100% proof and a 10% solution made by mixing one part of formaldehyde with 9 of water. Alternatively, buffered formalin or formol saline which are preferable to formalin may be available, already made up, from a laboratory. To ensure penetration of formalin the body wall should be *carefully* cut with a scalpel. The formalin should be discarded and replaced after 24 hours.

Specimens for *post-mortem* examination should not be preserved in alcohol unless nothing else is available.

Selected tissues from dead animals

Only small 1 cm "cubes" of a tissue are required, placed in 10% formalin. Do not squash them or squeeze them through the necks of bottles. Whenever this material is preserved in formalin there should be at least five, and preferably ten, times as much formalin as tissue present in the container. If this is not possible, the formalin should be changed after 24 hours.

The same principles apply to tissues as to whole animals. Again it is best if fresh material is submitted, chilled if necessary, providing it reaches the laboratory within 24 hours of death.

Bacteriological swabs must never be frozen nor fixed in formalin. Likewise, pus and faecal material must be submitted fresh.

Parasites from live or dead birds

Both external and internal parasites are best preserved in 70% ethyl or methyl alcohol. If neither of these is available, methylated spirits can be used or, in an emergency, gin or vodka!

In some cases a laboratory or research worker is anxious to receive live parasites and will issue his own instructions. Ticks and mites can usually be despatched dry, in a tube, but internal parasites usually require to be kept damp, preferably in a 0·9% saline solution.

References

It should be noted that some of the publications listed were subsequently reprinted or appeared in several editions. The edition referred to is the one used during the compilation of this book.

1 Altman, R. B. (1969). Conditions involving the integumentary system. In Petrak, M. L. Editor. *Diseases of Cage and Aviary Birds*. Lea and Febiger, Philadelphia.

2 Andrew, W, and Hickman, C. P. (1974). *Histology of the Vertebrates*. The C. V. Mosby Company, St. Louis.

3 Anon. (1953). Encephalitis in short-wings. *The Falconer* **11,** 28–30.

4 Anon. (1969). Report of the Joint Committee on the use of Antibiotics in Animal Husbandry and Veterinary Medicine. H.M.S.O., London.

5 Anon. (1969). Annual Report of the International Council for Bird Preservation, British Section, London.

6 Anon. (1970). Report on the Animal Health Services in Great Britain 1970. H.M.S.O., London.

7 Anon. (1972). Recommended Treatment of Oiled Seabirds. Research Unit on the Rehabilitation of Oiled Seabirds, Department of Zoology, University of Newcastle upon Tyne.

8 Anon. (1974). Fourth Annual Report, 1973. Research Unit on the Rehabilitation of Oiled Seabirds, Department of Zoology, University of Newcastle upon Tyne.

9 Anon. (1977). The Evaluation of Toxicological Data for the Protection of Public Health. Proceedings of the International Colloquium Luxembourg, 1976. Published for the Commission of the European Communities by Pergamon Press, Oxford.

10 Anon. (1977). The function of fever. *Lancet* **ii,** 178.

11 Antillon, A., Scott, M. L., Krook, L. and Wasserman, R. H. (1977). Metabolic response of laying hens to different dietary levels of calcium, phosphorus and vitamin D3. *Cornell Veterinarian* **67,** 413–444.

12 Apinis, A. E. and Pugh, G. J. F. (1967). Thermophilous fungi of birds' nests. Mycopathologia et Mycologia applicata **33,** 1–9.

13 Arnall, L. (1964). Aspects of anaesthesia in cagebirds. In Graham-Jones, O. Editor. *Small Animal Anaesthesia*. Pergamon Press, London.

14 Arnall, L. (1969). Diseases of the respiratory system. In Petrak, M. L. Editor. *Diseases of Cage and Aviary Birds*. Lea and Febiger, Philadelphia.

15 Arnall, L. and Keymer, I. F. (1975). *Bird Diseases*. Baillière Tindall, London.

16 Asakura, S., Nakagawa, S., Masui, M. and Yasuda, J. (1962). Immunological studies of aspergillosis in birds. *Mycopathologia et Mycologia applicata* **18,** 249–256.

17 Avicultural Society (1977). *Register of non-domesticated birds bred under controlled conditions in Britain during 1976*. Coordinated by B. Sayers, Chelmsford, Essex.

18 Baker, J. R. (1977). The results of post-mortem examination of 132 wild birds. *British Veterinary Journal* **133,** 327–333.

19 Balasch, J., Musquera, S., Palacios, L., Jimenez, M. and Palomeque, J. (1976). Comparative hematology of some falconiforms. *Condor* **78,** 258–259.

20 Barker, J. (1973). Epilepsy in the dog – a comparative approach. *Journal of Small Animal Practice* **14,** 281–289.

21 Bartholomew, G. A. and Cade, T. J. (1957). The body temperature of the American kestrel, *Falco sparverius*. *Wilson Bulletin* **69,** 149–154.

22 Bean, J. R. and Hudson, R. H. (1976). Acute oral toxicity and tissue residues of thallium sulphate in golden eagles, *Aquila chrysaetos*. *Bulletin of Environmental Toxicology* **15,** 118–121.

23 Beebe, F. L. (1976). *Hawks, Falcons and Falconry*. Hancock House Publishers Ltd., British Columbia.

24 Beebe, F. and Webster, H. (1964). *North American Falconry and Hunting Hawks*. World Press, Denver.

25 Beister, H. E. and Schwarte, L. H. (1975). Editors. *Diseases of Poultry*. 5th Edition. Iowa State University Press.

26 Bell, A. A. and Murton, R. K. (1977). Dieldrin residues in carcases of kestrels and barn owls. *Institute of Terrestrial Ecology, Annual Report* 1976, 22–25.

27 Benson, W. W., Pharoah, B. and Miller, P. (1974). Lead poisoning in a bird of prey. *Bulletin of Environmental Contamination and Toxicology* **II,** 105–108.

28 Berg, W., Johnels, A., Sjöstrand, B. and Westermark, T. (1966). Mercury content in feathers of Swedish birds from the past 100 years. *Oikos* **17,** 71–83.

29 Bergmann, F. and Dikstein, S. (1954). Studies on uric acid and related compounds. I. Quantitative determinations of uric acid in biological fluids. *Journal of Biological Chemistry* **211,** 149–153.

30 Berners, Dame Jullana (1486). *The Boke of St. Albans*. Printed at St. Albans by the Schoolmaster Printer. Reprinted with Introduction by William Blades. Elliott Stock, London, 1881.

31 Berry, R. B. (1972). Reproduction by artificial insemination in captive American goshawks. *Journal of Wildlife Management* **36,** 1283–1288.

32 Bert, E. (1619). *An Approved Treatise of Hawkes and Hawking*. Richard Moore. Reprinted in 1891 and again in 1969 by Bernard Quaritch Ltd., London.

33 Bicknell, E. J., Greichus, A., Greichus, Y. A., Bury, R. J. and Knudtson, W. U. (1971). Diagnosis and treatment of aspergillosis in captive cormorants. *Sabouraudia* **9,** 119–122.

34 Bigland, C. H. (1966). Common diseases of non-commercial and pet birds. *Canadian Veterinary Journal* **7,** 252–259.

35 Bigland, C. H., Liu, S-K. and Perry, M. L. (1964). Five cases of Serratospiculum amaculata (Nematoda: Filaroidea) infection in prairie falcons (Falco mexicanus). *Avian Diseases* **VIII,** 412–419.

36 Bilo, D., Best, G., Schönenberger I., and Nachtigall, W. (1972). Zur Methode der Halothan-Inhalationsnarkose bei Vögeln (Taube und Wellensittich). *Journal of Comparative Physiology* **79,** 137–152.

37 Bird, D. M. and Buckland, R. B. (1976). The onset and duration of fertility in the American kestrel. *Canadian Journal of Zoology* **54,** 1395–1397.

38 Bird, D. M. and Ho, S. K. (1976). Nutritive values of whole-animal diets for captive birds of prey. *Raptor Research* **10,** 45–49.

39 Bird, D. M. and Lague, P. C. (1975). Treatment of bumblefoot by radiotherapy. *Hawk Chalk* **XV,** 57–60.

40 Bird, D. M., Lague, P. C. and Buckland, R. B. (1976). Artificial insemination versus natural mating in captive American kestrels. *Canadian Journal of Zoology* **54,** 1183–1191.

41 Blackmore, D. K. (1965). The pattern of disease in budgerigars: a study in comparative pathology. Ph.D. thesis, London.

42 Blackmore, D. K. and Gallagher, G. L. (1964). An outbreak of erysipelas in captive wild birds and mammals. *Veterinary Record* **76**, 1161–1164.

43 Blackmore, D. K. and Keymer, I. F. (1969). Cutaneous diseases of wild birds in Britain. *British Birds* **62**, 316–331.

44 Blaine, G. (1936). *Falconry*. Reprinted in 1976 by Neville Spearman Ltd., London.

45 Blancou, J. and Rajaonarison, J. (1972). Note sur le rôle vecteur des rapaces dans la propagation de certaines maladies bactériennes. *Revue d' élevage et de médicine vétérinaire des pays tropicaux* **25**, 187–189.

46 Blome, R. (1686). *The Gentleman's Recreation*. Printed by S. Roycroft, London.

47 Board, R. G., Tullett, S. G. and Perrott, H. R. (1977). An arbitrary classification of the pore systems in avian eggshells. *Journal of Zoology*, London **182**, 251–265.

48 Bonath, K. (1972). Zur Inhalationsnarkose von Hühnern, Tauben, Enten und anderen Vögeln mit Halothan und Äther und deren Wirkung auf Blutdruck, Herz –, Atemfrequenz und Körpertemperatur. *Zentralblatt für Veterinärmedizin* **19**, 639–660.

49 Bonath, K. (1972). Inhalations –, Injektions– und Lokalanaesthesie der Vögel. Sonderdruck aus Verhandlungsbericht des XIV Internationalen Symposiums über die Erkrankungen der Zootiere. Akademie-Verlag. Berlin.

50 Borzio, F. (1973). Ketamine hydrochloride as an anesthetic for wild fowl. *Veterinary Medicine/Small Animal Clinician* **68**, 1364–1365.

51 Bougerol, C. (1967). *Essai sur la pathologie des oiseaux de chasse au vol*. Alfort, France.

52 Boyd, L. (1977). Hybridization of falcons by artificial insemination. Paper given at Symposium of the Zoological Society of London, September, 1977.

53 Boyd, L. L., Boyd, N. S. and Dobler, F. C. (1977). Reproduction of prairie falcons by artificial insemination. *Journal of Wildlife Management* **41**, 266–271.

54 Brisbin, I. L. (1970). A determination of live-weight caloric conversion factors for laboratory mice. *Ecology* **51**, 541–544.

55 Brisbin, L. and Wagner, C. K. (1970). Some health problems associated with the maintenance of American kestrels, *Falco sparverius*, in captivity. *International Zoo Yearbook* **10**, 29–30.

56 British Veterinary Association (1970). *Handbook on the Treatment of Exotic Pets (Part One: Cage Birds)*. British Veterinary Association, London.

57 Brown, L. H. (1976). *British Birds of Prey*. Collins, London.

58 Brown, L. H. (1976). *Birds of Prey; Their Biology and Ecology*. Hamlyn, London.

59 Brown, L. H. and Amadon, D. (1968). *Eagles, Hawks and Falcons of the World*. Country Life Books, Hamlyn House, Middlesex.

60 Bucke, D. and Mawdesley-Thomas, L. E. (1974). Tuberculosis in a barn owl (*Tyto alba*). *Veterinary Record* **95**, 373.

61 Buckley, P. A. (1969). Genetics. In Petrak, M. L. Editor. *Diseases of Cage and Aviary Birds*. Lea and Febiger, Philadelphia.

62 Burtscher, H. (1965). Die virusbedingte Hepatosplenitis infectiosa strigorum. I. Mitteilung: Morphologische Untersuchungen. *Pathologia Veterinaria* **2**, 227–255.

63 Burtscher, M. and Sibalin, M. (1975). Herpesvirus striges: host spectrum and distribution in infected owls. *Journal of Wildlife Diseases* **11**, 164–169.

64 Cade, T. J. (1975). Editor. *Captive Breeding – the 1975 Season*. Newsletter No. 3, The Peregrine Fund, Laboratory of Ornithology, Cornell University.

65 Cadle, D. R. and Martin, G. R. (1976). Metomidate as sole anaesthetic agent in tawny owls. *Veterinary Record* **98,** 91–92.

66 Calder, W. A. and Schmidt-Nielsen, K. (1968). Panting and blood carbon dioxide in birds. *American Journal of Physiology* **215,** 477–482.

67 Caldwell, L. D. and Connell, C. E. (1968). A precis on energetics of the old – field mouse. *Ecology* **49,** 542–548.

68 Campbell, J. A. (1934). Some observations relative to ailments of inmates in a zoological collection. *Journal of the American Veterinary Medical Association* **84,** 711–739.

69 Cerna, Z. and Louckova, M. (1977). *Microtus arvalis,* the intermediate host of a coccidian from the kestrel (*Falco tinnunculus*). *Vestnik Ceskoslov enske Spolecnosti Zoologicke* **XLI,** 1–4.

70 Chambers, W. B. and Pallagrosi, A. U. (1977). Gentamicin in the treatment of staphylococcal infections. *Journal of International Medical Research* **5,** 442–449.

71 Chiasson, R. B., Egge, A. S. and Lynch, B. (1973). The effect of ketalar on the adrenal gland of young white leghorn cockerels. *Poultry Science* **52,** 1014–1018.

72 Cho, B. R. and Kenzy, S. G. (1975). Virologic and serologic studies of zoo birds for Marek's disease virus infection. *Infection and Immunity* **11,** 809–814.

73 Chu, H. P., Trow, E. W., Greenwood, A. G., Jennings, A. R. and Keymer, I. F. (1976). Isolation of Newcastle disease virus from birds of prey. *Avian Pathology* **5,** 227–233.

74 Clarke, A. (1977). Contamination of peregrine falcons (*Falco peregrinus*) with fulmar stomach oil. *Journal of Zoology, London* **181,** 11–20.

75 Clausen, B. and Karlog, O. (1977). Thallium loading in owls and other birds of prey in Denmark. *Nordisk veterinaermedicin* **29,** 227–231.

76 Coatney, G. R. and West, E. (1937). Some notes on the effect of atrebrine on the gametocytes of the genus Leucocytozoon. *Journal of Parasitology* **23,** 227–228.

77 Cobb, S. (1960). Observations on the comparative anatomy of the avian brain. *Perspectives in Biology and Medicine* **3,** 383–408.

78 Comben, N. (1969). The early English printed literature on the diseases of poultry and other birds. *The Veterinarian* **6,** 17–25.

79 Conder, P. (1973). Illegal use of alphachloralose. *Veterinary Record* **92,** 325.

80 Cooper, J. E. (1965). Death of a trained falcon attributed to chlorinated hydrocarbon poisoning. *The Falconer* **IV,** 230–232.

81 Cooper, J. E. (1968). Tuberculosis in birds of prey. *Veterinary Record* **82,** 61.

82 Cooper, J. E. (1968). The trained falcon in health and disease. *Journal of Small Animal Practice* **9,** 559–566.

83 Cooper, J. E. (1968). Diseases of hawks. *The Falconer* **V,** 55–57.

84 Cooper, J. E. (1969). Some diseases of birds of prey. *Veterinary Record* **84,** 454–457.

85 Cooper, J. E. (1969). Oesophageal capillariasis in captive falcons. *Veterinary Record* **84,** 634–636.

86 Cooper, J. E. (1969). Two cases of pox in recently imported peregrine falcons (*Falco peregrinus*). *Veterinary Record* **85,** 683–684.

87 Cooper, J. E. (1970). Use of the hypnotic agent "Methoxymol" in birds of prey. *Veterinary Record* **87,** 751–752.

88 Cooper, J. E. (1970). Diseases of birds of prey. *Annual Report of the Hawk Trust* **1,** 22–31.

89 Cooper, J. E. (1971). First aid and preventive medicine for hawks. *The Falconer* **V**, 299–304.

90 Cooper, J. E. (1972). Feather conditions of birds of prey. *Journal of the North American Falconers' Association* **XI**, 39–44.

91 Cooper, J. E. (1972). Possible vaccination against aspergillosis. *Raptor Research* **6**, 105.

92 Cooper, J. E. (1972). Some haematological data for birds of prey. *Raptor Research* **6**, 133–136.

93 Cooper, J. E. (1973). Blood parasites from a red-chested owlet *Glaucidium tephronotum*. *Bulletin of British Ornithologists' Club* **93**, 25–26.

94 Cooper, J. E. (1973). Health and disease. In Mavrogordato, J. G. *A Hawk for the Bush*. 2nd Edition, Neville Spearman, London.

95 Cooper, J. E. (1973). Post-mortem findings in East African birds of prey. *Journal of Wildlife Diseases* **9**, 368–375.

96 Cooper, J. E. (1974). Metomidate anaesthesia of some birds of prey for laparotomy and sexing. *Veterinary Record* **94**, 437–440.

97 Cooper, J. E. (1974). Trichlorphon as a safe insecticide for use on birds of prey. *Veterinary Record* **94**, 455.

98 Cooper, J. E. (1975). Osteodystrophy in birds of prey. *Veterinary Record* **97**, 307.

99 Cooper, J. E. (1975). The role of vaccination in the maintenance of captive birds of prey. *Raptor Research* **9**, 21–26.

100 Cooper, J. E. (1975). Haematological investigations in East African birds of prey. *Journal of Wildlife Diseases* **11**, 389–394.

101 Cooper, J. E. (1975). First aid and veterinary treatment of wild birds. *Journal of Small Animal Practice* **16**, 579–591.

102 Cooper, J. E. (1976). Clinical conditions of East African birds of prey. *Tropical Animal Health and Production* **8**, 203–211.

103 Cooper, J. E. (1976). Health and diseases of hawks. Paper presented at the International Conference on Falconry and Conservation, Abu Dhabi, 10–18 December, 1976.

104 Cooper, J. E. (1977). Veterinary problems of captive breeding and possible reintroduction of birds of prey. *International Zoo Yearbook* **17**, 32–38.

105 Cooper, J. E. (1978). An adenocarcinoma in a buzzard (*Buteo buteo*). *Avian Pathology* **7**, 29–34.

106 Cooper, J. E. and Frank, L. (1973). Use of the steroid anaesthetic CT 1341 in birds. *Veterinary Record* **92**, 474–479.

107 Cooper, J. E. and Kenward, R. E. (1977). Editors. *Papers on the Veterinary Medicine and Domestic Breeding of Diurnal Birds of Prey*. Proceedings of the 1975 British Falconers' Club Conference. Published by the British Falconers' Club.

108 Cooper, J. E. and Kreel, L. (1976). Radiological examination of birds: report of a small series. *Journal of Small Animal Practice* **17**, 799–808.

109 Cooper, J. E. and Needham, J. R. (1976). An investigation into the prevalence of *S. aureus* on avian feet. *Veterinary Record* **98**, 172–174.

110 Cooper, J. E. and Redig, P. T. (1975). Unexpected reactions to the use of CT 1341 by red-tailed hawks. *Veterinary Record* **97**, 352.

111 Corbel, M. J. (1972). The serological response to *Aspergillus fumigatus* antigens in bovine mycotic abortion. *British Veterinary Journal* **128**, 73–75.

112 Corbel, M. J., Pepin, G. A. and Millar, P. G. (1973). The serological response to *Aspergillus fumigatus* in experimental mycotic abortion in sheep. *Journal of Medical Microbiology* **6**, 539–548.

113 Couch, J. R. and Ferguson, T. M. (1975). Nutrition and embryonic development in the domestic fowl. *Proceedings of the Nutrition Society* **34,** 1–3.

114 Cowan, P. F. (1968). Diseases of captive reptiles. *Journal of the American Veterinary Medical Association* **153,** 848–859.

115 Cowan, S. T. and Steel, K. J. (1975). *Manual for the Identification of Medical Bacteria.* Cambridge University Press.

116 Cox, H. and Lascelles, G. (1892). *Coursing and Falconry.* The Badminton Library, Longmans, Green & Co., London.

117 Craig, T. H. and Powers, L. R. (1976). Raptor mortality due to drowning in a livestock watering tank. *Condor* **78,** 412.

118 Cribb, P. H. and Haigh, J. C. (1977). Anaesthetic for avian species. *Veterinary Record* **100,** 472–473.

119 Crisp, E. (1854). Filaria in the heart of a peregrine falcon (*F. peregrinus*). *Transactions of the Pathological Society of London* **5,** 345.

120 Croxall, J. P. (in press). In Cooper, J. E. and Eley, J. T. Editors. *First Aid and Care of Wild Birds.* David and Charles, Newton Abbot.

121 Cummings, J. H., Duke, G. E. and Jegers, A. A. (1976). Corrosion of bone by solutions simulating raptor gastric juice. *Raptor Research* **10,** 55–57.

122 Czekala, N. M. and Lasley, B. L. (1977). A technical note on sex determination in monomorphic birds using faecal steroid analysis. *International Zoo Yearbook* **17,** 209–211.

123 Daghir, N. J. (1975). Studies on poultry by-product meals in broiler and layer rations. *World's Poultry Science Journal* **31,** 200–211.

124 Daniellson, B. (1977). Editor. *Cynegetic Anglica 1. William Twiti: The Art of Hunting 1327.* Almquist and Wiksell International, Stockholm.

125 Davis, T. A. W. (1975). Food of the kestrel in winter and early spring. *Bird Study* **22,** 85–91.

126 de Bastyai, L. (1968). *Hunting Bird from a Wild Bird.* Pelham Books, London.

127 Dedrick, M. L. (1965). Notes on a strigeid trematode – an intestinal parasite of a prairie falcon. *Journal of the North American Falconers' Association* **IV,** 12–14.

128 Devriese, L. A. and Devos, A. H. (1975). Suppressive effects of antibiotics on experimentally inoculated *Staphylococcus aureus* populations on the skin of poultry. *Avian Pathology* **4,** 295–302.

129 Dieter, M. P. (1973). Sex determination of eagles, owls and herons by analysing plasma steroid hormones. Special Scientific Report U.S. Fish and Wildlife Service No. 167.

130 Disbrey, B. D. and Rack, J. H. (1970). *Histological Laboratory Methods.* Livingstone, Edinburgh.

131 Drent, R. (1970). Adaptive aspects of the physiology of incubation. *Proceedings of the XV International Ornithological Congress* 258–280.

132 Du Bose, R. T. (1972). Rabies. In Hofstad, M. S. *et al.* Editors. *Diseases of Poultry.* 6th Edition, Iowa State University Press.

133 Duke, G. E., Ciganek, J. G. and Evanson, O. A. (1973). Food consumption and energy, water and nitrogen budgets in captive great-horned owls (*Bubo virginianus*). *Comparative Biochemistry and Physiology* **44A,** 283–292.

134 Duke, G. E., Jegers, A. A., Loff, G. and Evanson, O. A. (1975). Gastric digestion in some raptors. *Comparative Biochemistry and Physiology* **50A,** 649–656.

135 Durant, A. J. (1953). Removing the vocal cords of fowl. *Journal of the American Veterinary Medical Association* **122,** 14–17.

136 Ebedes, H. (1973). The capture of free-living vultures in the Etosha National Park with phencyclidine. *Journal of the South African Wildlife Management Association* **3,** 105–107.

137 Elliott, R. H., Smith, E. and Bush, M. (1974). Preliminary report on hematology of birds of prey. *Journal of Zoo Animal Medicine* **5,** 11–16.

138 Evans, H. ap (1960). *Falconry for You*. John Gifford Ltd., London.

139 Evans, H. E. (1969). Anatomy of the budgerigar. In Petrak, M. L., Editor. *Diseases of Cage and Aviary Birds*. Lea and Febiger, Philadelphia.

140 Evelyn, J. (1664). *The Diary of John Evelyn*. London.

141 F.A.O./W.H.O. (1974). *Pesticide Residues in Food*. Report of 1973 Joint F.A.O./W.H.O. Meeting. Technical Report Series 545. W.H.O., Geneva.

142 Farner, D. S. and King, J. R. (continuing). Editors. *Avian Biology*. Academic Press, New York and London.

143 Fiennes, R. N. T-W. (1969). Diseases of bacterial origin. In Petrak, M. L. Editor. *Diseases of Cage and Aviary Birds*. Lea and Febiger, Philadelphia.

144 Fiennes, R. N. T-W. (1971). Personal communication with Keymer (1972).

145 Fimreite, N., Fyfe, R. W. and Keith, J. A. (1970). Mercury contamination of Canadian prairie seed eaters and their avian predators. *Canadian Field-Naturalist* **84,** 269–276.

146 Fimreite, N. and Karstad, L. (1971). Effects of dietary methyl mercury on red-tailed hawks. *Journal of Wildlife Management* **35,** 293–300.

147 Finlayson, R. (1964). Vascular disease in captive animals. *Symposium of the Zoological Society of London* **11,** 99–106.

148 Fisher, H, (1972). The nutrition of birds. In Farner, D. S., King, J. R., and Parkes, K. C. Editors. *Avian Biology* Vol. II. Academic Press, New York and London.

149 Fisher, S. (1957). Loss of immunizing power of staphylococcal toxin during routine toxoiding with formalin. *Nature* **180,** 1479–1480.

150 Flegg, J. J. M., Glue, D. E. and Mead, C. J. (1974). Sexing birds of prey. *Veterinary Record* **94,** 625.

151 Fowler, N. G. and Hussaini, S. N. (1975). Clostridium septicum infection and antibiotic treatment in broiler chickens, *Veterinary Record* **96,** 14–15.

152 Fox, H. (1920). Arterial sclerosis in wild animals. *American Journal of the Medical Sciences* **49,** 821–825.

153 Fox, H. (1923). *Diseases in captive wild mammals and birds*. J. B. Lippincott Co., London.

154 Fox, N. (1976). Rangle. *Raptor Research* **10,** 61–64.

155 Fox, N. C. (1977). Some morphological data on the Australasian harrier (*Circus approximans gouldi*) in New Zealand. *Notornis* **24,** 9–19.

156 Frank, L. G. and Cooper, J. E. (1974). Further notes on the use of CT 1341 in birds of prey. *Raptor Research* **8,** 29–32.

157 Frank, L. G. and Cooper, J. E. (1974). A report on the use of a pectoral muscle biopsy in the field for organochlorine residue analysis. *Raptor Research* **8,** 33–36.

158 Frazer, J. F. D. (1977). Growth of young vertebrates in the egg or uterus. *Journal of Zoology, London* **183,** 189–201.

159 Freeman, B. M. (1976). Stress and the domestic fowl: a physiological re-appraisal. *World's Poultry Science Journal* **32,** 249–256.

160 Freeman, B. M. and Manning, A. C. C. (1976). Failure of procaine penicillin and zinc bacitracin to modify the response of the fowl to stressors. *British Poultry Science* **17,** 285–292.

161 Friedburg, K. M. (1962). Anesthesia of parakeets and canaries. *Journal of the American Veterinary Medical Association* **141**, 1157–1160.

162 Friend, M. and Trainer, D. O. (1969). Aspergillosis in captive herring gulls. *Bulletin of the Wildlife Disease Association* **5**, 271–275.

163 Fuller, M. R. (1975). A technique for holding and handling raptors. *Journal of Wildlife Management* **39**, 824–825.

164 Fuller, M. R., Redig, P. T. and Duke, G. E. (1974). Raptor rehabilitation and conservation in Minnesota. *Raptor Research* **8**, 11–19.

165 Furr, P. M., Cooper, J. E. and Taylor-Robinson, D. (1977). Isolation of mycoplasmas from three falcons (*Falco* spp.). *Veterinary Record* **100**, 72–73.

166 Garnham, P. C. C. (1966). *Malarial Parasites and Other Haemosporidia*. Blackwell, Oxford.

167 Gatehouse, S. N. and Markham, B. J. (1970). Respiratory metabolism of three species of raptor. *Auk* **87**, 738–741.

168 Gerdessen, A. (1956). Beitrag zur Entwicklung der Falknerei un der Falkenheilkunde. Inaugural Dissertation Tierärztliche Hochschule, Hannover.

169 Glees, P. (1961). *Experimental Neurology*. Clarendon Press, Oxford.

170 Gordon, R. F. (1977). Editor. *Poultry Diseases*. Baillière Tindall, London.

171 Goulding, R. and Volans, G. N. (1977). Emergency treatment of common poisons: emptying the stomach. *Proceedings of the Royal Society of Medicine* **70**, 766–769.

172 Gough, P. M. and Jorgensen, R. D. (1976). Rabies antibodies in sera of wild birds. *Journal of Wildlife Diseases* **12**, 392–395.

173 Graham, D. L. (1970).Nutrition and nutritional diseases. In "Raptor Pathology and Nutrition". *Hawk Chalk* **IX**, 30–37.

174 Graham, D. L., Maré, C. J., Ward, F. P. and Peckham, M. C. (1975). Inclusion body disease (Herpesvirus infection) of falcons (IBDF). *Journal of Wildlife Diseases* **11**, 83–91.

175 Green, C. J. (in press). *Animal Anaesthesia: A Handbook*. Laboratory Animal Science Association Handbook Number 8.

176 Green, R. G. and Shillinger, J. E. (1935). A virus disease of owls. *Journal of Immunology* **29**, 68–69.

177 Greenwood, A. G. (1973). Editor. *Veterinary Medicine of Birds of Prey*. Proceedings of the 1973 British Falconers' Club Conference.

178 Greenwood, A. G. (1974). Sexing birds of prey. *Veterinary Record* **95**, 69.

179 Greenwood, A. G. (1977). The role of disease in the ecology of British raptors. *Bird Study* **24**, 259–265.

180 Greenwood, A. G. and Blakemore, W. F. (1973). Pox infection in falcons. *Veterinary Record* **93**, 468.

181 Greiner, E. C. and Kocan, A. A. (1977). Leucocytozoon (Haemosporidia: Leucocytozoidae) of the Falconiformes. *Canadian Journal of Zoology* **55**, 761–770.

182 Grimm, R. J. and Whitehouse, W. M. (1963). Pellet formation in a great horned owl: a roentgenographic study. *Auk* **80**, 301–306.

183 Grossman, M. L. and Hamlet, J. (1965). *Birds of Prey of the World*. Cassell and Company Ltd., London.

184 Hacking, A. and Blandford, T. A. (1971). Aspergillosis in five-to-16 week-old turkeys. *Veterinary Record* **88**, 519–520.

185 Hafez, E. S. E. (1975). Editor. *The Behaviour of Domestic Animals*. 3rd Edition. Baillière Tindall, London.

186 Halliwell, W. H. (1967). Bumblefoot in raptorial birds. *Journal of the North American Falconers' Association* **VI**, 49–53.

187 Halliwell, W. H. (1971). Lesions of Marek's disease in a great horned owl. *Avian Diseases* **15**, 49–55.

188 Halliwell, W. H. (1972). Avian pox in an immature red-tailed hawk. *Journal of Wildlife Diseases* **8**, 104–105.

189 Halliwell, W. H., Graham, D. L. and Ward, F. P. (1973). Nutritional diseases in birds of prey, *Journal of Zoo Animal Medicine* **4**, 18–20.

190 Halloran, P. O'C. (1955). *A Bibliography of References to Diseases in Wild Mammals and Birds*. American Veterinary Medical Association.

191 Hamerstrom, F. and Skinner, J. L. (1971). Cloacal sexing of raptors. *Auk* **88**, 173–174.

192 Hamerton, A. E. (1935). Report on the deaths in the Society's Gardens during 1934. *Proceedings of the Zoological Society of London* **105**, 443–474.

193 Hamerton, A. E. (1938). Report on the deaths in the Society's Gardens during 1937. *Proceedings of the Zoological Society of London* **108**, 489–526.

194 Hamerton, A. E. (1939). Review of mortality rates and report on the deaths occurring in the Society's Gardens during the year 1938. *Proceedings of the Zoological Society of London* **109**, 281–287.

195 Hamerton, A. E. (1941). Report on the deaths occurring in the Society's Gardens during the years 1939–1940. *Proceedings of the Zoological Society of London* **111**, 151–187.

196 Hamerton, A. E. (1943). Report on the deaths occurring in the Society's Gardens during the years 1941–1942. *Proceedings of the Zoological Society of London* **112**, 120–137.

197 Hamm, D. and Hicks, W. J. (1975). A new oral electrolyte in calf scours therapy. *Veterinary Medicine/Small Animal Clinician* **70**, 279–282.

198 Hare, T. (1939). Notes on two diseases of hawks; capillariasis and coccidiosis. *The Falconer* **V**, 4–7.

199 Harting, J. E. (1891). *Bibliotheca Accipitraria, A Catalogue of Books Ancient and Modern relating to Falconry*. Reprinted by the Holland Press. London, 1964.

200 Harting, J. E. (1898). *Hints on the Management of Hawks and Practical Falconry*. Reprinted in 1971 by the Thames Valley Press, Maidenhead.

201 Hasholt, J. (1960). Diseases of the nervous system. In Petrak, M. L. Editor. *Diseases of Cage and Aviary Birds*. Lea and Febiger, Philadelphia.

202 Hegner, R. W. (1925). *Giardia felis* n.sp. from the domestic cat and Giardias from birds. *American Journal of Hygiene* **5**, 258–273.

203 Heintzelman, D. S. (1971). Observations on the role of nest box sanitation in affecting egg hatchability of wild sparrowhawks in Eastern Pennsylvania. *Raptor Research News* **5**, 100–103.

204 Hesser, E. F. (1960). Methods for routine fish hematology. *Progressive Fish Culturist* **22**, 164–171.

205 Hickey, J. J. (1969). Editor. *Peregrine Falcon Populations*. University of Wisconsin Press.

206 Higuchi, K. (1976). *PCB Poisoning and Pollution*. Academic Press, New York and London.

207 Hill, H. M. and Work, T. H. (1947). Protocalliphora larvae infesting nestling birds of prey. *Condor* **49**, 74–75.

208 Hitchner, S. B., Domermuth, C. H., Purchase, H. G. and Williams, J. E. (1975). Editors. *Isolation and Identification of Avian Pathogens*. American Association of Avian Pathologists, Texas A & M University.

209 Hodges, R. D. (1974). *The Histology of the Fowl*. Academic Press, New York and London.

210 Hodges, R. D. (1977). Avian haematology. In Archer, R. K. and Jeffcott, L. B. Editors. *Comparative Clinical Haematology*. Blackwell Scientific Publications, Oxford.

211 Hodgetts, B., Jones, D. R. and Binstead, J. A. (1977). The response of broiler chicks to vitamin drenches immediately after hatching. *Veterinary Record,* **101,** 268.

212 Hoerlein, B. F. (1971). *Canine Neurology*. W. B. Saunders Company, Philadelphia.

213 Hofstad, M. S., Calnek, B. W., Helmboldt, C. F., Reid, W. M. and Yoder, H. W. (1972). Editors. *Diseases of Poultry*. 6th Edition. Iowa State University Press.

214 Holliday, T. A., Van Meter, J. R., Julian, L. M. and Asmundson, V. S. (1965). Electromyography of chickens with inherited muscular dystrophy. *American Journal of Physiology* **209,** 871–876.

215 Holt, P. E. (1977). The use of a steroid anaesthetic in a long-eared owl (*Asio otus*). *Veterinary Record* **101,** 118.

216 Hoogstraal, H., Oliver, R. M. and Guirgis, S. S. (1970). Larva, nymph and life cycle of *Ornithodoros* (*Alectorobius*) *muesebecki* (Ixodoidea: Argasidae), a virus-infected parasite of birds and petroleum industry employees in the Arabian Gulf. *Annals of the Entomological Society of America* **63,** 1762–1763.

217 Houston, D. C. (1972). The ecology of Serengeti vultures. D. Phil. thesis, University of Oxford.

218 Houston, D. C. and Cooper, J. E. (1973). Use of the drug metomidate to facilitate the handling of vultures. *International Zoo Yearbook* **13,** 269–271.

219 Houston, D. C. and Cooper, J. E. (1975). The digestive tract of the whiteback griffon vulture and its role in disease transmission among wild ungulates. *Journal of Wildlife Diseases* **11,** 306–313.

220 Howard, B. R. (1972). Sleep in the domestic fowl. *Proceedings of the Royal Society of Medicine* **65,** 177–179.

221 Humphreys, P. N. (1977). Debilitating syndrome in budgerigars. *Veterinary Record* **101,** 248–249.

222 Hunter, C. G., Robinson, J. and Jager, K. W. (1967). Aldrin and dieldrin – the safety of present exposures of the general populations of the United Kingdom and United States. *Food and Cosmetics Toxicology* **5,** 781–787.

223 Hurrell, L. H. (1967). Wild raptor casualties. *The Falconer* **V,** 30–37.

224 Hurrell, L. H. (1973). On breeding the sparrow-hawk in captivity. In Mavrogordato, J. G. *A Hawk for the Bush*. 2nd Edition, Neville Spearman, London.

225 Inskipp, T. P. and Thomas, G. J. (1976). *Airborne Birds*. Royal Society for the Protection of Birds, Sandy, Bedfordshire.

226 Irving, L. (1955). Nocturnal decline in the temperature of birds in cold weather. *Condor* **57,** 362–365.

227 Jack, T. A. M. (1972). A goshawk recovers. *The Falconer* **VI,** 57–58.

228 Jack, T. A. M. (1977). A reply to the challenge. *Birds* **6,** 62.

229 Jaksch, W. (1960). Fussballengeschwulst bei Hühnern als Folge eines Mangelfutters. *Wiener tierärztliche Monatsschrift* **47,** 388–396.

230 Jefferies, D. J. and Prestt, I. (1966). Post-mortems of peregrines and lanners with particular reference to organochlorine residues. *British Birds* **59,** 49–64.

231 Jennings, A. R. (1959). Diseases in wild birds. Fifth Report. *Bird Study* **6**, 19–22.
232 Jennings, A. R. (1961). An analysis of 1,000 deaths in wild birds. *Bird Study* **8**, 25–31.
233 Jennings, A. R. (1969). Tumours of free-living wild mammals and birds in Great Britain. *Symposium of the Zoological Society of London* **24**, 273–287.
234 Jesiotr, M. (1973). Treatment of aspergillosis with emetine hydrochloride. *Scandinavian Journal of Respiratory Diseases* **54**, 326–332.
235 Johnson, D. C., Cooper, R. S. and Osborn, J. S. (1974). Velogenic viscerotropic Newcastle disease virus isolated from mice. *Avian Diseases* **18**, 633–634.
236 Johnson, I. M. (1969). Electrolyte and water balance of the red-tailed hawk, *Buteo jamaicensis*. Abstract, *American Society of Zoologists* **9**, 587.
237 Johnston, R. E. (1972). Water medication with sulphadiazine and trimethoprim for the treatment of staphylococcal osteomyelitis in poultry. *Australian Veterinary Journal* **48**, 578.
238 Jones, D. M. (1977). The occurrence of dieldrin in sawdust used as a bedding material. *Laboratory Animals* **11**, 137.
239 Jones, D. M. (1977). The sedation and anaesthesia of birds and reptiles. *Veterinary Record* **101**, 340–342.
240 Jorgenson, R. D., Gough, P. M. and Graham, D. L. (1976). Experimental rabies in a great horned owl. *Journal of Wildlife Diseases* **12**, 444–447.
241 Kaleta, E. F. and Drüner, K. (1976). Hepatosplenitis infectiosa strigum und andere Krankheiten der Greifvögel und Eulen. *Fortschritte der Veterinärmedizin* **25**, 173–180.
242 Kaliner, G. and Cooper, J. E. (1973). Dual infection of an African fish eagle with acid-fast bacilli and an *Aspergillus* sp. *Journal of Wildlife Diseases* **9**, 51–55.
243 Kalmbach, E. R. (1939). American vultures and the toxin of Clostridium botulinum. *Journal of the American Veterinary Medical Association* **94**, 187–197.
244 Karstad, L. and Sileo, L. (1971). Causes of death in captive wild waterfowl in the Kortright Waterfowl Park, 1969–70. *Journal of Wildlife Diseases* **7**, 236–241.
245 Kenward, R. E. (1974). Mortality and fate of trained birds of prey. *Journal of Wildlife Management* **34**, 751–756.
246 Kenward, R. E. (1976). The numbers of birds of prey obtained and possessed by falconers in the United Kingdom. Paper presented at Hawk Trust Conference, October, 1976.
247 Kenward, R. E. (1976). The effect of goshawk, *Accipiter gentilis*, predation on wood pigeon, *Columba palumbus*, populations. D. Phil. thesis, University of Oxford.
248 Keymer, I. F. (1969). Parasitic diseases. In Petrak., M. L. Editor. *Diseases of Cage and Aviary Birds*. Lea and Febiger, Philadelphia.
249 Keymer, I. F. (1972). Diseases of birds of prey. *Veterinary Record* **90**, 579–594.
250 Keymer, I. F. (1974). Ornithosis in free-living and captive birds. *Proceedings of the Royal Society of Medicine* **67**, 733–735.
251 Keymer, I. F. (1977). Diseases of birds other than domestic poultry. In Gordon, R. F. Editor. *Poultry Diseases*. Baillière Tindall, London.
252 Keymer, I. F. (1977). The importance of pathological examinations of birds of prey. In Cooper, J. E. and Kenward, R. E. Editors. *Papers on the Veterinary Medicine and Domestic Breeding of Diurnal Birds of Prey*. Published by the British Falconers' Club.
253 Keymer, I. F. (1977). Cataracts in birds. *Avian Pathology* **6**, 335–341.
254 Keymer, I. F. and Dawson, P. S. (1971). Newcastle disease in birds of prey.

Veterinary Record **88,** 432.

255 Khan, R. A. (1965). Development of Leucocytozoon ziemanni (Laveran). *Journal of Parasitology* **61,** 449–457.

256 King, A. S. and McLelland, J. (1975). *Outlines of Avian Anatomy.* Baillière Tindall, London.

257 Kingston, N., Remple, J. D., Burnham, W., Stabler, R. M. and McGhee, R. B. (1976). Malaria in a captively-produced F1 gyrfalcon and in two F1 peregrine falcons. *Journal of Wildlife Diseases* **12,** 562–565.

258 Kish, F. (1970). Egg laying and incubation by American golden eagles *Aquila chrysaetos canadensis* at Topeka Zoo. *International Zoo Yearbook* **10,** 26–29.

259 Kisling, V. N. (1974). A review of pesticide residues in commercial zoo feeds. *International Zoo Yearbook* **14,** 187–189.

260 Kocan, A. A. and Gordon, L. R. (1976). Fatal air sac infection with *Serratospiculum amaculata* in a prairie falcon. *Journal of the American Veterinary Medical Association* **169,** 908.

261 Kocan, A. A., Potgieter, L. N. D. and Kocan, K. M. (1977). Inclusion body disease of falcons (herpesvirus infection) in an American kestrel. *Journal of Wildlife Diseases* **13,** 199–201.

262 Kocan, A. A., Snelling, J. and Greiner, E. C. (1977). Some infectious and parasitic diseases in Oklahoma raptors. *Journal of Wildlife Diseases* **13,** 304–306.

263 Koeman, J. H., Garsson-Hoekstra, J., Pels, E. and de Goeij, J. J. M. (1971). Poisoning of birds of prey by methyl mercury compounds. *Mededelingen van de Faculteit Landbouwwetenschappen Rijksuniversiteit Gent* **36,** 43–49.

264 Köhler, B. and Baumgart, W. (1970). Toxi-Infektionen durch Clostridium perfringens Typ A. *Monatschefte für Veterinärmedizin* **25,** 348–352.

265 Kösters, J. (1974). Haltungsbedingte Krankheiten bei Greifvögeln. Der *Praktische Tierarzt (Supplement)* **55,** 31–33.

266 Kruijt, J. P. (1962). Imprinting in relation to drive interactions in Burmese red jungle fowl. *Symposium of the Zoological Society of London* **8,** 219–226.

267 Lancaster, D. A. and Johnson, J. R. (1975). Editors. *Peregrine Falcons Reintroduced.* Cornell Laboratory of Ornithology Newsletter **78,** 3.

268 Lane, J. G. and Warnock, D. W. (1977). The diagnosis of *Aspergillus fumigatus* infection of the nasal chambers of the dog, with particular reference to the value of the double diffusion test. *Journal of Small Animal Practice* **18,** 169–177.

269 Latham, S. (1615). *Falconry, or the Faulcons Lure and Cure.* Printed by J. B., London.

270 Lawson, P. T. and Kittle, E. L. (1970). Induced molt. *Raptor Research News* **4,** 138.

271 Leake, L. D. (1975). *Comparative Histology.* Academic Press, New York and London.

272 Leese, A. S. (1927). *A Treatise on the One-humped Camel in Health and Disease.* Haynes and Son, Stamford, Lincolnshire.

273 Leonard, J. L. (1969). Clinical laboratory examinations. In Petrak, M. L. Editor. *Diseases of Cage and Aviary Birds.* Lea and Febiger, Philadelphia.

274 Levinger, I. M., Kedem, J. and Abram, M. (1973). A new anaesthetic-sedative agent for birds. *British Veterinary Journal* **129,** 296–300.

275 Lincer, J. L. and Peakall, D. B. (1970). Metabolic effects of polychlorinated biphenyls in the American kestrel. *Nature* **228,** 783–784.

276 Lloyd, C. S., Thomas, G. J., MacDonald, J. W., Borland, E. D., Standring, K. and Smart, J. L. (1976). Wild bird mortality caused by botulism in Britain, 1975.

Biological Conservation **10**, 119–129.

277 Locke, L. N., Bagley, G. E., Frickie, D. N. and Young, L. T. (1969). Lead poisoning and aspergillosis in an Andean condor. *Journal of the American Veterinary Medical Association* **155**, 1052–1056.

278 Loken, A. C. (1971). Vitamin deficiencies. In Minckler, J. Editor. *Pathology of the Nervous System*. Volume II, McGraw-Hill Book Company, New York.

279 Longbottom, J. L. and Pepys, J. (1964). Pulmonary aspergillosis: diagnostic and immunological significance of antigens and c-substance in *Aspergillus fumigatus*. *Journal of Pathology and Bacteriology* **88**, 141–151.

280 Lorenz, K. Z. (1935). Der Kumpan in der Umwelt des Vogels. *Journal für Ornithologie* **83**, 137–213, 289–413.

281 Lucas, A. M. and Jamroz, C. (1961). *Atlas of Avian Hematology*. U.S. Dept. of Agriculture, Washington, D.C.

282 Lumb, W. V. and Jones, E. W. (1973). *Veterinary Anesthesia*. Lea and Febiger, Philadelphia.

283 McDiarmid, A. (1948). The occurrence of tuberculosis in the wild wood-pigeon. *Journal of Comparative Pathology* **58**, 128–133.

284 McDowell, E. M. and Trump, B. F. (1977). Practical fixation techniques for light and electron microscopy. *Comparative Pathology Bulletin* **IX**, 1 and 4.

285 McGill, A. E. J., Robinson, J. and Stein, M. (1969). Residues of dieldrin (HEOD) in complete prepared meals in Great Britain during 1967. *Nature* **221**, 761–762.

286 MacPhail, R. M. (1964). A goshawk's death attributed to carbon monoxide poisoning. *The Falconer* **IV**, 174–175.

287 Markham, G. (1631). *Country Contentments or, the Husbandmans Recreations*. London.

288 Markham, G. (1655). *Hungers Prevention: or The whole Art of Fowling by Water and Land*. London.

289 Marks, J. and Birn, K. J. (1963). Infection due to Mycobacterium avium. *British Medical Journal* **ii**, 1503–1506.

290 Markus, M. B. and Oosthuizen, J. H. (1972). Pathogenicity of *Haemoproteus columbae*. *Transactions of the Royal Society of Tropical Medicine and Hygiene* **66**, 186–187.

291 Martin, G. R. and Gordon, I. E. (1974). Increment-threshold spectral sensitivity in the tawny owl (*Strix aluco*). *Vision Research* **14**, 615–621.

292 Martin, G. R. and Gordon, I. E. (1974). Visual acuity in the tawny owl (*Strix aluco*). *Vision Research* **14**, 1393–1397.

293 Martin, G. R., Gordon, I. E. and Cadle, D. R. (1975). Electretinographically determined spectral sensitivity in the tawny owl (*Strix aluco*). *Journal of Comparative and Physiological Psychology* **89**, 72–78.

294 Matthews, P. R. J. and McDiarmid, A. (1977). *Mycobacterium avium* infection in free-living hedgehogs (*Erinaceus europaeus* L.). *Research in Veterinary Science* **22**, 388.

295 Mavrogordato, J. G. (1960). *A Hawk for the Bush*. 1st Edition, F. H. and G. Witherby, London, 2nd Edition (1973). Neville Spearman, London.

296 Mavrogordato, J. G. (1966). *A Falcon in the Field*. Knightly Vernon Ltd., London.

297 Mendelssohn, H. and Marder, U. (1970). Problems of reproduction in birds of prey in captivity. *International Zoo Yearbook* **10**, 6–11.

298 Mengden, C. A. and Stock, A. D. (1976). A preliminary report on the application of current cytological techniques to sexing birds. *International Zoo Yearbook* **16**,

138–141.

299 Michell, E. B. (1900). *The Art and Practice of Hawking*. The Holland Press, London.

300 Möller, D. (1976). Arabic treatises on falconry. Paper presented at the International Conference on Falconry and Conservation, Abu Dhabi, 10–18 December, 1976.

301 Moore, L. G. and Ronniger, P. A. (1966). Raptorial foot disease. *Journal of the North American Falconers' Association* **V,** 29–37.

302 Morley, C. J. (1977). Falconry – the facts. *Birds* **6,** 58.

303 Morrow, T. L. and Glover, F. A. (undated). *Experimental Studies on Post-Mortem Changes in Mallards*. Bureau of Sport Fisheries and Wildlife. Special Scientific Report Wildlife No. 134 Washington D.C.

304 Mosher, J. A. (1976). Raptor energetics; a review. *Raptor Research* **10,** 97–107.

305 Mumcuoglu, Y, and Müller, R. (1974). Parasitische Milben und Würmer als Todesursache eines Uhus *Bubo bubo. Der Ornithologische Beobachter* **71,** 289–292.

306 Mundy, P. J. and Ledger, J. A. (1976). Griffon vultures, carnivores and bones. *South African Journal of Science* **72,** 106–110.

307 Munger, L. L. and McGavin, M. D. (1972). Sequential post-mortem changes in chicken liver at 4, 20 or 37 C. *Avian Diseases* **16,** 587–605.

308 Munger, L. L. and McGavin, M. D. (1972). Sequential post-mortem changes in chicken kidney at 4, 20 or 37 C. *Avian Diseases* **16,** 606–621.

309 Nair, M. K. (1973). The early inflammatory reaction in the fowl. *Acta Veterinaria Scandinavica Supplementum* **42,** 1–103.

310 Nalin, D. R., Cash, R. A., Rahman, M., and Yunus, M. D. (1970). Effect of glycine and glucose on sodium and water absorption in patients with cholera. *Gut* **11,** 768–772.

311 Needham, J. R. (1974). A study of the coagulase and deoxyribonuclease tests applied to staphylococci fron non-human sources. *Medical Laboratory Technology* **31,** 141–143.

312 Needham, J. R. (1976). Control of animal health in a modern experimental unit: laboratory and microbiological investigations. Thesis for Fellowship of Institute of Medical Laboratory Sciences, London.

313 Needham, J. R. (1977). The collection of animal faeces for laboratory examination. *Journal of the Institute of Animal Technicians* **28,** 63–66.

314 Nelson, M. W. and Nelson, P. (1976). Power lines and birds of prey. *Idaho Wildlife Review,* March–April 1976, 1–5.

315 Nelson, N., Elgart, S. and Mirsky, I. A. (1942). Pancreatic diabetes in the owl. *Endocrinology* **31,** 119–123.

316 Nelson, R. W. (1967). A post-frounce complication. *Hawk Chalk* **VI,** 20.

317 Nelson, R. W. (1977). On the diagnosis and "cure" of imprinting in falcons which fail to breed in captivity. In Cooper, J. E. and Kenward, R. E. Editors. *Papers on the Veterinary Medicine and Domestic Breeding of Diurnal Birds of Prey.* Published by the British Falconers' Club.

318 Newton, I. (1976). Raptor research and conservation during the last five years. *Canadian Field-Naturalist* **90,** 225–227.

319 Newton, I, and Bogan, J. (1974). Organochlorine residues, eggshell thinning and hatching success in British sparrowhawks. *Nature* **249,** 582–583.

320 Newton, C. D. and Zeitlin, S. (1977). Avian fracture healing. *Journal of the American Veterinary Medical Association* **170,** 620–625.

321 Norberg, R. A. (1977). Occurrence and independent evolution of bilateral ear asymmetry in owls and implications on owl taxonomy. *Philosophical Transactions of*

the Royal Society, Series B, Volume 280, Issue Number 973.

322 Nunn, G. L., Klem, D., Kimmel, T. and Merriman, T. (1976). Surplus killing and caching by American kestrels (*Falco sparverius*). *Animal Behaviour* **24,** 759–763.

323 Okumura, J. and Tasaki, I. (1969). Effect of fasting, refeeding and dietary protein levels on uric acid and ammonia content of blood, liver and kidney in chickens. *Journal of Nutrition* **97,** 316–320.

324 Olney, P., Schmidt, C. R. and Lint, K. C. (1970). Longevity of birds of prey and owls in captivity. *International Zoo Yearbook* **10,** 36–37.

325 Owen, M. and Cook, W. A. (1977). Variations in body weight, wing length and condition of mallard *Anas platyrhynchos platyrhynchos* and their relationship to environmental changes. *Journal of Zoology, London* **183,** 377–395.

326 Palomeque, J. and Planas, J. (1977). Dimensions of the erythrocytes of birds. *Ibis* **119,** 533–535.

327 Palmer, A. C. (1976). *Introduction to Animal Neurology.* 2nd Edition. Blackwell Scientific Publications, Oxford.

328 Parsons, A. J. (1974). Condition of imported birds. *Veterinary Record* **95,** 155.

329 Patt, D. I. and Patt, G. R. (1969). *Comparative Vertebrate Histology.* Harper and Roe, New York.

330 Peakall, Γ. B. (1976). The peregrine falcon (*Falco peregrinus*) and pesticides. *Canadian Field-Naturalist* **90,** 301–307.

331 Pearson. R. (1972). *The Avian Brain.* Academic Press, New York and London.

332 Peckham, M. C. (1972). Poisons and toxins. In Hofstad, M. S. *et al.* Editors. *Diseases of Poultry.* 6th Edition. Iowa State University Press.

333 Peckham, M. C. (1975). Herpesviruses of pigeons, owls and falcons. In Hitchner, S. B. *et al* Editors. *Isolation and Identification of Avian Pathogens.* American Association of Avian Pathologists, Texas A & M University.

334 Peirce, M. A. and Cooper, J. E. (1977). Haematozoa of birds of prey in Great Britain. *Veterinary Record* **100,** 493.

335 Peirce, M. A. and Cooper, J. E. (1977). Haematozoa of East African birds. V. Blood parasites of birds of prey. *East African Wildlife Journal* **15,** 213–216.

336 Peirce, M. A. and Mead, C. J. (1977). Haematozoa of British birds. II. Blood parasites of birds from Hertfordshire. *Journal of Natural History* **11,** 597–600.

337 Pellérdy, L. P. (1974). *Coccidia and Coccidiosis.* Verlag Paul Parey, Berlin and Hamburg.

338 Peters, J. L. (1940). *Check-list of Birds of the World.* Volume 4, Harvard University Press.

339 Petrak, M. L. (1969). Editor. *Diseases of Cage and Aviary Birds.* Lea and Febiger, Philadelphia.

340 Pierson, G. P. and Pfow, C. J. (1975). Newcastle disease surveillance in the United States. *Journal of the American Veterinary Medical Association* **167,** 801–803.

341 Porter, R. D. and Wiemeyer, S. N. (1970). Propagation of captive American kestrels. *Journal of Wildlife Management* **34,** 594–604.

342 Porter, R. D. and Wiemeyer, S. N. (1972). DDE at low dietary levels kills captive American kestrels. *Bulletin of Environmental Contamination and Toxicology* **8,** 193–199.

343 Premovich, M. S. and Chiasson, R. B. (1976). Reproductive tissue activity in hypothyroid or heat stressed hens. *Poultry Science* **55,** 906–910.

344 Prestwich, A. A. (1955). *Records of Birds of Prey Bred in Captivity.* 2nd Edition. Arthur A. Prestwich, London.

345 Pugh, G. J. F. (1966). Associations between birds' nests, their pH, and keratinophilic fungi. *Sabouraudia* **5,** 49–53.

346 Rad, M. A. (1976). Treatment of moulting in psittacines with medroxyprogesterone acetate. *Avian Pathology* **5,** 155.

347 Ratcliffe, D. A. (1963). The status of the peregrine in Great Britain. *Bird Study* **10,** 56–90.

348 Ratcliffe, D. A. (1965). The peregrine situation in Great Britain, 1963–64. *Bird Study* **12,** 66–82.

349 Ratcliffe, D. A. (1967). Decrease in eggshell weight in certain birds of prey, *Nature* **215,** 208–210.

350 Ratcliffe, D. A. (1970). Changes attributable to pesticides in egg breakage frequency and eggshell thickness in some birds. *Journal of Applied Ecology* **7,** 67–116.

351 Redig, P. T. (1977). Raptor rehabilitation: diagnosis, prognosis and moral issues. Paper presented at Conference on Bird of Prey Management Techniques, Oxford, 3–5 October, 1977.

352 Redig, P. T. (in press). Infectious diseases. In Cooper, J. E. and Eley, J. T. Editors. *First Aid and Care of Wild Birds.* David and Charles, Newton Abbot.

353 Redig. P. T. and Duke, G. E. Intravenously administered ketamine HCl and diazepam for anesthesia of raptors. *Journal of the American Veterinary Medical Association* **169,** 886–888.

354 Reed, C. I. and Reed, B. P. (1928). The mechanism of pellet formation in the great horned owl (*Bubo virginianus*). *Science, Washington* **68,** 359–360.

355 Reid, H. W. and Boyce, J. B. (1974). Louping-ill virus in red grouse in Scotland. *Veterinary Record* **95,** 156.

356 Rewell, R. E. (1950). Report of the Society's Pathologist for the year 1949. *Proceedings of the Zoological Society of London* **120,** 486–595.

357 Roberts, J. C. and Straus, R. (1965). Editors. *Comparative Atherosclerosis.* Harper and Row, New York and London.

358 Robinson, P. T. (1975). Unilateral Patagiectomy: a technique for deflighting large birds. *Veterinary Medicine/Small Animal Clinician* **70,** 143–143.

359 Ryder-Davies, P. (1973). The use of metomidate, an intramuscular narcotic for birds. *Veterinary Record* **92,** 507–509.

360 Ryder-Davies, P. (1974). Some practical aspects of anaesthesia and surgery in exotic animals. *Veterinary Annual* 15th Issue, 235–237.

361 Salvin, F. H. and Brodrick, W. (1855). *Falconry in the British Isles.* John Van Voorst, London.

362 Sawby, S. W. and Gessaman, J. A. (1974). Telemetry of electrocardiograms from free-living birds: a method of electrode placement. *Condor* **76,** 479–481.

363 Schlumberger, H. G. (1954). Neoplasia in the parakeet. 1. Spontaneous chromophobe pituitary tumors. *Cancer Research* **14,** 237–245.

364 Schlumberger, H. G. and Henschke, U. K. (1956). Effect of total body X-irradiation on the parakeet. *Proceedings of the Society for Experimental Biology and Medicine* **92,** 261–266.

365 Scholander, P. F., Hock, R., Walters, V., and Irving, L. (1950). Adaptation to cold in Arctic and tropical mammals and birds in relation to body temperature, insulation and basal metabolic rate. *Biological Bulletin* **99,** 259–271.

366 Schwarte, L. H. (1967). Poultry surgery. In Biester, H. E. and Schwarte, L. H. Editors. *Diseases of Poultry.* 5th Edition, Iowa State University Press.

367 Schwartz, A., Weaver, J. D., Scott, N. R. and Cade, T. J. (1977). Measuring the

temperature of eggs during incubation under captive falcons. *Journal of Wildlife Management* **41**, 12–17.

368 Scott, W. A. (1971). Treatment of parasitic pneumonia in Californian sealions. *Veterinary Record* **88**, 588

369 Scott, M. L. and Krook, L. (1972). Nutritional deficiency diseases. In Hofstad, M. S. *et al* Editors. *Diseases of Poultry*. 6th Edition, Iowa State University Press.

370 Seegar, W. S., Schiller, E. L., Sladen, W. J. L. and Trpis, M. (1976). A Mallophaga, *Trinoton anserinum*, as a cyclodevelopmental vector for a heartworm parasite of waterfowl. *Science* **194**, 739–741.

371 Seidensticker, J. C. and Reynolds, H. V. (1969). Preliminary studies on the use of a general anesthetic in falconiform birds. *Journal of the American Veterinary Medical Association* **155**, 1044–1045.

372 Seneviratna, P. (1969). *Diseases of Poultry*. John Wright and Sons Ltd., Bristol.

373 Severino, M. A. (1645). *Zootomia Democritaea*. Noribergae.

374 Shlosberg, A. (1976). Treatment of monocrotophos-poisoned birds of prey with pralidoxime iodide. *Journal of the American Veterinary Medical Association* **169**, 989–990.

375 Sileo, L., Carlson, H. C. and Crumley, S. C. (1975). Inclusion body disease in a great horned owl. *Journal of Wildlife Diseases* **11**, 92–96.

376 Sileo, L., Karstad, L., Frank, R., Holdrinet, M. V. H., Addison, E. and Braun, H. E. (1977). Organochlorine poisoning of ring-billed gulls in Southern Ontario. *Journal of Wildlife Diseases* **13**, 313–322.

377 Smit, F. G. A. M. (1957). *Handbook for the Identification of British Insects:* **1**, *(16)*, *Siphonaptera*. Royal Entomological Society of London.

378 Smith, G. R., Hime, J. M. Keymer, I. F., Graham, J. M., Olney, P. J. S. and Brambell, M. R. (1975). Botulism in captive birds fed commercially bred maggots. *Veterinary Record* **97**, 204–205.

379 Smith, I. M. and Licence, S. T. (1977). Observations on the use of a semi-automatic system for haematological measurements in birds. *British Veterinary Journal* **133**, 585–592.

380 Snelling, J. C. (1975). Raptor rehabilitation at the Oklahoma City Zoo. *Raptor Research* **9**, 33–45.

381 Snow, D. W. (1968). Movements and mortality of British kestrels (*Falco tinnunculus*). *Bird Study* **15**, 65–83.

382 Stabler, R. M. (1954). *Trichomonas gallinae* – a review. *Experimental Parasitology* **III**, 368–402.

383 Stabler, R. M. and Holt, P. A. (1965). Hematozoa from Colorado birds. II. Falconiformes and Strigiformes. *Journal of Parasitology* **51**, 927–928.

384 Stauber, E. (1973). Suspected riboflavin deficiency in a golden eagle. *Journal of the American Veterinary Medical Association* **163**, 645–646.

385 Stehle, S. (1965). *Krankheiten bei Greifvögeln (Accipitres) und bei Eulen (Striges) mit Ausnahme der parasitären Erkrankungen*. Inaugural Dissertation Tierärztliche Hochschule, Hannover.

386 Stevenson, D. E. and Carter, B. I. (1975). Pesticides and domestic animals. *Veterinary Record* **97**, 164–169.

387 Stone, W. B. and Janes, D. E. (1969). Trichomoniasis in captive sparrowhawks. *Bulletin of the Wildlife Disease Association* **5**, 147.

388 Sutherland, R., Croydon, E. A. P. and Rolinson, G. N. (1970). Flucloxacillin, a new isoxazolyl penicillin, compared with oxacillin, cloxacillin, and dicloxacillin. *British*

Medical Journal **4,** 455–460.

389 Sutter, E. (1951). Growth and Differentiation of the brain in nidifugous and nidicolous birds. *Proceedings of the Xth International Ornithological Congress,* 636–644.

390 Tanabe, M. (1925). The cultivation of trichomonads from man, rat and owl. *Journal of Parasitology* **12,** 101–104.

391 Thacker, R. (1971). Estimations relative to birds of prey in captivity in the United States of America. *Raptor Research News* **5,** 108–122.

392 Thienpont, D. C., Vanparijs, O. F. J. and Hermans, L. C. (1973). Mebendazole, a new potent drug against *Syngamus trachea* in turkeys. *Poultry Science* **52,** 1712–1714.

393 Townsend, G. H. (1969). The grading of commercially-bred laboratory animals. *Veterinary Record* **85,** 225–226.

394 Trainer, D. O., Folz, S. D. and Samuel, W. M. (1968). Capillariasis in the gyrfalcon. *Condor* **70,** 276–277.

395 Turbervile, G. (1575). *The Booke of Faulconrie or Hawking.* Christopher Barker, London.

396 Turner, K. G., Hackshaw, R., Papadimitriou, J. and Perrott, J. (1976). The pathogenesis of experimental pulmonary aspergillosis in normal and cortisone-treated rats. *The Journal of Pathology* **118,** 65–73.

397 Tyler, C. (1966). A study of the egg shells of the Falconiformes. *Journal of Zoology, London* **150,** 413–425.

398 Urbain, A. and Nouvel, J. (1946). Possibilité de dispersion des bacilles tuberculeux et des spores charbonneuses par les déjections d'oiseaux carnivores. *Bulletin de L'Académie Vétérinaire de France* **XIX,** 237–239.

399 van Miert, A. S. J. P. A. M., van Gogh, J. and Wit, J. G. (1976). The influence of pyrogen induced fever on absorption of sulpha drugs. *Veterinary Record* **99,** 480–481.

400 van Nie, G. J. (1975). Mogelijke chloralose vergiftiging bij buizerds. *Tijdschrift voor Diergeneeskunde* **100,** 1052–1053.

401 Vincent, J. (1966). Editor. *Red Data Book. Volume 2 – Aves.* I.U.C.N. Morges.

402 Voitkevich, A. A. (1966). *The Feathers and Plumage of Birds.* Sidgwick and Jackson, London.

403 von Faber, H. (1964). Stress and general adaptation syndrome in poultry. *World's Poultry Science Journal* **20,** 175–182.

404 Wallis, A. S. and Parker, A. J. (1974). Formulation of poultry rations. *Veterinary Record* **95,** 301.

405 Wallach, J. D. (1970). Nutritional diseases of exotic animals. *Journal of the American Veterinary Medical Association* **157,** 583–599.

406 Wallach, J. D. and Flieg, G. M. (1969). Frostbite and its sequelae in captive exotic birds. *Journal of the American Veterinary Medical Association* **155,** 1035–1038.

407 Wallach, J. D. and Flieg, G. M. (1970). Cramps and fits in carnivorous birds. *International Zoo Yearbook* **10,** 3–4.

408 Ward, F. P. (1971). Thiamine deficiency in a peregrine falcon. *Journal of the American Veterinary Medical Association* **159,** 599–601.

409 Ward, F. P. and Fairchild, D. G. (1972). Air sac parasites of the genus *Serratospiculum* in falcons. *Journal of Wildlife Diseases* **8,** 165–168.

410 Ward, F. P., Fairchild, D. G. and Vuicich, J. V. (1970). Pulmonary aspergillosis in prairie falcon nest mates. *Journal of Wildlife Diseases* **6,** 80–83.

411 Ward, F. P. and Slaughter, L. J. (1968). Visceral gout in a captive Cooper's hawk. *Bulletin of the Wildlife Disease Association* **4,** 91–93.

412 Wasielewski, T. von and Wülker, G. (1918). Eigene Untersuchungen a) Die Parasiten in den roten Blutkörperchen. *Beihefte zum Archiv für Schiffs und Tropen Hygiene* **XXII,** 18–51, 89–100.

413 Wenyon, C. M. (1926). *Protozoology.* Baillière, Tindall and Cox, London.

414 Wheeldon, E. B., Bogan, J. A. and Taylor, D. J. (1975). Dieldrin poisoning in a captive bird of prey. *Veterinary Record* **97,** 412.

415 Williams, M. H. and Cooper, J. E. (1976). Veterinary report. *Annual Report of the Hawk Trust* **7,** 10–11.

416 Williams Smith, H. (1954). Serum levels of penicillin, dihydrostreptomycin, chloramphenicol, aureomycin and terramycin in chickens. *Journal of Comparative Pathology* **64,** 225–233.

417 Wilson, R. (1976). Fulmar oils lanneret. *The Falconer* **VI,** 263–264.

418 Wingfield, W. E. and DeYoung, D. W. (1972). Anesthetic and surgical management of eagles with orthopedic difficulties. *Veterinary Medicine/Small Animal Clinician* **67,** 991–993.

419 Winteröll, G. (1976). Newcastle-Disease bei Greifen und Eulen. *Der praktische Tierarzt* **57,** 76–78.

420 Wobeser, G. and Saunders, J. R. (1975). Pulmonary oxalosis in association with Aspergillus niger infection in a great horned owl (Bubo virginianus). *Avian Diseases* **19,** 388–392.

421 Wolfson, F. (1936). *Plasmodium oti* n. sp., a Plasmodium from the eastern screech owl (*Otus asio naevius*), infective to canaries. *American Journal of Hygiene* **24,** 94–101.

422 Woodford, M. H. (1960). *A Manual of Falconry.* A. & C. Black, London.

423 Woodford, M. H. and Glasier, P. E. (1955). Sub-committee's report on disease in hawks, 1954. *The Falconer* **111,** 63–65.

424 Young, E. (1967). Leg paralysis in the greater flamingo and lesser flamingo following capture and transportation. *International Zoo Yearbook* **7,** 226–227.

425 Zaid, Bin Sultan Al Nahayan. (1976). *Falconry as a Sport: Our Arab Heritage.* Compiled by Yahya Badr. Published for the International Conference on Falconry and Conservation, Abu Dhabi, 10–18 December, 1976.

426 Zeigler, H. P. and Karten, H. J. (1973). Brain mechanisms and feeding behavior in the pigeon (*Columba livia*). *The Journal of Comparative Neurology* **152,** 59–78, 83–101.

Index

This index does not include the names of authors of references, species of raptors (unless particularly pertinent to the text) or detailed items from the Appendices.

"Veterinary Aspects of Captive Birds of Prey"

1985 Supplement to the 1978 Edition

JOHN E. COOPER
BVSc, DTVM, MRCVS, FIBiol.

The Standfast Press, Gloucestershire

This Supplement is not intended to be fully comprehensive. Nevertheless, it includes reference to many of the papers relevant to raptor disease published since 1978 together, where appropriate, with a synopsis or comments. Although occasional notes on cases are added I have not incorporated analyses of my own clinical or *post-mortem* data and have not referred in any detail to 1978–85 correspondence on the subject.

Page of
1978
Edition

CHAPTER 1 *Introduction*

1   There is increasing interest in the history of hawk medicine and a short paper on this subject has been published (Cooper, 1979) but there remains a need for a detailed study. References to falconers and to diseases of birds of prey are regularly located in mediaeval texts: a rather nice one, dating back to 1586, occurs in a Puritan survey of Warwickshire clergy and describes the vicar of Temple Grafton, John Frith, as "an old priest and unsound in religion, he can neither prech nor read well, his chiefest trade is to cure hawkes that are hurt or diseased, for which purpose manie doe usuallie repaire to him" (Schoenbaum, 1975).

2   Although the output of literature on falconry declined after the 17th century some contributions to our knowledge of the biology and pathology of raptors were made by anatomists and zoologists. John Hunter (1728–93) did some experimental work on hawks in connection with his studies on the air-sacs and the Hunterian Museum (housed in the Royal College of Surgeons of England) contains 14 surviving specimens from birds of prey (Cooper, 1982a).

4   The past seven years have seen a great increase in captive breeding of birds of prey and in studies on their behaviour, physiology and ecology. Useful examples and data are to be found in Bird and Rehder (1981), in the section on birds of prey in Olney (1984) and in journals such as "Raptor Research". The "state of the art" was summarised by Olendorff *et al* (1980) while practical advice on captive breeding was provided by Weaver and Cade (1983). The role of captive breeding in the management of endangered species has been recognised and has become an integral part of many programmes – for example, on the Mauritius kestrel (*Falco punctatus*) and Philippine eagle (*Pithecophaga jefferyi*).

5   An increasingly active part is being played by the veterinary profession. In Britain the Wildlife and Countryside Act 1981 and the Zoo Licensing Act 1981 have both provided new opportunities for veterinarians to inspect premises where raptors are kept and to advise on health and welfare. Work on casualties has, to a certain extent, been facilitated by the provisions of the Wildlife and Countryside Act. Under this Act all falconiform species are on Schedule 4 and may only be kept if ringed and registered: there are, however, special provisions for veterinary surgeons and for "licensed rehabilitation keepers" (LRKs) who are tending sick and injured specimens. One condition of the licence which permits such work is that proper records should be kept: as a result it is proving easier to obtain and collate data.

5–6   Since 1978 many scientific papers have appeared which are either concerned with the health of raptors or relevant to it. Some of these are referred to later in this Supplement. Two books devoted to the subject have been published. *Recent Advances in the Study of Raptor Diseases* (Cooper and Greenwood, 1981) comprises the Proceedings of the First International Symposium on Diseases of Birds of Prey, held in London in 1980 and many of the papers in that volume remain the most up-to-date and authoritative texts on the subject. *Care and Rehabilitation of Injured Owls* (McKeever, 1979) is described as "a user's guide to the medical treatment of raptorial birds and the housing, release training and captive breeding of native (Canadian; JEC) owls". It is a useful text but has the great disadvantage that it lacks references. Sections and chapters on raptor diseases are also to be found in a number of other books including Fowler (1978), Cooper and Eley (1979) and Wallach and Boever (1983). The second edition of Petrak's book (1982) on cagebirds makes reference to raptors in a number of places. Review articles include those by Cooper (1980a) and Halliwell (1979) while an increasing trend has been in-depth studies on morbidity and mortality in individual species – for example, the sparrow-hawk (Cooper, 1980b), goshawk (Cooper, 1982b) and merlin (Cooper and Forbes, 1985). Dr. Murray Fowler has produced an extensive bibliography on raptors but this has not yet been published.

References

Bird, D. M. and Rehder, N. B. (1981). The science of captive breeding of falcons. *Avicultural Magazine* **89,** 208–212.

Cooper, J. E. (1979). The history of hawk medicine. *Veterinary History* NS **1,** 11–18.

Cooper, J. E. (1980a). Medicine and diseases of birds of prey. *Annual Proceedings of the American Association of Zoo Veterinarians, Washington, DC,* 73–75.

Cooper, J. E. (1980b). Diseases of the sparrowhawk (*Accipiter nisus*). *The Falconer* **VII**, 252–256.

Cooper, J. E. (1982a). Some aspects of John Hunter's work on the diseases of birds of prey. *Annals of the Royal College of Surgeons of England*, **64**, 345–347.

Cooper, J. E. (1982b). A historical review of goshawk training and disease. In Kenward, R. E. and Lindsay, I. eds. *Understanding the Goshawk*. International Association for Falconry and Conservation of Birds of Prey.

Cooper, J. E. and Eley, J. T. (1979). Editors. *First Aid and Care of Wild Birds*. David and Charles, Newton Abbot.

Cooper, J. E. and Forbes, N. (1985). Studies on morbidity and mortality in the merlin (*Falco columbarius*). *Veterinary Record*. In press.

Cooper, J. E. and Greenwood, A. G. (1981). Editors. *Recent Advances in the Study of Raptor Diseases*. Chiron Publications, Keighley, Yorkshire.

Fowler, M. E. (1978). Editor. *Zoo and Wild Animal Medicine*. W. B. Saunders, Philadelphia.

Halliwell, W. H. (1979). Diseases of birds of prey. *Veterinary Clinics of North America* **9**, 541–568.

McKeever, J. (1979). *Care and Rehabilitation of Injured Owls*. W. F. Rannie, Lincoln, Ontario.

Olendorff, R. R., Motroni, R. S. and Call, M. W. (1980). *Raptor Management – the State of the Art in 1980*. Technical Note No. 343. US Department of the Interior – Bureau of Land Management.

Olney, P. J. S. (1984). Editor. Birds of Prey. *International Zoo Yearbook* **23**, Zoological Society of London, London.

Petrak, M. L. (1982). Editor. *Diseases of Cage and Aviary Birds*. Lea and Febiger, Philadelphia.

Schoenbaum, S. (1975). *William Shakespeare, a Documentary Life*. Clarendon Press, Oxford.

Wallach, J. D. and Boever, W. J. (1983). *Diseases of Exotic Animals*. W. B. Saunders, Philadelphia.

Weaver, J. D. and Cade, T. J. (1983). *Falcon Propagation*. The Peregrine Fund, Ithaca, New York.

*Page of
1978
Edition*

CHAPTER 2   *Nomenclature*

11   The only new terms of any note that have found their way into raptor work are those associated with captive breeding – for example, eggs are "set" in an incubator and embryos may die "at pipping" etc., etc.

CHAPTER 3   *Methods of investigation and treatment*

15   Data on the numbers and species of birds of prey maintained in captivity in Britain are becoming available as a result of registration under the Wildlife and Countryside Act.

16   Guidelines on accommodation for birds of prey are being formulated in Britain by the Department of the Environment.

            The list of British legislation relevant to veterinary work is updated later (see Appendix XI)

18–19   The effect of handling on a ferruginous hawk was investigated by Busch *et al* (1978) who monitored the bird's heartrate under different conditions. The rate was greatly accelerated when the hawk was restrained but it is noteworthy that hooding resulted in a slowing to 51–66% of the "maximal" rate.

            A large bird, such as an eagle, is often more easily handled by grasping its legs and then holding it upside down on its back. The wings can then be drawn in and the bird wrapped in a cloth or blanket for examination and treatment.

19   Examination of a raptor can be facilitated by use of an Arab device called a "Guba" (Cooper and Al-Timimi, in prep). This consists of a cloth jacket which can be tied round the bird's body. Its use permits singlehanded swabbing, cleaning of wounds and dosing.

20   It is important to examine the beak carefully. If it is overgrown or damaged the bird may have difficulty in feeding.

21   The clinical examination of casualty birds prior to release presents particular problems (Humphreys, 1981): criteria for assessing the health of such birds were given by Cooper *et al* (1980).

22   Heart rate increases significantly during handling (see pp. 18–19). Data on "normal" heart rate in a captive red-tailed hawk were given by Busch *et al* (1984).

22–23   Contrast media (barium preparations) can be of great value when investigating the alimentary tract. The introduction of air plus a small quantity of barium will greatly facilitate examination of the crop and cloaca.

            Various other aids to clinical examination have come into prominence in the past few years. Endoscopy is a particular example: rigid endoscopes (e.g. human arthroscopes) can be used to examine the oesophagus, trachea, cloaca and (via a laparoscopy incision) internal organs (Böttcher, 1982; Bush, 1980). Flexible instruments have great potential but at the time of writing have been used relatively infrequently. Even if fibre-optic instruments are not available useful results can be obtained using an auroscope or the battery operated "Focuscope" (Medical Diagnostic Services, U.S.A.).

A particularly impressive report was that by Furley and Greenwood (1982) who described computerised axial tomography (CAT) in birds of prey in the Middle East: using such scanning they were able to demonstrate lesions of aspergillosis.

23–26　The value in clinical diagnosis of correctly taken samples has become increasingly recognised. Further information is to be found in Cooper (1985).

30–31　Wholebody radiographs can be a valuable aid to *post-mortem* examination, especially in young birds – in which skeletal disease may be present – or in older ones where traumatic injury is suspected. Suggested additions to *post-mortem* and egg examination forms are to be found later in this Supplement.

33–34　There has been an upsurge of interest in, and publications on, the haematology of raptors and other non-domesticated birds: relevant references include those by Gerlach (1978), Kirkwood *et al* (1979), Gee *et al* (1981), Lepoutre (1982), Rehder *et al* (1982) and Rehder and Bird (1983). The paper by Gerlach contains coloured photographs of leucocytes of raptors while in all four the importance of establishing baseline data, preferably over a period of time in view of possible variations, is emphasised.

34–35　Interest in the clinical chemistry of raptors has also increased in recent years. Halliwell (1981) provided a useful introduction and valuable data are included in the paper by Gee *et al* (1981). More information on normal values is required and it is encouraging to note that a number of laboratories in Britain will perform blood biochemical analysis at a relatively low cost.

A micromethod for plasma uric acid determination in "companion" birds was described by McFarland *et al* (1979).

35　Cytology has great potential in birds (Campbell, 1984; Cooper, 1985) and I have used it on many occasions in raptors.

Much remains to be learned of the normal histology of birds of prey. From time to time structures are seen which appear to be unreported or the significance of which is unclear: for example, Borst *et al* (1976) reported ectopic bone in the lungs of birds, including the European kestrel.

36   Electron microscopy is an important tool in the investigation of disease in raptors. A number of papers (see Chapter 5) testify to its value in the detection of viral infections.

37   It is generally only the smaller birds that have a higher metabolic rate than mammals. However, body size affects the rate at which drugs are absorbed, metabolised and excreted and Kirkwood (1983) recommended the use of the formula bodyweight$^{0.75}$ for the estimation of dose rate. The principle here is that smaller birds need relatively higher doses of drugs than their larger counterparts or the same dose repeated more frequently.

A number of drugs appear to be contra-indicated or excessively toxic in birds of prey. Few controlled studies have been carried out but one exception was research on the toxicity of gentamicin in great horned owls by Bauck and Haigh (1984). These authors showed that the response varies greatly, even within the one species. Reactions in owls receiving gentamicin ranged from death within three days to no clinical signs at any stage.

Homeopathic remedies have been suggested for certain conditions in birds of prey (P. A. Culpin, personal communication) but I have not yet had an opportunity to try them.

40–41   The nursing of sick and injured raptors is of the greatest importance, especially if they are wild bird casualties. Further information is given in *First Aid and Care of Wild Birds* (Cooper and Eley, 1979) and in a number of papers – for example, Cooper (1979) and Coles (1984).

References

Bauck, L. A. and Haigh, J. C. (1984). Toxicity of gentamicin in great horned owls (*Bubo virginianus*). *Journal of Zoo Animal Medicine* **15**, 62–66.

Borst, G. H. A., Zwart, P., Mullink, H. W. M. A. and Vroege, C. (1976). Bone structures in avian and mammalian lungs. *Veterinary Pathology* **13**, 98–103.

Böttcher, M. (1982). Erfahrungen mit der diagnostischen endoskopie beim vogel. *Tierärztl. Prax.* **10**, 183–188.

Busch, D. A., de Graw, W. A. and Clampitt, N. C. (1978). Effects of handling-disturbance stress on heartrate in the ferruginous hawk (*Buteo regalis*). *Raptor Research* **12**, 122–125.

Busch, D. E., de Graw, W. A. and Clampitt, N. C. (1984). Biotelemetered daily heart rate cycles in the red-tailed hawk (*Buteo jamaicensis*). *Raptor Research* **18**, 74–77.

Bush, M. (1981). Diagnostic avian laparoscopy. In Cooper, J. E. and Greenwood, A. G., editors, *Recent Advances in the Study of Raptor Diseases*. Chiron Publications, Keighley, Yorkshire.

Campbell, T. W. (1984). Diagnostic cytology in avian medicine. *Veterinary Clinics of North America* **14**, 317–344.

Coles, B .H. (1984). Some considerations when nursing birds in veterinary premises. *Journal of Small Animal Practice* **25**, 275–288.

Cooper, J. E. (1979). Veterinary care of birds. *Animal Regulation Studies* **2**, 21–29.

Cooper, J. E. (1985). Diagnostic techniques in birds. *The Veterinary Annual* **25**, 236–244.

Cooper, J. E. and Eley, J. T. (1979). Editors. *First Aid and Care of Wild Birds*. David and Charles, Newton Abbot.

Cooper, J. E., Gibson, L. and Jones, C. G. (1980). The assessment of health in casualty birds of prey intended for release. *Veterinary Record* **10**, 340–341.

Furley, C. W. and Greenwood, A. G. (1982). Treatment of aspergillosis in raptors (Order Falconiformes) with miconazole. *Veterinary Record* **111**, 584–585.

Gee, G. F., Carpenter, J. W. and Hensler, G. L. (1981). Species differences in hematological values of captive cranes, geese, raptors and quail. *Journal of Wildlife Management* **45**, 463–483.

Gerlach, H. (1978). Grundlagen der Blutdiagnostik bei Greifvögeln. *Der Praktische Tierarzt* **9**, 642–650.

Halliwell, W. (1981). Serum chemistry profiles in the health and disease of birds of prey. In Cooper, J. E. and Greenwood, A. G., editors, *Recent Advances in the Study of Raptor Diseases*. Chiron Publications, Keighley, Yorkshire.

Humphreys, P. N. (1981). The problems of rehabilitation. In Cooper, J. E. and Greenwood, A. G., editors, *Recent Advances in the Study of Raptor Diseases*. Chiron Publications, Keighley, Yorkshire.

Kirkwood, J. K. (1983). Treatment of aspergillosis in raptors. *Veterinary Record* **112**, 182.

Kirkwood, J. K., Cooper, J. E. and Brown, G. (1979). Some haematological data for the European kestrel (*Falco tinnunculus*). *Research in Veterinary Science* **26**, 263–264.

Lepoutre, D. R. (1982). Contribution à l'étude de l'hematologie, la biochimie sanguine et la pathologie infectieuse et parasitaire des rapaces europeens. These, Ecole Nationale Veterinaire de Toulouse, France.

McFarland, D. C., Kenzy, S. G. and Coon, C. N. (1979). Research note – A micromethod for plasma uric acid determinations in companion birds. *Avian Diseases* **23**, 772–774.

Rehder, N. B. and Bird, D. M. (1983). Annual profiles of blood packed cell volumes of captive American kestrels. *Canadian Journal of Zoology* **61**, 2550–2555.

Rehder, N. B., Bird, D. M., Laguë, P. C. and Mackay, C. (1982). Variation in selected hematological parameters of captive red-tailed hawks. *Journal of Wildlife Diseases* **18**, 105–109.

Page of
1978
Edition

CHAPTER 4 *Physical diseases*

42 Studies on skeletal preparations have shown that birds with severe cere damage may also have underlying lesions in the skull.

46–47   A useful review of orthopaedic techniques in raptors was given by Patrick Redig (1982) who discussed the types of fracture that may be encountered and the different methods of treatment available. He concluded that intramedullary pinning remains one of the methods of choice but the development of the Kirschner- -Ehmer device has provided an inexpensive, lightweight and flexible means of stabilising wing fractures.

Fowler (1981) presented a preliminary report on the long bones in raptors while Bush (1981) described results obtained in treating fractures by external fixation. The subject was reviewed by Withrow (1982).

49   A number of reports of the fitting of prosthetic limbs to raptors have appeared in recent years, including the fitting of two false feet to a peregrine that was badly electrocuted (Anon, 1981). Particular attention has focussed on the provision of prostheses for injured birds in order to facilitate copulation and captive breeding.

50–51   The assessment of health in casualty birds prior to release was discussed in a paper by Cooper *et al* (1980).

References

Anon (1981). Injured peregrine fitted with false feet. *Cage and Aviary Birds* (May 23), 7.

Bush, M. (1981). Avian fracture repair using external fixation. In Cooper, J. E. and Greenwood, A. G., editors, *Recent Advances in the Study of Raptor Diseases*. Chiron Publications, Keighley, Yorkshire.

Cooper, J. E., Gibson, L. and Jones, C. G. (1980). The assessment of health in casualty birds of prey intended for release. *Veterinary Record* **106**, 340–341.

Fowler, M. E. (1981). Ossification of long bones in raptors. In Cooper, J. E. and Greenwood, A. G., editors, *Recent Advances in the Study of Raptor Diseases*. Chiron Publications, Keighley, Yorkshire.

Redig, P. T. (1982). A clinical review of orthopedic techniques used in the rehabilitation of raptors. *Annual Proceedings of the American Association of Zoo Veterinarians, New Orleans*, 8–13.

Withrow, S. J. (1982). General principles of fracture repair in raptors. *Compendium on Continuing Education for the Practicing Veterinarian* **4**, 116–121.

Page of
1978
Edition

CHAPTER 5   *Infectious diseases*

56   Occasional cases of ornithosis (chlamydiosis) in free-living or recently captured birds of prey continue to be reported – for example in a buzzard (Sabisch, 1977).

A serological survey of 71 captive and free-living raptors by Riemann *et al* (1977) showed 30% to be positive for Q fever (*Coxiella burnetii*) antibodies (and, incidentally, 8% positive for *Toxoplasma* and one bird only positive for infectious bursal disease virus).

Mycoplasmas have now been isolated by other workers from birds of prey – from buzzards (Bölske and Mörner, 1981) and from a prairie falcon (Halliwell and Graham, 1978). Their role remains uncertain, however.

57   Data on hygiene, including recommended disinfectants, are given in a chapter on preventive medicine in birds of prey in *Zoo and Wild Animal Medicine* (Cooper, 1978).

59   A differential diagnosis in cases of chronic dermatitis should be neoplasia. I have diagnosed (on biopsy) a squamous cell carcinoma in a Barbary falcon which had a long-standing skin lesion in its groin.

60   "Blain" continues to occur and is on occasion a problem for no obvious reason in young captive bred raptors. It usually responds to drainage but research is urgently needed on its aetiology and pathogenesis.

61   Studies on the bacterial flora of the cloaca were carried out by Cooper *et al* (1980) and of the nasal mucosa by Richter and Gerlach (1981).

65–69   Aspergillosis remains an important disease in raptors and one that is commonly the cause of death. It has been investigated in some detail by Patrick Redig who reported some of his findings at the International Symposium in 1980 (Redig, 1981). Diagnosis is facilitated by serology, air sac lavage or laparoscopy. A potentially useful diagnostic aid is haematology. Hawkey *et al* (1984) described morphologically abnormal heterophils in the circulating blood of a king shag (*Phalacorax albivenier*) with aspergillosis: it remains to be seen whether similar changes occur in raptors. The prospects of vaccination against aspergillosis have improved following work by Redig and, in turkeys, by Richard *et al* (1982). Advances have also been made in treatment: nebulisers are increasingly being used to treat avian respiratory disease (Miller, 1984) while success using miconazole ("Daktarin": Janssen) intramuscularly at a dose of 10 mg/kg has been reported in raptors by Furley and Greenwood (1982). The role of stressors in precipitating aspergillosis in free-living goshawks was emphasised by Redig *et al* (1980).

69   Studies on the gut flora of raptors have been carried out by a number of investigators – for example, Needham *et al* (1979) and Cooper *et al* (1980).

          A haemorrhagic enteritis associated with adenovirus-like particles was described by Sileo *et al* (1983).

70   A pseudomembranous gastritis compatible with a *Clostridium* infection was reported by Enderson and Berthrong (1980).

72–74   Useful review papers on tuberculosis in raptors are those by van Nie *et al* (1982) and Lumeij and van Nie (1982). In the latter paper the value in diagnosis of laparoscopy – if necessary followed by liver biopsy – is emphasised.

75   *Salmonella* infections are occasionally reported in birds of prey – for example, in a captive peregrine by Sykes *et al* (1981), who emphasised that salmonellosis could pose a threat to birds in large breeding facilities. A clinical case on which I advised showed clinical signs of diarrhoea and weight loss and proved very intractable to treatment.

76   Raptors imported into Britain now have to be quarantined for 35 days.

79   *Herpesvirus* infections have now been reported in Britain. An account of the disease in a group of falcons was probably the first formal record (Greenwood and Cooper, 1982) but at about the same time I diagnosed a case in an imported great horned owl and subsequently Andrew Greenwood and I have seen it in a captive merlin – a histological diagnosis confirmed by Dr. David Graham.

          Hepatitis in raptors may also be associated with an adenovirus infection (Sileo *et al*, 1983) – see earlier.

          The need to search for viral infections in raptors – by electron microscopy, cultivation and serology – cannot be overemphasised. It is highly probable that some of the unexplained morbidity and mortality in captive birds may be due to, or associated with, viral infections.

References

Bölske, G. and Mörner, T. (1981). Case Report – Isolation of a mycoplasma sp. from three buzzards (*Buteo* spp.). *Avian Diseases* **26,** 406–411.

Cooper, J. E. (1978). Preventive medicine in birds of prey. In Fowler, M. E., editor. *Zoo and Wild Animal Medicine*. W. B. Saunders, Philadelphia.

Cooper, J. E., Redig, P. T. and Burnham, W. (1980). Bacterial isolates from the pharynx and cloaca of the peregrine falcon (*Falco peregrinus*) and gyrfalcon (*F. rusticolus*). *Raptor Research* **14,** 6–9.

Enderson, J. H. and Berthrong, M. (1984). Pseudomembraneous gastritis compatible with (*Clostridium* sp.) in a captive peregrine falcon. *Raptor Research* **18,** 72–74.

Furley, C. W. and Greenwood, A. G. (1982). Treatment of aspergillosis in raptors (Order Falconiformes) with miconazole. *Veterinary Record* **111,** 584–585.

Greenwood, A. G. and Cooper, J. E. (1982). Herpesvirus infections in falcons. *Veterinary Record* **111,** 514.

Halliwell, W. H. and Graham, D. L. (1978). Bacterial diseases of birds of prey. In Fowler, M. E., editor. *Zoo and Wild Animal Medicine.* W. B. Saunders, Philadelphia.

Hawkey, C. M., Pugsley, S. L. and Knight, J. A. (1984). Abnormal heterophils in a king shag with aspergillosis. *Veterinary Record* **114,** 322–324.

Lumeij, J. T. and van Nie, G. J. (1982). Tuberculosis in raptorial birds. Review of the literature and suggestions for clinical diagnosis and vaccination. *Tijdschr. Diergeneesk* **107,** 573–579.

Miller, T. A. (1984). Nebulization for avian respiratory disease. *Carnation Research Digest,* 7–8.

Needham, J. R., Kirkwood, J. K. and Cooper, J. E. (1979). A survey of the aerobic bacteria in the droppings of captive birds of prey. *Research in Veterinary Science* **27,** 125–126.

Redig, P. T. (1981). Aspergillosis in raptors. In Cooper, J. E. and Greenwood, A. G., editors, *Recent Advances in the Study of Raptor Diseases.* Chiron Publications, Keighley, Yorkshire.

Redig, P. T., Fuller, M. R. and Evans, D. L. (1980). Prevalence of *Aspergillus fumigatus* in free-living goshawks (*Accipiter gentilis atricapillus*). *Journal of Wildlife Diseases* **16,** 169–174.

Richard, J. L., Thurston, J. R., Cutlip, R. C. and Peir, A. C. (1982). Vaccination studies of aspergillosis in turkeys: subcutaneous inoculation with several vaccine preparations followed by aerosol challenge exposure. *American Journal of Veterinary Research* **43,** 488–492.

Richter, T. and Gerlach, H. (1981). The bacterial flora of the nasal mucosa of birds of prey. In Cooper, J. E. and Greenwood, A. G., editors, *Recent Advances in the Study of Raptor Diseases.* Chiron Publications, Keighley, Yorkshire.

Riemann, H., Behymer, D., Fowler, M., Ley, D., Schultz, T., Ruppanner, R. and King, J. (1977). Serological investigation of captive and free living raptors. *Raptor Research* **11,** 104–110.

Sabisch, G. von (1977). Ornithose bei einem Mäsebussard (Buteo buteo). *Berl. Münch, Tierärztl. Wschr.*, **90,** 441–442.

Sileo, L., Franson, J. C., Graham, D. L., Domermuth, C. H., Rattner, B. A. and Pattee, O. H. (1983). Hemorrhagic enteritis in captive American kestrels (*Falco sparverius*). *Journal of Wildlife Diseases* **19,** 244–247.

Sykes, G. P., Murphy, C. and Hardaswick, V. (1981). *Salmonella* infection in a captive peregrine falcon. *Journal of the American Veterinary Medical Association* **179,** 1269–1271.

van Nie, G. J., Lumeij, J. T., Dorrestein, G. M., Wolvekam, W. Th. C., Zwart, P. and Stam, J. W. E. (1982). Tuberculosis in raptorial birds. Clinical cases and differential diagnosis. *Tijdschr. Diergeneesk* **107,** 563–572.

CHAPTER 6   *Parasites*

82–83   Ticks may be of more relevance in birds of prey than has hitherto been recognised. A paper by Schilling *et al* (1981) reported a high mortality rate in (free-living) nestling peregrines in West Germany associated with the tick *Ixodes arboricola*. A similar situation could occur in captive birds in "skylight and seclusion" aviaries or outdoor enclosures containing natural vegetation.

p. 85   Myiasis is a potential problem in the rare Mauritius kestrel. A captive bird which I examined with Carl Jones in 1984 had larvae, subsequently identified as *Passeromyia heterochaeta*, in its nares. The latter had to be removed manually. *Protocalliphora* larvae have been reported in nestlings (Crocoll and Parker, 1981).

p. 86   Flukes (trematodes) are probably of more significance in raptors than I suggested in 1978. Since then clinical trematodiasis has been reported by Greenwood *et al* (1984) who advocated rafoxanide at 10–15 mg/kg by stomach tube – and I have investigated other cases in Britain in which heavy fluke burdens appeared to be significant.

p. 88   A *Cyathostoma* infestation of the orbital sinuses of a British kestrel has been reported (Anon, 1983).

89–90   Fenbendazole ("Panacur": Hoechst) at a single dose of 100 mg/kg is a safe and effective drug for the treatment of nematodes in birds, including raptors (Lawrence, 1983).

95–96   I am in no doubt that coccidiosis can be a cause of ill-health and death in captive raptors, especially nestlings. I have diagnosed it in merlins and barn owls. The best way to prevent coccidiosis is (a) strict hygiene, including cleaning and disinfection of incubators and nestboxes and (b) screening of faeces of parent birds prior to egg-laying and treatment with sulphonamides until oocysts are no longer detectable. Useful papers on coccidian lifecycles are those by Cerna and Louckova (1976) and Cerna (1984).

96   Birds of prey can be intermediate hosts for *Sarcocystis* (Crawley *et al*, 1982; Munday, 1977; Tuggle and Schmeling, 1982).

References
Anon (1983). Nematodes found in the orbital sinuses of a kestrel (*Falco tinnunculus*). *Veterinary Record* **112,** 24.
Cerna, Z. (1984). Role of birds as definite hosts and intermediate hosts of heteroxenous coccidia. *Journal of Parasitology* **31,** 579–581.
Cerna Z. and Louckova, M. (1976). *Microtus arvalis* as the intermediate host of a coccidian from the kestrel (*Falco tinnunculus*). *Folia Parasitologia* **23,** 110.
Crawley, R. R., Ernst, J. V. and Milton, J. L. (1982). *Sarcocystis* in a bald eagle (*Haliaeetus leucocephalus*). *Journal of Wildlife Diseases* **18,** 253–255.
Crocoll, S. and Parker, J. W. (1981). Protocalliphora infestation in broad-winged hawks. *Wilson Bulletin* **93,** 110
Greenwood, A. G., Furley, C. W. and Cooper, J. E. (1984). Intestinal trematodiasis in falcons (Order Falconiformes). *Veterinary Record* **114,** 477–478.
Lawrence, K. (1983). Efficacy of fenbendazole against nematodes of captive birds. *Veterinary Record* **112,** 433–434.
Munday, B. L (1977). A species of *Sarcocystis* with owls as definitive hosts. *Journal of Wildlife Diseases* **13,** 205–207.
Schilling, F. von, Böttcher, M. and Walter, G. (1981). Probleme des Zeckenbefalls bei Nestlingen des Wanderfalken. *Journal für Ornithologie* **112,** 359–367.
Tuggle, B. N. and Schmeling, S. K. (1982). Parasites of the bald eagle of North America. *Journal of Wildlife Diseases* **18,** 501–506.

Page of
1978
Edition

CHAPTER 6 *Foot conditions*

97–111   Advances have been made in our understanding of the pathogenesis of bumblefoot (Cooper, 1980a; Cooper and Needham, 1981; Riddle, 1981) but the methods of treatment have remained relatively unchanged (Cooper, 1980b). Further work is needed on the possible value of vaccination and immunomodulation (Satterfield and O'Rourke, 1981a,b).

Bumblefoot remains an important disease of captive birds of prey which warrants far more research. A recent review of a book on current veterinary therapy stated, *inter alia,* "On the other hand, bumblefoot in raptors would have a limited appeal" (Murdoch, 1984). This view is not borne out by colleagues in veterinary practice who confirm that bumblefoot is one of the most common conditions on which they are consulted over birds of prey.

References
Cooper, J. E. (1980a). Pathologie und Therapie von Ballenentzündungen bei Greifvögeln. *Der Praktische Tierarzt* **11,** 966.

Cooper, J. E. (1980b). Surgery of the foot in falcons: a historic operation. *Annals of the Royal College of Surgeons of England* **62**, 445–448.

Cooper, J. E. and Needham, J. R. (1981). The starling (*Sturnus vulgaris*) as an experimental model for staphylococcal infection of the avian foot. *Avian Pathology* **10**, 273–279.

Murdoch, D. B. (1984). (Book review). *Veterinary Record* **115**, 471.

Riddle, K. E. (1981). Surgical treatment of bumblefoot in raptors. In Cooper, J. E. and Greenwood, A. G., editors, *Recent Advances in the Study of Raptor Diseases.* Chiron Publications, Keighley, Yorkshire.

Satterfield, W. C. and O'Rourke, K. I. (1981a). Staphylococcal bumblefoot: vaccination and immunomodulation in the early treatment and management. *Journal of Zoo Animal Medicine* **12**, 95–98.

Satterfield, W. C. and O'Rourke, K. I. (1981b). Immunological considerations in the management of bumblefoot. In Cooper, J. E. and Greenwood, A. G., editors, *Recent Advances in the Study of Raptor Diseases.* Chiron Publications, Keighley, Yorkshire.

Page of
1978
Edition

CHAPTER 8 *Nervous disorders*

112–123   Few advances have been made in the field of nervous diseases of birds of prey.

The water soluble benzodiazepine midazolam ("Hypnovel": Roche) has proved useful in raptors and can be given intramuscularly or intravenously. When administered by the former route it appears to be less painful and more effective than diazepam.

A case of right cranial nerve paralysis in a (casualty) red-tailed hawk was described by Chubb (1982): the bird was successfully treated and could be released after five weeks.

Epileptiform seizures of unknown aetiology were reported in captive African vultures by Mundy and Foggin (1981). They suspected an infectious disease but bacteriological and virological investigations proved negative.

119   *Cryptococcus* is a fungus, not a protozoon.

References

Chubb, K. (1982). A case of right cranial nerve paralysis in a red-tailed hawk. *Ontario Field Biologist* **36**, 96.

Mundy, P. J. and Foggin, C. M. (1981). Epileptiform seizures in captive African vultures. *Journal of Wildlife Diseases* **17**, 259–265.

CHAPTER 9   *Nutritional diseases, including poisons*

124   Valuable research on the nutrition of raptors has been carried out
           by James Kirkwood, including comparative studies on energy
           requirements of the kestrel and barn owl in captivity (Kirkwood,
           1979), and of the young free-living kestrel (Kirkwood, 1980), and
           a review of data on various other raptorial species (Kirkwood,
           1981).
               A study pertinent to the nursing and treatment of raptors was
           that by Shapiro and Weathers (1981).

126   Overfeeding and obesity can result in the deposition of excessive
           quantities of fat under the skin and within the body cavity and
           fatty change in various organs (Wadsworth *et al*, 1984). In addition
           a "fatty liver-kidney syndrome of merlins" has been recognised
           and reported (Cooper and Forbes, 1983). The cause is unclear
           but factors that are currently being investigated include excessive
           feeding of day-old chicks and inbreeding.

131   Biotin deficiency may be involved in conditions in which the beak
           (and sometimes talons) are of poor consistency and tend to break
           or crumble easily. A dietary supplement may be tried.

133   Further work on (free-living) Cape vultures has been carried out
           by Evans and Piper (1981) who described the bone abnormalities
           seen in those birds as "juvenile osteoporosis" or "nutritional osteo-
           dystrophy" and attributed the condition to a calcium/phosphorus
           imbalance following a lack of calcium intake.

133–134   Perosis similar to "slipped tendon" in poultry was reported in pere-
           grine falcons by Sykes *et al* (1982) who suspected that marginal
           manganese levels in the whole pigeon diet might be responsible.
           I have seen similar cases in peregrines and eagle owls in Britain:
           again the cause has been unclear. In other birds e.g. ratites and
           cranes, excessive growth rate has been implicated. More research
           is clearly needed.

136–137   Poisoning remains a significant cause of death in raptors (Cooke
           et al, 1982). A useful text which provides data on the toxicity of
           pesticides to wildlife but is also very relevant to captive birds of
           prey is that by Hudson *et al* (1984).
               Chlorinated hydrocarbon insecticides certainly may accumulate

in captive raptors: such chemical burdens are probably acquired from the diet but this is often difficult to prove. Birds which die unexpectedly and which show no *post-mortem* evidence of disease should be analysed. Clinical diagnosis may be facilitated by the use of blood tests (Henny and Meeker, 1981).

138   Other poisons which may prove lethal to raptors and which should be borne in mind in diagnosis include strychnine (Redig *et al*, 1982) and anticoagulant rodenticides (Mendenhall and Pank, 1980; Townsend *et al*, 1981); these may be acquired as a result of feeding on other species which have been accidentally or intentionally poisoned.

139   Lead poisoning is now recognised as a significant cause of illness and death in captive birds of prey in both North America and Britain (Redig *et al*, 1980; Macdonald *et al*, 1983) and has been studied experimentally by a number of researchers including Meister (1981), Pattee *et al* (1981) and Reiser and Temple (1981). It is increasingly being recognised as a cause of death in bald eagles and other species in the wild (Hoffman *et al*, 1981).

Radiography (in conjunction with toxicological and haematological investigations) plays an important part in diagnosis or lead poisoning but care must be taken to distinguish shot in the gastrointestinal tract from any lodged in the muscle. A useful way of detecting tiny particles of lead in stomach contents *post mortem* is to radiograph the latter in a Petri dish.

The effect of ingested oil on American kestrels was studied experimentally by Pattee and Franson (1982) who concluded that crude oil from a spill posed little hazard to this and other falconiform species.

142   The feeding of hand-reared raptors can present problems: a number of papers have appeared on this subject, especially in the International Zoo Yearbook – for example, Zwart and Louwman (1980), Brown (1984) and Samour *et al* (1984). General information is to be found in Weaver and Cade (1983).

References

Brown, C. (1984). Breeding and hand-rearing the common kestrel *Falco tinnunculus* and other bird of prey species. *International Zoo Yearbook* **23**, 71–75.

Cooke, A. S., Bell, A. A. and Haas, M. B. (1982). *Predatory Birds, Pesticides and Pollution*. Institute of Terrestrial Ecology, Huntingdon.

Cooper, J. E. and Forbes, N. (1983). A fatty liver-kidney syndrome of merlins. *Veterinary Record* **112**, 182–183.

Evans, L. B. and Piper, S. (1981). Bone abnormalities in the Cape vulture (*Gyps coprotheres*). *Journal of the South African Veterinary Association* **52**, 67–68.

Henny, C. J. and Meeker, D. L. (1981). An evaluation of blood plasma for monitoring DDE in birds of prey. *Environmental Pollution (Series A)* **25**, 291–304.

Hoffman, D. J., Pattee, O. H., Wiemeyer, S. N. and Mulhern, B. (1981). Effects of lead shot ingestion on δ-aminolevulinic acid dehydratase activity, hemoglobin concentration, and serum chemistry in bald eagles. *Journal of Wildlife Diseases* **17**, 423–431.

Hudson, R. H., Tucker, R. K. and Haegele, M. A. (1984). *Handbook of Toxicity of Pesticides to Wildlife*. United States Department of the Interior Resource Publication 153. Washington DC.

Kirkwood, J. K. (1979). The partition of food energy for existence in the kestrel (*Falco tinnunculus*) and the barn owl (*Tyto alba*). *Comparative Biochemistry and Physiology* **63A**, 495–498.

Kirkwood, J. K. (1980). Energy and prey requirements of the young free-flying kestrel. *Hawk Trust Report* **10**, 12–14.

Kirkwood, J. K. (1981). Maintenance energy requirements and rate of weight loss during starvation in birds of prey. In Cooper, J. E. and Greenwood, A. G., editors, *Recent Advances in the Study of Raptor Diseases*. Chiron Publications, Keighley, Yorkshire.

Macdonald, J. W., Randall, C. J., Moon, G. M. and Ruthven, A. D. (1983). Lead poisoning in captive birds of prey. *Veterinary Record* **113**, 65–66.

Meister, B. (1981). Untersuchungen zur Alimentären Bleivergiftung bei Greifvögeln. Inaugural Dissertation, Universität zu Giessen.

Mendenhall, V. M. and Pank, L. F. (1980). Secondary poisoning of owls by anticoagulant rodenticides. *Wildlife Society Bulletin* **8**, 311–315.

Pattee, O. H., Wiemeyer, S. N., Mulhern, B. M., Sileo, L. and Carpenter, J. W. (1981). Experimental lead-shot poisoning in bald eagles. *Journal of Wildlife Management* **45**, 806–810.

Pattee, O. H. and Franson, J. C. (1982). Short-term effects of oil ingestion on American kestrels (*Falco sparverius*). *Journal of Wildlife Diseases* **18**, 235–241.

Redig, P. T., Stowe, C. M. and Barnes, D. M. (1980). Lead toxicosis in raptors. *Journal of the American Veterinary Medical Association* **177**, 941–943.

Redig, P. T. and Arendt, T. D. (1982). Relay toxicity of strychnine in raptors in relation to a pigeon eradication program. *Veterinary and Human Toxicology* **24**, 335–336.

Reiser, M. H. and Temple, S. A. (1981). Effects of chronic lead ingestion in birds of prey. In Cooper, J. E. and Greenwood, A. G., editors, *Recent Advances in the Study of Raptor Diseases*. Chiron Publications, Keighley, Yorkshire.

Samour, H. J., Olney, P. J. S., Herbert, D., Smith, F., White, J. and Wood, D. (1984). Breeding and hand-rearing the Andean condor *Vultur gryphus*. *International Zoo Yearbook* **23**, 7–11.

Shapiro, C. J. and Weathers, W. W. (1981). Metabolic and behavioral responses of American kestrels to food deprivation. *Comparative Biochemistry and Physiology* **68A**, 111–114.

Sykes, G., Hardaswick, V. and Heck, W. (1982). Nutritional deficiency and perosis in peregrine falcons. *Hawk Chalk* **21**, 33–36.

Townsend, M. G., Fletcher, M. R., Odam, E. M. and Stanley, P. I. (1981). An assessment of the secondary poisoning hazard of warfarin to tawny owls. *Journal of Wildlife Management* **45**, 242–248.

Wadsworth, P. F, Jones, D. M. and Pugsley, S. L. (1984). Fatty liver in birds at the Zoological Society of London. *Avian Pathology* **13**, 231–239.

Weaver, J. D. and Cade, T. (1983). *Falcon Propagation*. The Peregrine Fund, Ithaca, New York.

Zwart, P. and Louwman, J. W. W. (1978). Feeding a hard-reared Andean condor and king vulture (*Vulture gryphus* and *Sarcoramphus papa*) at Wassenaar Zoo. *International Zoo Yearbook* **20**, 276–277.

Page of
1978
Edition

CHAPTER 10   *Anaesthesia and surgery*

143–151   The anaesthetic agents of choice in raptors remain (a) (inhalation) halothane and methoxyflurane and (b) (injection) ketamine and alphaxalone-alphadolone ("Saffan": Glaxovet; formerly called CT 1341). Ketamine is best given in combination with xylazine, diazepam or the water-soluble benzodiazepine midazolam ("Hypnovel": Roche). The duration of action of the injectable agents increases with body size: thus, a large bird, such as an eagle, will take significantly longer to absorb, metabolise and eliminate a drug than a small sparrow-hawk or kestrel. Samour *et al* (1984) compared ketamine, xylazine and alphaxalone-alphadolone in over a thousand birds, some of them raptors. They reported satisfactory results with ketamine in most species but vultures showed marked salivation, excitation and convulsions and it did not prove possible to achieve adequate surgical anaesthesia. This, however, was not my experience when I used ketamine in black vultures on Mallorca in 1983.

Methohexitone is an ultra short-acting barbiturate. Its successful use in the domestic fowl was reported 13 years ago (Scott and Stewart, 1972): I have used it, by the intravenous route, as an alternative to alphaxalone alphadolone, in a number of species of bird (Cooper, 1984). The administration of this and other agents by the intravenous route is facilitated if a butterfly attachment is strapped into position with tape: incremental doses can be given as and when required.

149   The manufacturers (Veterinary Instruments) of the "Imp Respiration Monitor" advertise the latter as being suitable for animals from "Raptors to Ridgebacks". I have used the monitor in birds of prey and can confirm that it works well, permitting respiration to be detected audibly – a useful safeguard during surgery.

151   When submitting a raptor for *post-mortem* examination a note

should be made, where appropriate, of the method of euthanasia. If this is not done problems can result and the pathologist may have difficulty in interpreting the sequence of events. Pentobarbitone given intraperitoneally shows as crystalline deposits on the serosal surface of organs: this can be mistaken for visceral gout. Likewise, physical methods of euthanasia will produce signs of haemorrhage and trauma.

151–155   A wide variety of surgical procedures can be carried out in birds of prey. Orthopaedic techniques are discussed under Chapter 4 and laparoscopy in Chapters 3 and 11. Ophthalmological operations have increasingly been reported – for example, enucleation (Greenwood and Barnett, 1981) and lens extraction by ultrasonic pharmacoemulsification by Kern *et al* (1984). Many examples of new and developing techniques in avian surgery are described by Harrison (1984).

152   Pumice stone is very useful for manicuring the beak and talons.

Pinioning techniques, which may under certain circumstances be necessary or acceptable in captive birds of prey, are described by Humphreys (1985).

Falconiform birds kept in captivity in Britain now have to be ringed and registered. Individuals born in captivity are marked with a government (Department of the Environment) closed ring, imported birds with a plastic "cable tie". The search for reliable methods of marking and recognising birds goes on, however. Havelka (1984) discussed the merits of various methods, including tattooing and he suggested that "footprinting" (evaluation of dorsal scale patterns on the third digit) has particular potential. The latter was also advocated by Beyerbach (1980). DNA studies are likely to provide an exact method in the not too distant future (D. Parkin, personal communication).

References

Beyerbach, U. (1980). Kennzeichnung und Identifikation von Greifvögeln. *Der Praktische Tierarzt* **61**, 936–940.

Cooper, J. E. (1984). Avian anaesthesia. *Veterinary Record* **114**, 283.

Greenwood, A. G. and Barnett, K. C. (1981). The investigation of visual defects in raptors. In Cooper, J. E. and Greenwood, A. G., editors, *Recent Advances in the Study of Raptor Diseases*. Chiron Publications, Keighley, Yorkshire.

Havelka, P. (1983). Registration and marking of captive birds of prey. *International Zoo Yearbook* **23**, 125–132.

Harrison, G. J. (1984). New aspects of avian surgery. *Veterinary Clinics of North America: Small Animal Practice* **14**, 363–380.

Humphreys, P. N. (1985). Water-Birds. In Cooper, J. E. and Hutchison, M. F., editors, *A Manual of Exotic Pets*. British Small Animal Veterinary Association, London.

Kern, T. J., Murphy, C. J. and Riis, R. C. (1984). Lens extraction by phacoemulsification in two raptors. *Journal of the American Veterinary Medical Association* **185,** 1403–1406.

Samour, J. H., Jones, D. M., Knight, J. A. and Howlett, J. C. (1984). Comparative studies of the use of some injectable anaesthetic agents in birds. *Veterinary Record* **115,** 6–11.

Scott, H. and Stewart, J. M. (1972). A new anaesthetic for birds. *British Poultry Science* **13,** 105–106.

Page of
1978
Edition

CHAPTER 11   *Miscellaneous and emerging diseases*

Many of the headings in this section would now warrant chapters to themselves, so great have been the developments over the past 7–8 years.

156   Further examples of longevity of captive birds of prey were given by Minnemann and Busse (1983).

156–157   Important advances have been made in our understanding of feather conditions in psittacine birds and some of these may be relevant to raptors – for example, McOrist *et al* (1984) investigated "feather and beak disease syndrome" in sulphur-crested cockatoos (*Cacatua galerita*) and demonstrated virus-like particles in the epidermis. They concluded that a viral infection may be responsible for this condition. Similarly, Lemahieu *et al* (1985) reported feather abnormalities associated with paramyxovirus-1 pigeon variant in pigeons and chickens.

Electron-microscopy (e-m) is of value in the study of feather abnormalities. Transmission e-m permits the investigation of intracellular abnormalities and demonstration of viral particles while I have found scanning e-m to be an excellent way of studying lesions of the shaft, barbs and barbules (Cooper, in preparation).

157   Further evidence as to the effect of fulmar oil on peregrines was presented by Mearns (1983) while Miller-Mundy (1984) described the clinical treatment of a golden eagle (which had been found heavily oiled) using eucalyptus oil and "Fairy Liquid".

A useful paper on feather disorders, which includes a flow chart for differential diagnosis, is that by Harrison (1984). This includes discussion of the use of hormones – mainly thyroxine and testosterone – in the treatment of feather loss. There is a need for controlled studies in birds of prey.

162–163   There has been an upsurge of interest in ocular conditions of raptors, much of it prompted by Andrew Greenwood. Greenwood and Barnett (1981) drew attention to the largely overlooked book *The Fundus Oculi of Birds* by Casey Wood (1917) and discussed the functional anatomy and clinical examination of the eye of raptors. They described a number of conditions encountered in these species, many of them assumed to be traumatic in origin. Greenwood and Barnett's own observations bear out Wood's comment that many otherwise normal owls are affected with chorioretinitis: the cause is unknown but nutritional deficiencies and toxoplasmosis are both possibly involved.

     Papers by other authors on this subject include reports of bilateral keratopathy in a barred owl (Murphy *et al*, 1981) and retinal dysplasia in a prairie falcon (Dukes and Fox, 1983). Studies on the retinal structure of owls, using electroretinography, were carried out by Ault (1984).

163–164   The paper on cardiac lesions in raptors has now been published (Cooper and Pomerance, 1982).

     Electrocardiography is now frequently used on raptors, especially in North America (Haigh, 1981).

165   As was mentioned under Chapter 3, improved clinical chemical tests are now available, including microassay techniques for uric acid, which can assist in the diagnosis of urinary disease. However, there is an urgent need for baseline values for the more common raptorial species to be ascertained.

166–167   Surprisingly little progress has been made in our understanding of the immune process of birds of prey. Lawler and Redig (1984) examined the response to foreign red blood cells of the red-tailed hawk and great-horned owl and Satterfield and O'Rourke (1981) discussed the possible role of immune mechanisms in bumblefoot.

     Havelka (1983) stated that birds of prey may be "allergic" to metal rings but my own view, based upon examination of similar cases, is that the skin lesions associated with these rings are due to trauma.

167   A number of neoplasms have been recognised and reported in recent years in birds of prey. Papers of relevance include those describing a renal carcinoma in an augur buzzard (Wadsworth and Jones, 1980), a mixed cell tumour in a Seychelles kestrel (Cooper *et al*, 1978), a oviduct adenocarcinoma in a Mauritius kestrel (Cooper, 1979) and a mesothelioma in a ferruginous hawk (Cooper and Pugsley, 1984). The last of these is of particular interest in

that, subsequent to the publication of the paper, a second case occurred, also in a captive ferruginous hawk which originated from the same part of Britain.

In addition, I have diagnosed two squamous cell carcinomas – one removed surgically and successfully from the skin over the breast of a European eagle owl, the other the cause of death following extensive dermal ulceration in a Barbary falcon.

170–173 A useful review of psychological disturbances is given by Jones (1981).

173–174 With the upsurge of interest in captive breeding reproductive disorders are seen more frequently. Keymer (1980) reported disorders of the female reproductive tract in 2/41 falconiform birds and 4/38 strigiforms: conditions seen were obstruction of oviduct or cloaca, oophoropathy and presence of a functional right ovary. The last of these is normal in many of the Falconiformes but not generally a feature of owls.

174–175 Accurate sexing remains a problem in breeding establishments: a useful review of the methods currently available is provided by Fry (1983). Faecal steroid analysis (Stavy *et al*, 1979) is no longer carried out at the Zoological Society of London and my attempts to interest commercial laboratories in this technique – for psittacine as well as raptorial birds – have proved unsuccessful.

Chromosomal investigation (karyotyping) has much to commend it and is relatively inexpensive (Stock and Worthen, 1980). However, at the time of writing such techniques are not readily available. Exciting developments involving the study of DNA patterns have been made by Dr. David Parkin and others and are likely to provide a reliable method of sexing and identification in the not too distant future.

In the meantime sex determination by endoscopy (laparoscopy) remains a reliable and increasingly widely used technique. Jones *et al* (1984) reported on fibreoptic endoscopy in over 1000 birds of 144 different species, including 62 falconiform and 96 strigiform raptors. I routinely use a human arthroscope (Thackray) but have found the American Focuscope (Medical Diagnostic Services, U.S.A.) of value in sexing as well as being a useful diagnostic instrument, especially in the field. Laparoscopy is a relatively safe procedure: Smith (1983) reported a death rate of 0.4% in a series of over 2000 birds. The possibility that tissue damage associated with laparoscopy might cause problems in egg-laying was raised by Frankenhuis and Kappert (1980) but does not appear to have been substantiated in practice.

176–177 Inbreeding may be of relevance to the conservation of raptors in the wild since, once a population is small, the inbreeding coefficient increases (Lovejoy, 1978) and, *inter alia*, susceptibility to disease may be enhanced. This may, for example, be the case with the Mauritius kestrel (Cooper *et al*, 1981). The possible role of inbreeding in the "fatty liver-kidney syndrome of merlins" (Cooper and Forbes, 1983) is also being investigated.

Insofar as developmental abnormalities are concerned, I have examined cases of hydrocephalus in captive bred peregrines and received reports of a number of other conditions. Cade (1980) described a "Drooping alula" syndrome in captive bred peregrines but this may have been nutritional rather than genetic in aetiology. Two cases of developmental abnormalities in birds in the wild in Britain were reported recently (Cooper, 1984) – peregrine which had duplication of a hind toe and extra vestigial digits on a carpus, and a merlin with syndactyly. The possibility of an increased incidence of such abnormalities because of the population "bottleneck" which occurred in British raptors in the 1960s should be explored. In this context it should be noted that vestigial wing claws are a feature of a few species including the great gray owl (*Strix nebulosa*) (Nero and Loch, 1984) and that supernumerary digits on the legs of a yellow-billed kite in Africa were described by Brooke (1975).

A short article in *The Times* (October 1981) reported a golden eagle with "two pairs of claws on each leg" but no further information on this bird has been traced.

177–180 Captive breeding is now an accepted and important aspect of raptor management. It has great potential in terms of conservation and research. Indeed, Cade (1982) has pointed out that the expertise now available in this field means that no raptor species need ever become extinct. Nevertheless, remarkably little information has been published on techniques – a notable exception being the book *Falcon Propagation* by J. D. Weaver and T. J. Cade (1983) and review articles, for example by Cade (1980). Artificial insemination was also discussed by Boyd (1978) and Gee and Temple (1978).

The pathological examination of eggs is of great importance (see Chapter 3 and Appendix) and even apparently normal infertile eggs should be submitted for investigation so that baseline data on appearance, size and thickness can be established. Papers on raptor eggs which have appeared recently include those by Jenkins (1984), Pattee *et al* (1984) and Bird *et al* (1984). The last of these describes the normal embryonic development of the American kestrel and refers to similar work on the pariah kite by Desai and Malhotra (1980). There is no doubt that comparable studies are needed on other raptor species. Until this is done interpretation of findings in eggs which have failed to hatch will continue to prove difficult.

Cryogenic preservation of spermatozoa of the American kestrel was reported by Brock *et al* (1983) who used a diluent containing 13.64% glycerol. Fertility was low, however, and the authors concluded that "the method obviously needs further refinement".

A little information on the problems of the newly hatched chick was provided by Weaver and Cade (1983) but this section, and that on "Pharmacology" are disappointing in their scope and lack of references.

180   The importance of keeping records must again be emphasised. In this respect the requirement in Britain (under the Wildlife and Countryside Act, 1981) for captive raptors to be ringed and registered has meant that "keepers" have been obliged to maintain records of their birds and breeding results. It is to be hoped that some of these data will, in due course, be made available for scientific study. Computerised records have much to commend them and can have the added advantage of increased confidentiality.

References

Ault, S. J. (1984). Electroretinograms and retinal structure of the eastern screech owl (*Otus asio*) and great horned owl (*Bubo virginianus*). *Raptor Research* **18,** 62–66.

Bird, D. M., Gautier, J. and Montpetit, V. (1984). Embryonic growth of American kestrels. *Auk* **101,** 392–396.

Brock, M. K., Bird, D. M. and Ansah, G. A. (1983). Cryogenic preservation of spermatozoa of the American kestrel. *International Zoo Yearbook* **23,** 67–71.

Brooke, R. K. (1975). A pathological yellow-billed kite. *Honeyguide* **82,** 39.

Boyd, L. L. (1978). Artificial insemination of falcons. *Symposium of the Zoological Society of London* **43,** 73–80.

Cade, T. J. (1980). The husbandry of falcons for return to the wild. *International Zoo Yearbook* **20,** 23–35.

Cade, T. (1982). *The Falcons of the World.* Collins, London.

Cooper, J. E. (1979). An oviduct adenocarcinoma in a Mauritius kestrel (*Falco punctatus*). *Avian Pathology* **8,** 187–191.

Cooper, J. E. (1984). Developmental abnormalities in two British falcons (*Falco* spp.). *Avian Pathology* **13,** 639–645.

Cooper, J. E. and Forbes, N. (1983). A fatty liver-kidney syndrome of merlins. *Veterinary Record* **112,** 182.

Cooper, J. E. and Pomerance, A. (1982). Cardiac lesions in birds of prey. *Journal of Comparative Pathology* **92,** 161–168.

Cooper, J. E. and Pugsley, S. L. (1984). A mesothelioma in a ferruginous hawk (*Buteo regalis*). *Avian Pathology* **13,** 797–801.

Cooper, J. E., Watson, J. and Payne, L. N. (1978). A mixed cell tumour in a Seychelles kestrel (*Falco araea*). *Avian Pathology* **7,** 651–658.

Cooper, J. E., Jones, C. G. and Owadally, A. W. (1981). Morbidity and mortality in the Mauritius kestrel (*Falco punctatus*). In Cooper, J. E. and Greenwood, A. G., editors, *Recent Advances in the Study of Raptor Diseases*. Chiron Publications, Keighley, Yorkshire.

Desai, J. H. and Malhotra, A. K. (1980). Embryonic development of pariah kite *Milvus migrans govinda*. *Journal of the Yamishina Institute of Ornithology* 12, 82–86.

Dukes, T. W. and Fox, G. A. (1983). Blindness associated with retinal dysplasia in a prairie falcon, *Falcon mexicanus*. *Journal of Wildlife Diseases* 19, 66–69.

Frankenhuis, M. T. and Kappert H. J. (1980). Infertility due to surgery on body cavity in female birds – cause and prevention. Sonderdruck aus Verhandlungsbericht, des XXII Internationalen Symposiums über die Erkrankungen der Zootiere. Akademie-Verlag, Berlin.

Fry, D. M. (1983). Techniques for sexing monomorphic vultures. In Wilbur, S. R. and Jackson, J. A., editors, *Vulture Biology and Management*. University of California Press.

Gee, G. F. and Temple, S. A. (1978). Artificial insemination for breeding non-domestic birds. *Symposium of the Zoological Society of London* 43, 51–72.

Greenwood, A. G. and Barnett, K. C. (1981). The investigation of visual defects in raptors. In Cooper, J. E. and Greenwood, A. G., editors, *Recent Advances in the Study of Raptor Diseases*. Chiron Publications, Keighley, Yorkshire.

Haigh, J. C. (1981). Anaesthesia of raptorial birds. In Cooper, J. E. and Greenwood, A. G., editors, *Recent Advances in the Study of Raptor Diseases*. Chiron Publications, Keighley, Yorkshire.

Harrison, G. J. (1984). Feather disorders. *Veterinary Clinics of North America: Small Animal Practice* 14, 179–199.

Havelka, P. (1983). Registration and marking of captive birds of prey. *International Zoo Yearbook* 23, 125–132.

Jenkins, M. A. (1984). A clutch of unusually small peregrine falcon eggs. *Raptor Research* 18, 151–153.

Jones, C. G. (1981). Abnormal and maladaptive behaviour in captive raptors. In Cooper, J. E. and Greenwood, A. G., editors, *Recent Advances in the Study of Raptor Diseases*. Chiron Publications, Keighley, Yorkshire.

Jones, D. M., Samour, J. H., Knight, J. A. and Ffinch, J. M. (1984). Sex determination of monomorphic birds by fibreoptic endoscopy. *Veterinary Record* 115, 596–598.

Keymer, I. F. (1980). Disorders of the avian female reproductive system. *Avian Pathology* 9, 405–519.

Lawler, E. M. and Redig, P. T. (1984). The antibody responses to sheep red blood cells of the red-tailed hawk and great-horned owl. *Developmental and Comparative Immunology* 8, 733–738.

Lemahieu, P., De Vriese, L, and Bijnens, B. (1985). Feather abnormalities associated with paramyxovirus-1 pigeon variant in pigeons and chickens. *Veterinary Record* 116, 591.

Lovejoy, T. E. (1978). Genetic aspects of dwindling populations. A review. In Temple, S. A., editor, *Endangered Birds. Management Techniques for Preserving Threatened Species*. University of Wisconsin, Madison.

McOrist, S., Black, D. G., Pass, D. A., Scott, P. C. and Marshall, J. (1984). Beak and feather dystrophy in wild sulphur-crested cockatoos (*Cacatua galerita*). *Journal of Wildlife Diseases* 2, 120–124.

Mearns, R. (1983). Breeding peregrines oiled by fulmars. *Bird Study* 30, 243–244.

Miller-Mundy, A. (1984). Hawking in the Hebrides. *The Falconer* 47–51.

Minnemann, D. and Busse, H. (1983). Longevity of birds of prey and owls at East Berlin Zoo. *International Zoo Yearbook* **23,** 108–110.

Murphy, C. J., Kern, T. J. and MacCoy, D. M. (1981). Bilateral keratopathy in a barred owl. *Journal of the American Veterinary Medical Association* **179,** 1271–1273.

Nero, R. W. and Loch, S. L. (1984). Vestigial wing claws on great gray owls, *Strix nebulosa. Canadian Field Naturalist* **98,** 45–46.

Pattee, O. H., Mattox, W. G. and Seegar, W. S. (1984). Twin embryos in a peregrine falcon egg. *The Condor* **86,** 352–353.

Satterfield, W. C. and O'Rourke, K. I. (1981). Immunological considerations in the management of bumblefoot. In Cooper, J. E. and Greenwood, A. G., editors, *Recent Advances in the Study of Raptor Diseases.* Chiron Publications, Keighley, Yorkshire.

Smith, G. (1983). Avian sex determination. *Veterinary Record* **112,** 182.

Stauber, E. H. (1984). Footprinting of raptors for identification. *Raptor Research* **18,** 67–71.

Stavy, M., Gilbert, D. and Martin, R. D. (1979). Routine determination of sex in monomorphic bird species using faecal steroid analysis. *International Zoo Yearbook* **19,** 209–214.

Stock, A. D. and Worthen, G. L. (1980). Identification of the sex chromosomes of the red-tailed hawk (*Buteo jamaicensis*) by C- and G-banding. *Raptor Research* **14,** 65–68.

Wadsworth, P. F. and Jones, D. M. (1980). A renal carcinoma in an augur buzzard (*Buteo rufofuscus augur*). *Avian Pathology* **9,** 219–223.

Weaver, J. D. and Cade, T. J. (1983). *Falcon Propagation.* The Peregrine Fund, Ithaca, New York.

Wood, C. A. (1917). *The Fundus Oculi of Birds.* Lakeside Press, Chicago.

Page of
1978
Edition

CHAPTER 12   *Discussion and Conclusions*

Birds of prey are increasingly being studied in captivity: for example, Kirkwood (1980) described the establishment of a colony of common kestrels for research on nutrition and bio-energetics and Bird and Rehder (1981) outlined work using the American kestrel.

An important step in the development and recognition of bird of prey pathology as a bona fide discipline has been the establishment of a Sub-Group on Pathology and Disease of the ICBP World Working Group on Birds of Prey and the production and publication by that Sub-Group of a Register of persons working on raptor pathology and disease (Cooper, 1983a,b). Closer liaison has also been established between avian biologists, aviculturists and veterinary surgeons.

Scientific meetings devoted to raptor disease have done much to promote the subject and to disseminate information. These have been held in Britain, the United States, West Germany and elsewhere.

183   The "dramatic developments" anticipated in 1978 have indeed taken place. As earlier parts of this Addendum indicate, there have been important advances in many fields and an upsurge in general interest in raptor biology and disease has been accompanied by a degree of specialisation by members of the veterinary profession. The final paragraph of the book, emphasising the need for more research, remains as true as it was when first published in 1978.

References

Bird, D. M. and Rehder, N. B. (1981). The science of captive breeding of falcons. *Avicultural Magazine* **87,** 208–209.

Cooper, J. E. (1983a). Disease studies in endangered species. *IUCN SSC Newsletter* **2,** 18.

Cooper, J. E. (1983b). Sub-Group on Pathology and Disease. *Bulletin of the ICBP World Working Group on Birds of Prey* **1,** 190–193.

Kirkwood, J. K. (1980). Management of a colony of common kestrels (*Falco tinnunculus*) in captivity. *Laboratory Animals* **14,** 313–316.

Page of
1978
Edition

    APPENDIX II   *Bird of prey record card*

188–190   Extra data which may be added to the record card include ring numbers and more detailed breeding records.

    APPENDIX III   *Clinical examination*

191   Extra data may include ring number, carpus measurement and a column for sequential weights/measurements. In addition, the time that the bird has been in captivity should be recorded.

    APPENDIX IV   **Post-mortem** *examination*

192–193   Extra data include ring number, carpus measurements, organ weights and columns for "Samples stored" and "Samples submitted elsewhere". In addition the bird's condition should be *graded*; I use a grading system of 1–4 which covers a range from emaciated to plump.

Whole body radiography is a useful aid to *post-mortem* examination and the findings should be recorded.

Special investigations may be necessary in legal cases.

APPENDIX V   *Egg examination*

194

A far more extensive egg examination form is desirable. Much of this relates to "History and relevant data" – for example, whether incubated by parents, fostered or artificially incubated, incubator type and whether the egg was dipped, turned and candled. In addition, however, the "Results of examination" should include shell thickness, appearance on candling, comments on embryo, air cell, blood vessels, yolk sac and fluids, crown-rump length and a note of samples stored.

APPENDIX VI   *Drugs and other agents used in treatment*

210–218

Many additional agents have proved useful in raptors and some of these are mentioned in previous sections of the Addendum.

Insofar an antibacterial agents are concerned, clavulanate-potentiated amoxycillin and the various potentiated sulphonamides (many of them licensed for use in poultry) are particularly recommended.

I have modified the dosages of a number of agents in the light of experience. For instance, diazepam is effective at 1–5 mg/kg intramuscularly.

APPENDIX XI   *Relevant law*

221

The Wildlife and Countryside Act, 1981 supersedes the Protection of Birds Acts. Useful summaries of the 1981 Act are to be found in Cooper and Cooper (1984) and Cooper (1986).

One of the most important points is that falconiform birds of prey are all on Schedule 4 of the Act and as such have to be registered and ringed if held in captivity. Open general licences permit the care of sick and injured specimens for up to six weeks by veterinary surgeons and "licensed rehabilitation keepers". The latter are subject to inspection before being licensed.

222   The Diseases of Animals Act, 1950 has been replaced by the Animal Health Act, 1981.

223   The Endangered Species (Import and Export) Act, 1976 has been supplemented by the Wildlife and Countryside Act, 1981.
         The Importation of Captive Birds Order (1976) has been replaced by the Importation of Birds, Poultry and Hatching Eggs Order, 1979.

References
Cooper, M. E. and Cooper, J. E. (1984). Wildlife and non-domesticated species. In RCVS *Legislation Affecting the Veterinary Profession in the United Kingdom.* Royal College of Veterinary Surgeons, London.
Cooper, M. E. (1986). *An Introduction to Animal Law.* Academic Press, London.